Teaching Evidence-Based Practice in Nursing

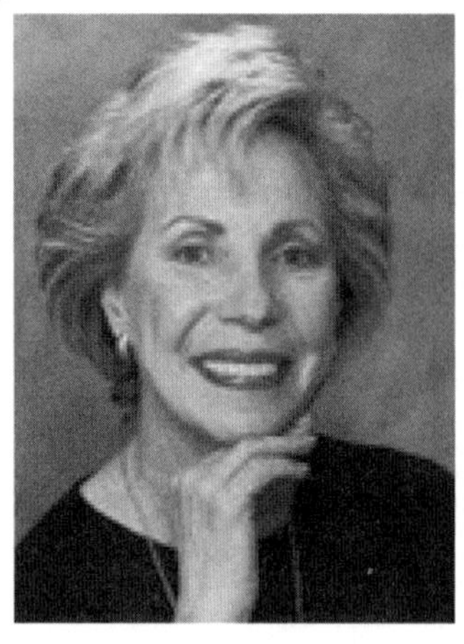

Rona F. Levin, PhD, RN, is an internationally known consultant in evidence-based practice (EBP). She is currently serving as adjunct professor at New York University and adjunct visiting professor at the University of Medicine and Dentistry of New Jersey. Dr. Levin teaches nursing research and EBP at all educational levels and in the practice setting, mentors nurses in clinical practice and doctoral students, and provides guest lectures in classes at both the graduate and undergraduate levels as well as for clinical agencies. During the last 10 years, she held varied full-time positions at Pace University, Lienhard School of Nursing (LSN), which is now the College of Nursing. From 2003 until 2006 she was project director of the Joan M. Stout, RN Evidence-Based Practice (EBP) Initiative, and created shared appointments with two clinical agencies for the purpose of integrating EBP into the nursing services. She also served as chair of graduate studies in the LSN and visiting faculty at the Visiting Nurse Service of New York. Dr. Levin is also professor emeritus of Felician College, where she served as director, Division of Nursing and then director, Division of Health Sciences and professor for 12 years (1988–1999). Professor Levin served as chair of the Foundation of New York State Nurses Center for Nursing Research and Planning Committee for several years and remains an active member of the Foundation. In 2008 she received the Jesse M. Scott award for exemplary integration of research, education, and practice by the American Nurses Association.

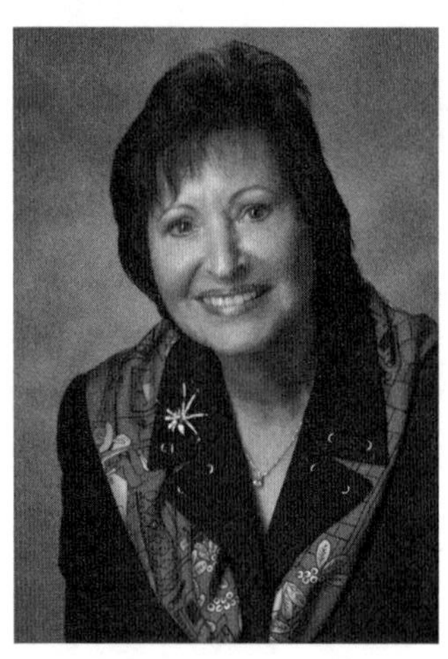

Harriet R. Feldman, PhD, RN, FAAN, served as interim provost and executive vice president for Academic Affairs at Pace University until May 2012. She assumed the position as dean of the College of Health Professions and dean of the Lienhard School of Nursing at Pace University on July 1, 2012. Dr. Feldman is a leading figure in nursing education with numerous publications and presentations nationally and internationally. She is also an expert in nursing accreditation, having served in a number of capacities with the Commission on Collegiate Nursing Education, and as an accreditation consultant to nursing programs in South Korea and Ghana. She cofounded and coedited the *Scholarly Inquiry for Nursing Practice* and was editor of *Nursing Leadership Forum.* Her other publications include the first edition of the current book, *Teaching Evidence-Based Practice in Nursing, Nursing Leadership: A Concise Encyclopedia, Nurses in the Political Arena: The Public Face of Nursing, Educating Nurses for Leadership,* and more. Dr. Feldman has worked extensively with faculty and other colleagues to provide mentorship in writing for publication, establishing scholarship trajectories, and developing their leadership skills. She has received numerous awards, for example, the American Association of Colleges of Nursing "STAR" award for grassroots political advocacy, the Westchester YWCA Women and Racial Justice Award for Science/Medicine/Technology, and the Grace Davidson Award for leadership in nursing education.

Teaching Evidence-Based Practice in Nursing

Second Edition

Rona F. Levin, PhD, RN
Harriet R. Feldman, PhD, RN, FAAN
Editors

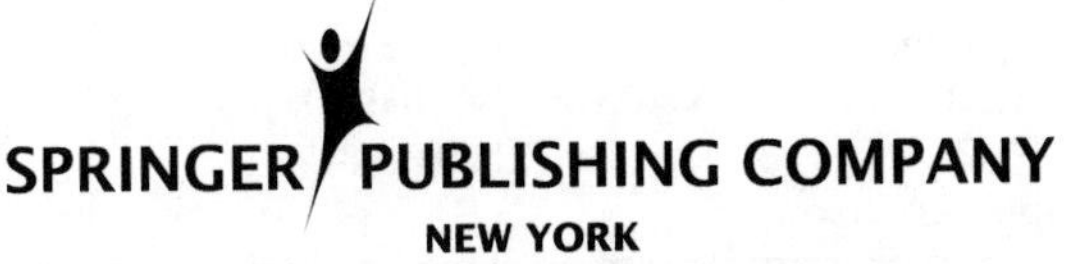

Springer Publishing Company, LLC
11 West 42nd Street
New York, NY 10036
www.springerpub.com

Acquisitions Editor: Allan Graubard
Composition: Techset

ISBN 978-0-8261-4812-4
E-book ISBN: 978-0-8261-4813-1

12 13 14/ 5 4 3 2 1

Library of Congress Cataloging-in-Publication Data
Teaching evidence-based practice in nursing/[edited by] Rona F. Levin,
Harriet R. Feldman. — 2nd ed.
p. ; cm.
Includes bibliographical references and index.
ISBN 978-0-8261-4812-4 — ISBN 978-0-8261-4813-1 (e-book)
I. Levin, Rona F. II. Feldman, Harriet R.
[DNLM: 1. Evidence-Based Nursing–education. 2. Mentors—education.
3. Evidence-Based Nursing–methods. WY 18]
610.73071'1–dc23

2012027749

Printed in the United States of America by Bang Printing.

For Riannah Sage, Anderson Samuels, and Mikey—
You can make fairy tales come true.
And to David, for being the prince in my fairy tales.
—Mimi

In memory of my late husband, Ron—
You encouraged and supported me to keep expanding my horizons, and to grow as a professional and a person. I will always love you.
—HRF

Contents

Contributors

Kathryn H. Bowles PhD, RN, FAAN, Professor and Ralston House Endowed Term Chair in Gerontological Nursing, Associate Director, New Courtland Center for Transitions and Health, University of Pennsylvania School of Nursing, Beatrice Renfield Visiting Scholar, Visiting Nurse Service of New York

Robert E. Burke, DNP, RN, FNP-BC, LAc, Family Nurse Practitioner, Montefiore Medical Center, Bronx, NY; Adjunct Clinical Professor, Lienhard School of Nursing, College of Health Professions, Pace University

Harriet R. Feldman, PhD, RN, FAAN, Dean and Professor, College of Health Professions and the Lienhard School of Nursing, Pace University

Lorraine Ferrara, RN-BC, MA, AE-C, Education Coordinator Visiting Nurse Service of New York, Faculty Beatrice Renfield Fellows Program, Adjunct Clinical Instructor College of Nursing, New York University

Lucille Ferrara, EdD, RN, FNP-BC, MBA, Assistant Professor, Lienhard School of Nursing, College of Health Professions, Pace University

Ellen Fineout-Overholt, PhD, RN, FNAP, FAAN, Dean and Professor, Groner School of Professional Studies, Chair, Department of Nursing, East Texas Baptist University

Janice B. Foust, PhD, RN, Assistant Professor, College of Nursing and Health Sciences, University of Massachusetts Boston; Nurse Research Associate, Center for Home Care Policy and Research, Visiting Nurse Service of New York

Jeanne Grace RN, PhD, Chair, Research Subjects Review Board 03 Biomedical, Emeritus Professor of Clinical Nursing, University of Rochester School of Nursing

Judith Haber, PhD, APRN-BC, FAAN, The Ursula Springer Leadership Professor in Nursing, Associate Dean for Graduate Programs, New York University College of Nursing

Cheryl Holly, EdD, RN, Director of Faculty and Scholarly Development – Capacity Building Systems, Associate Professor and Co-Director of the New Jersey Center for Evidence-Based Practice School of Nursing, University of Medicine and Dentistry of New Jersey

Paule V. Joseph, MSN, FNP-BC, RN, CRRN, BCLNC-C, CTN-B, PhD Student, University of Pennsylvania School of Nursing

Jeffrey M. Keefer, MA, MEd, MA, Doctoral Student, Lancaster University, Northern UK; Project Manager, Instructional Design, Visiting Nurse Service of New York; Adjunct Instructor, Doctor of Nursing Practice (DNP) Program, Lienhard School of Nursing, College of Health Professions, Pace University

Barbara Krainovich-Miller, EdD, PMHCNS-BC, ANEF, FAAN, Associate Dean, Academic & Clinical Affairs, Professor, New York University College of Nursing

Bonnie Lauder MIS, RN, CPHQ, Director of Measurement and Quality Improvement, Visiting Nurse Service of New York

Patricia Lavin, MS, RN, Director of Outcomes Management, New York University Hospital for Joint Diseases

Rona F. Levin, PhD, RN, Professor Emeritus, Felician College, Lodi, New Jersey, Consultant in Evidence-Based Practice Improvement and Program Design, Adjunct Professor, New York University, Adjunct Associate Professor, Northeastern University

Seon Lewis-Holman, MSN, ACNS-BC, Director, Education and Clinical Development, Visiting Nurse Service of New York

Joan M. Marren, MEd, MA, RN, Chief Operating Officer, VNSNY & President, Visiting Nurse Service of New York Home Care

Bernadette Mazurek Melnyk, PhD, RN, CPNP/PMHNP, FNAP, FAAN, Associate Vice President for Health Promotion, University Chief Wellness Officer and Dean, College of Nursing, The Ohio State University

Ellen R. Rich, PhD, RN, FNP, FAANP, Professor, Molloy College and Nurse Researcher, New York University Hospital for Joint Diseases

Susan W. Salmond, EdD, RN, Professor and Dean, School of Nursing, University of Medicine and Dentistry of New Jersey

Lillie M. Shortridge-Baggett, EdD, RN, FAAN, Professor, Department of Graduate Studies, Lienhard School of Nursing, College of Health Professions, Pace University

Jason T. Slyer, DNP, RN, FNP-BC, Clinical Assistant Professor, Lienhard School of Nursing, College of Health Professions, Pace University

Joanne K. Singleton, PhD, RN, FNP, BC, Professor, Chairperson, Department of Graduate Studies, Director FNP-Doctor of Nursing Practice Program, Lienhard School of Nursing, College of Health Professions, Pace University

Mary Jo Vetter, MS, RN, A/GNP-BC, Vice President, Clinical Product Development, Visiting Nurse Service of New York

Priscilla Sandford Worral, PhD, RN, Coordinator of Nursing Research, Upstate University Hospital, Clinical Associate Professor, Upstate College of Nursing, Upstate University Health System; Adjunct Professor, Lienhard School of Nursing, Pace University

Fay Wright, MS, RN, ACNP-BC, New York University College of Nursing Doctoral Student; Former Assistant Director Evidence-Based Practice & Nursing Research at Northern Westchester Hospital

FOREWORD

Findings from multiple studies have indicated that evidence-based practice (EBP) improves the quality and reliability of health care, enhances patient outcomes, and reduces costs for the U.S. health care system. Despite this evidence, EBP is not consistently practiced by professionals in health care systems across the nation and globe. Multiple factors are responsible for this slow paradigm shift to EBP as standard of care, including lack of time and competing clinical priorities, cultures that do not support EBP, insufficient administrative support, lack of EBP mentorship, as well as inadequate search and critical appraisal skills. Another major barrier to advancing EBP is that educators in many institutions across the country continue to teach research courses in baccalaureate and master's programs in the traditional manner with detailed emphasis on strategies necessary for the generation of external evidence (i.e., findings from rigorous research) instead of the use and application of evidence to practice. Lengthy critique processes of single studies also continue to be taught in academic programs instead of rapid critical appraisal of a body of evidence designed to answer a clinical question. One result of teaching research the traditional way is that students often acquire a negative attitude toward research and leave their professional programs with little desire to continue to read, critically appraise, use, and apply evidence from research to their everyday clinical practices.

To accelerate the paradigm shift, educators need to ignite a passion for EBP in their students and teach them an evidence-based approach to clinical care that facilitates a "spirit of inquiry" long after graduation from their educational programs. Aside from core courses in EBP, it is necessary to integrate evidence-based decision-making processes throughout all courses in baccalaureate and master's programs in order to facilitate this lifelong approach to learning and high-quality clinical practice. In DNP programs, students should be prepared to be the best translators of evidence into clinical care to improve patient outcomes, as well as the greatest producers of internal evidence (i.e., findings from quality improvement/outcomes management projects) that can be integrated into evidence-based clinical decision making.

This outstanding book by Rona F. Levin and Harriet R. Feldman draws upon several years of educational experience to capture creative approaches for teaching EBP. The book includes comprehensive and unique strategies for teaching EBP for all types of learners across a variety of educational and clinical practice settings. The concrete examples of innovative teaching assignments provided in the book bring the content alive and serve as a useful, detailed guide for how to incorporate this material into meaningful exercises for learners. Levin and Feldman's book is a truly wonderful and essential resource for educators working in all health professional programs as well as clinical settings. Use of the strategies highlighted in this book will no doubt play a key role in accelerating the paradigm shift to EBP that will lead to the highest quality of care and best patient outcomes in health care systems across the nation and globe.

Bernadette Mazurek Melnyk
PhD, RN, CPNP/PMHNP, FNAP, FAAN

PREFACE

The second edition of this book evolved from 6 years of experience in helping academic and clinical agencies understand and implement evidence-based practice (EBP). An important lesson we have learned through research and experience is the crucial part that mentorship plays in creating EBP champions and a culture of EBP in both the academic and clinical settings. Preliminary research that Levin, Melnyk, Fineout-Overholt, Barnes, and Vetter (2011) conducted with the Visiting Nurse Service of New York has indicated that didactic workshops on EBP were not sufficient to change nurses' attitudes toward EBP or their implementation of evidence-based interventions. Thus, new to the second edition is the concept of mentorship. We think this is so important that we are starting off the second edition with mentorship as the first section, emphasizing the concept of mentorship and how mentorship is designed and implemented to promote EBP.

Also different in this edition is the greatly enhanced sharing of successful experiences of implementing EBP into academic curricula and clinical projects. When we wrote the first edition of this book, the trend for integrating EBP into academic nursing and clinical practice was just beginning. In the past 7 years the nursing profession has progressed a long way toward this goal. As we are now beginning to evaluate data on the success of our implementation efforts, there is a lot more to tell.

A number of chapters that appeared in the first edition have been eliminated, as we believe they are either less relevant to readers, or that they are not germane to what faculty and our clinical partners are asking for today. Thus, this new edition integrates a new perspective: Not only do we discuss important issues for educators, we also value and include the results of feedback from clinical partners at all levels of the organization—from chief operating officer (COO) and the clinical educator to the staff nurse responsible for implementing EBP projects. In the process, we highlight administrative leadership support efforts in both academic and clinical organizations. Without such support, integrating any change in an organizational culture is simply not possible.

Finally, we highlight the beginning of the establishment of creative, collaborative endeavors to share and spread the knowledge gained to improve nursing practice at all levels. One reason that new information takes so long to implement in practice is the difficulty some of our colleagues have in sharing information as it becomes available (i.e., prior to publication). We hope that one day such personal and special interests will be overshadowed by the altruistic goal of improving clinical, educative, and administrative practices much more expediently and regardless of attribution.

REFERENCE

Levin, R. F., Melnyk, B. M., Fineout-Overholt, E., Barnes, M., & Vetter, M. (2011). Fostering evidence-based practice to improve nurse and cost outcomes in a community health setting: A pilot test of the ARCC model. *Nursing Administration Quarterly*, *35*(1), 1–13.

ACKNOWLEDGMENTS

We would first like to acknowledge each other. As a writing team for these many years, we have somehow managed to agree and disagree, to embrace each other's strengths and accept each other's limitations, and to still remain steadfast colleagues and friends. We are committed educators and scholars, devoted to improving patient care through writing and mentoring current and future generations of nurses, and that includes mentoring each other.

Our families and friends have contributed through their support and love, and by never complaining about the time we spent in thinking and writing instead of focusing on them. Equally important are those who partner and collaborate with us daily: students, clinicians, and faculty alike.

We also extend a heartfelt thank you to the contributors, whose expertise has enriched the content of this book. Not only did they submit their thoughtful work, they also responded positively to the many suggestions we had for change. Their varied experiences enhanced the relevance of their chapters, and we hope will help readers to teach the valuable concepts of evidence-based practice.

Part I

Mentorship: An Essential Component of Creating Evidence-Based Practice Champions

The four chapters in Part I set the stage for teaching in general, teaching in academic and clinical settings, and collaborating beyond the academic and clinical settings to enhance the teaching of evidence-based practice. The importance of mentoring cannot be overemphasized. Unless we prepare others—in this case "champions"—to advance ideas, change will not take place and those ideas will cease to exist. Faculty, clinicians, and those serving in preceptor roles are integral in preparing nurses to provide practice that is evidence based so that the ultimate goal of improving patient care is met.

1

Defining Mentorship for EBP

Ellen Fineout-Overholt, Rona F. Levin, and Bernadette Mazurek Melnyk

Mentoring is a brain to pick, an ear to listen, and a push in the right direction.

—John Crosby

Our research and experience with promoting evidence-based practice (EBP) since the first edition of this book has revealed important lessons. Foremost among them is this: mentoring and coaching are key ingredients for achieving successful EBP outcomes at all levels—nurse, patient, and system (Levin, Fineout-Overholt, Melnyk, Vetter, & Barnes, 2011; Melnyk & Fineout-Overholt, 2010, 2011). Didactic presentations or interactive workshops on EBP without follow-up support for nurses by coaches or mentors are simply not sufficient to change EBP beliefs or implementation behaviors (Levin et al., 2011).

Although we believed these statements to be true as demonstrated by the initial version of the Advancing Research and Clinical Practice Through Close Collaboration (ARCC) Model in 1999 (Melnyk, Fineout-Overholt, Stone, & Ackerman, 2000), it was not until we began testing the model that we garnered sufficient scientific support (Levin et al., 2011; Melnyk et al., 2004; Melnyk, Fineout-Overholt, Feinstein, Sadler, & Green-Hernandez, 2008; Melnyk, Fineout-Overholt, & Mays, 2008; Melnyk, Fineout-Overholt, Giggleman, & Cruz, 2010). In addition, our experiences with implementing EBP in hospital and home care organizations have consistently supported the significance of coaching and mentorship in order to integrate and sustain EBP in an organizational culture. Both the ARCC Model and research that has supported the mentorship component of the model are given in Figure 1.1.

Before describing these, however, it is important to clarify the difference between coaching and mentoring so as to understand how best to use each to assist novices in gaining confidence when implementing clinical practice improvements.

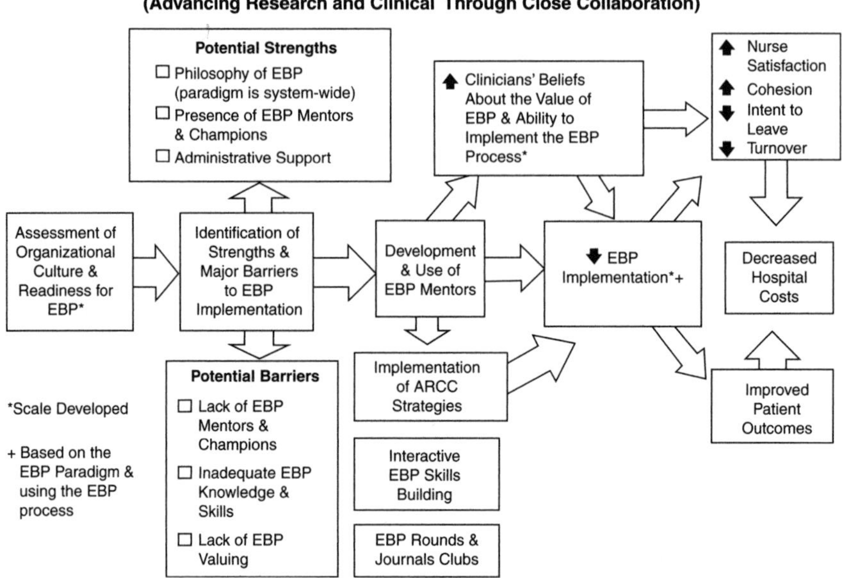

Source: © Melnyk & Fineout-Overholt, 2005.

FIGURE 1.1 The ARCC Model.

MENTORING

Historically speaking, the word *mentor,* when used to describe an individual, comes from a character in Homer's *Odyssey*. Odysseus's son, Telemachus, on his journey to maturity has a guide, Athene, a Greek god. In his human form, however, Athene is called Mentor (Lattimore, 1965). History informs us then that a mentor is someone who is a guide and takes a journey with a mentee "to maturity."

Differentiating Mentoring From Similar Concepts

Because the term *mentoring* tends to be used in many types of relationships other than that depicted by Homer, clarifying what we mean by mentoring and differentiating it from other closely related terms (especially coaching) are essential. In brief, a mentoring relationship takes place between two individuals in some planned form (Dorsey & Baker, 2004). A review of several definitions of mentoring (Allen, Eby, & Lentz, 2006; Barker, 2006; Davis, Little, & Thornton, 1977; Dorsey & Baker, 2004; Madison & Huston, 1996) identifies common components:

- The mentor and mentee choose each other
- The relationship is planned

- The stated goal of the relationship is personal and professional development
- Desired outcomes of the relationship are identified
- Mutual learning takes place during the relationship

This definition differentiates mentoring from other closely related terms: *precepting, role modeling,* and *coaching*. Precepting is an educational approach to teaching neophytes a particular role, set of skills, and behaviors. It usually has specific preset objectives and takes place within the short term between the novice who is learning a skill set and the expert nurse who serves as the learning guide (Barker, 2006). Role modeling is defined as engaging in behaviors that serve as exemplars for others, primarily novices or younger individuals (Dictionary.com Unabridged, n.d.). Homa et al. (2008) differentiate coaching from mentoring as well as facilitating. They define a coach as one who is "... assigned by organizations or programs to promote the development and internalization of knowledge and skills" (p. 38). This is in contrast to a mentor, who is a "trusted advisor" sought out by a potential mentee for mutually determined goals. Homa and others also differentiate both coaches and mentors from facilitators, who they define as "... those that make work easy ..." (p. 38). Neither a coach nor a mentor is expected to ease the work of the mentee; they are expected to help the mentee reach one's goals with support.

Phases of a Mentoring Relationship

Barker (2006) discussed how a mentoring relationship changes over time, which by the nature of the relationship is longer term than the prior relationships discussed. She identified four phases of such a relationship: *initiation, cultivation, separation,* and *redefinition*. The *initiation* phase—an important differentiator between a mentoring relationship and the other types of relationships as identified—consists of mutual selection by the mentor and mentee. During the *cultivation* phase, the peak mentoring function occurs. When the goals of the mentor/mentee relationship are reached, the mentoring comes to an end. This does not mean, however, that the relationship between mentor and mentee ends. The last phase of a successful mentoring relationship is one of redefinition and often results in a "peer friendship," in which mentor and mentee become equal colleagues and even personal friends. Wright brings this theoretical model of mentorship to life in Chapter 2, *Mentoring Clinical Champions*, by telling her story of being an EBP mentee. She also provides an exemplar of the difference between the mentoring and coaching relationship as she relates how she and her mentor coached many nurses to become EBP champions.

Regardless of whether one is a mentor or a coach, however, there are certain characteristics that the individual fulfilling either of those roles needs to bring to the relationship.

Mentor/Coach Characteristics

Mentors and coaches must be experienced in the particular role for which they are grooming their mentees or students (whether those students are in a formal academic program in or are health professionals in a clinical agency) (Madison & Huston, 1996). For mentoring, there must be a strong commitment to a long-term relationship (Allen et al., 2006). This is not the case in a coaching or precepting relationship, where the commitment is more short than long term and usually proceeds over a defined period of time. During this period of time, however, the preceptor or coach does need to be committed to educating the next generation in EBP. These relationships are just as important to creating EBP champions as is the mentor relationship (see Chapters 2, 3, and 4). Important for any of these relationships is the ability of the mentor, coach, or preceptor to nurture the novice.

Nurturing involves creating a safe place for the mentee to learn and grow (Davis et al., 1977). Creating a safe place entails: (1) a mutual understanding that making mistakes is acceptable because mistakes lead to learning; (2) building the mentee's or novice's self-confidence in one's ability; (3) acting as a sounding board for any and all challenges and frustrations; and (4) serving as a constant support in any and all of the mentee's role functions in an effort to achieve their goals for professional development. Trust, of course, is a foundational principle for a mentor–mentee relationship. In his treatise on the seven roles of a mentor (i.e., teacher, sponsor, advisor, agent, role model, coach, and confidante), Tobin (2004) indicated that "mentorship is more an affair of the heart than it is of the head … it is a two-way relationship based on trust" (p. 115). As such, each EBP mentor is charged with understanding his or her role(s) and their impact. The ARCC Model provides a successful framework for EBP mentors to actualize their role and to positively impact sustainable health care outcomes.

ARCC MODEL

The Advancing Research and Clinical Practice through Close Collaboration (ARCC) Model was created to assist organizations and individuals to implement and sustain a best practice culture. The model is dynamic, evolving over the past decade due to ongoing research and experiences

(Fineout-Overholt & Melnyk, 2011; Levin et al., 2011). There are four major assumptions that underpin the model:

1. There are barriers to and facilitators of EBP for individuals and within health care systems.
2. Barriers to EBP must be removed or mitigated and facilitators put in place for both individuals and health care systems to implement EBP as standard of care.
3. In order for clinicians to change their practices to be evidence-based, cognitive beliefs about the value of EBP and their confidence in their ability to implement it must be strengthened.
4. A culture of EBP that includes mentors (i.e., clinicians with advanced knowledge of EBP, mentorship, and individual as well as organizational change) is necessary in order to advance and sustain evidence-based care in individuals and health care systems.

These foundational assumptions provide the framework for the tenets of the ARCC Model that must be in place for the model to be successful:

a. Inquiry is a daily part of the health care environment
b. Quality outcomes and decrease costs are the overall goals of an organization
c. Process exists for the purpose of achieving the best outcomes
d. Outcome and process data are transparent
e. Clinicians are change agents who work within systems to initiate collaborative change
f. Health care is dynamic

The extent to which EBP can be successfully integrated into an organization depends on the degree to which these tenets are consistently maintained in a health care organization. Circumstances in which system barriers prevent the actualization of these basic tenets, EBP is less successful and health care outcomes are compromised. Hypotheses that represent how the model operationalizes these tenets have been raised and tested as the model has been refined:

- There are positive relationships among EBP culture, clinicians' beliefs about EBP, and their implementation of EBP
- There is a positive relationship between clinicians' beliefs about EBP and their implementation of EBP
- There are positive relationships among clinicians' beliefs about EBP, implementation of EBP, and their role satisfaction

- Clinicians who practice in organizations with stronger EBP cultures, versus those who practice in organizations with weaker EBP cultures, will have stronger EBP beliefs and greater implementation of EBP
- Clinicians who practice in organizations with stronger EBP cultures, versus those who practice in organizations with weaker EBP cultures, will report greater role satisfaction and less intent to leave
- Health care systems that implement the ARCC Model in which there is a cadre of EBP mentors will have stronger EBP cultures, greater implementation of EBP, higher nurse satisfaction, and less nurse turnover
- Health care systems in which clinicians report greater implementation of EBP versus those in which clinicians report lower implementation of EBP will have less turnover rates and better quality indicators

All of these hypotheses have been fully or partially supported through research. Studies are ongoing to further substantiate the impact of the ARCC Model (Figure 1.1). In the ARCC Model, EBP mentors evaluate and use the results of an organizational assessment focused on determining its culture and readiness for system-wide implementation of EBP. These mentors are integral in the development of a strategic plan to engage in innovative, creative strategies designed to advance clinicians' knowledge and skills in EBP. As EBP mentors enhance point-of-care providers' beliefs about the value of EBP and their ability to implement it, clinicians engage greater EBP implementation (Melnyk et al., 2004) that promotes improved health care outcomes and cost.

Research Evidence to Support the ARCC Model

Research to support the relationships depicted in the ARCC Model has been conducted and is ongoing. The initial study to evaluate relationships in the ARCC Model was a descriptive survey with a convenience sample of 160 nurses who were attending EBP conferences or workshops in four states located within the eastern region of the United States. The purposes of this study were to: (a) describe nurses' knowledge, beliefs, skills, and needs regarding EBP, (b) determine whether relationships exist among these variables, and (c) describe major barriers and facilitators to EBP (Melnyk et al., 2004). Although participant beliefs about the benefit of EBP were high, knowledge of EBP was relatively low. Significant relationships were found between the extent to which the nurses' practice was evidence-based and: (a) nurses' knowledge of EBP, (b) nurses' beliefs about the benefits of EBP, (c) having an EBP mentor, and (d) using the Cochrane database of systematic reviews and the National Guidelines Clearinghouse. Findings from this study provided additional support for barriers and facilitators in the ARCC Model as well as evidence to support the relationship between EBP beliefs and EBP implementation.

From this initial study, separate EBP beliefs and EBP implementation scales were developed in order to more fully study these constructs within the context of the ARCC Model. The second study to substantiate the relationships described in the ARCC Model (Melnyk, Fineout-Overholt, & Mays, 2008) was designed to determine the psychometric properties of these EBP beliefs and the EBP implementation scales. A total of 394 volunteer nurses who attended continuing education workshops completed the scales. Data were analyzed to evaluate the validity and the reliability of both instruments. Principal components analyses indicated that each scale measured a unidimensional construct. The Cronbach's alpha for each scale was above .90. Moreover, findings indicated that the strength of nurses' EBP beliefs and EBP implementation increased as their educational level and responsibility in workplace roles increased. As expected, EBP beliefs and EBP implementation scores were highly positively correlated.

The third study that supported the relationships in the ARCC Model, a randomized controlled pilot study, was conducted with 47 nurses from three regions of a home health care service in downstate New York (Levin et al., 2011). The regions were randomly assigned to either receive the phased ARCC intervention (i.e., education about EBP plus having an EBP mentor) or an attention control intervention that focused on teaching the nurses in-depth physical assessment skills. The EBP mentor provided the nurses in the ARCC group with: (a) didactic content on EBP basics, (b) an EBP toolkit, (c) environmental prompts (e.g., posters that encourage the nurses to use EBP), and (d) on-site and email consultation about implementing an EBP project to improve patient outcomes. The ARCC EBP intervention program lasted 16 weeks, beginning with a 4-week training period that was followed by the EBP mentor being on site with the nurses for 2 hours, 1 day a week for 12 weeks. Findings indicated that the ARCC group, compared to the attention control group, had higher EBP beliefs, greater EBP implementation, and less nurse attrition/turnover. In addition, there was no significant difference between the ARCC and control groups on the outcome variable of nurses' productivity, indicating that learning how to integrate EBP into daily practice along with implementing an EBP project during work time did not affect the number of home visits made by the nurses. Findings from this study support the positive outcomes of implementing the ARCC Model in clinical practice, specifically, the essential value of having an ARCC mentor in a health care system and subsequent nurse outcomes.

The fourth study conducted was a quasi-experimental study of the effectiveness of a structured multifaceted mentorship program that was based on the ARCC Model (Wallen et al., 2010). The program was designed to implement EBP in a clinical research-intensive environment. This study also evaluated factors that defined the readiness of an organization to embrace EBP as well as the impact of an EBP mentor program. The mentorship program included structured workshops, focused discussions with nursing leadership and shared governance staff, as well as a pre- ($N = 159$) and post- ($N = 99$) evaluation trial via online surveys that measured organizational culture and readiness for system-wide EBP, EBP beliefs, EBP implementation, job satisfaction, group cohesion, and intent to leave nursing and their current job. The authors of this study found that those attending the EBP mentorship program had a larger pre to post increase in perceived organizational culture and readiness for EBP and EBP Beliefs than those who did not participate. Furthermore, study findings suggested that collaboration among staff, advanced practice EBP mentors, and leadership may be important regarding the EBP implementation and culture (Wallen et al., 2010). This study further corroborates other studies that have found that EBP beliefs of nurses are significantly correlated with EBP implementation, and that having an EBP mentor leads to stronger beliefs and greater EBP implementation by nurses as well as greater group cohesion, which is a major predictor of nursing turnover rates.

The fifth study (Melnyk, Fineout-Overholt, Giggleman, & Cruz, 2010), a descriptive correlational study, was designed to examine the relationships among EBP beliefs, implementation, organizational culture, group cohesion, and job satisfaction. The 58 interdisciplinary participants were staff in a community hospital system in the western region of the United States. The 10-month incremental ARCC program prepared interdisciplinary teams, each with an EBP mentor, to engage in evidence-based decision making. Clinicians' EBP beliefs were significantly correlated with perceived organizational culture for EBP, their implementation of EBP, group cohesion, and job satisfaction. Furthermore, organizational EBP culture was significantly and positively related to EBP implementation. From the findings of this study, hospitals need to assess how their current cultures support EBP and implement interventions to strengthen clinicians' beliefs about their value of and ability to engage evidence-based decision making.

Cumulative findings from these studies support the relationships in the ARCC Model; an evidence-based framework that can guide organizations in the implementation and sustainability of EBP as they embrace the role of the EBP mentor. Further testing of the ARCC Model will strengthen its evidential base and increase confidence that mission critical outcomes will be reliably produced when the model is implemented in health care organizations. As organizations formally embrace the role of the EBP mentor (e.g., use the title in organizational role descriptions and subsequent performance evaluation criteria), they will experience broader impact of these special clinicians on health care outcomes.

REFERENCES

Allen, T. D., Eby, L. T., & Lentz, E. (2006). The relationship between mentoring characteristics and perceived program effectiveness. *Personnel Psychology, 59,* 125–153.

Barker, E. (2006, February). Mentoring—A complex relationship. *Journal of the American Academy of Nurse Practitioners, 18*(2), 56–61.

Davis, L., Little, M., & Thornton, W. (1977). The art and angst of the mentoring relationship. *Academic Psychiatry, 21,* 61–67.

Dorsey, L., & Baker, C. (2004). The art and angst of the mentoring relationship. *Academic Psychiatry, 21,* 61–67.

Fineout-Overholt, E., & Melnyk, B. M. (2011). ARCC evidence-based practice mentors: The key to sustaining evidence-based practice. In B. M. Melnyk, & E. Fineout-Overholt (Eds.), *Evidence-based practice in nursing and health care: A guide to best practice* (2nd ed., pp. 344-352). Philadelphia: Lippincott, Williams & Wilkins.

Homa, K., Regan-Smith, M., Foster, T., Nelson, E. C., Liu, S., Kirland, K. B. et al. (2008). Coaching physicians in training to lead improvement in clinical microsystems: A qualitative study on the role of the clinical coach. *The International Journal of Clinical Leadership, 16,* 37–48.

Lattimore, R. (Trans.). (1965). *Homer: The odyssey.* New York: Harper & Row.

Levin, R. F., Melnyk, B. M., Fineout-Overholt, E., Barnes, M., & Vetter, M. (2011). Fostering evidence-based practice to improve nurse and cost outcomes in a community health setting: A pilot test of the ARCC model. *Nursing Administration Quarterly, 35*(1), 1–13.

Madison, J., & Huston, C. (1996). Faculty–faculty mentoring relationships: An American and Australian perspective. *NASPA Journal, 33*(4), 316–328.

Melnyk, B., Fineout-Overholt, E., Stone, P., & Ackerman, M. (2000). Evidence-based practice: The past, the present, and recommendations for the millennium. *Pediatric Nursing, 26,* 77–80.

Melnyk, B. M., & Fineout-Overholt, E. (2010). ARCC (Advancing research and clinical practice through close collaboration): A model for system-wide implementation & sustainability of evidence-based practice. In J. Rycroft-Malone, & T. Bucknall (Eds.), *Models and frameworks for implementing evidence-based practice.* Indianapolis: Wiley-Blackwell & Sigma Theta Tau International.

Melnyk, B. M., & Fineout-Overholt, E. (2011). *Evidence-based practice in nursing and health care: A guide to best practice* (2nd ed.). Philadelphia: Lippincott, Williams & Wilkins.

Melnyk, B. M., Fineout-Overholt, E., Feinstein, N., Li, H. S., Small, L., Wilcox, L. et al. (2004). Nurses' perceived knowledge, beliefs, skills, and needs regarding evidence-based practice: Implications for accelerating the paradigm shift. *Worldviews on Evidence-Based Nursing, 1*(3), 185–193.

Melnyk, B. M., Fineout-Overholt, E., Feinstein, N. F., Sadler, L. S., & Green-Hernandez, C. (2008). Nurse practitioner educators' perceived knowledge, beliefs, and teaching strategies regarding evidence-based practice: Implications for accelerating the integration of evidence-based practice into graduate programs. *Journal of Professional Nursing, 24*(1), 7–13.

Melnyk, B. M., Fineout-Overholt, E., Giggleman, M., & Cruz, R. (2010). Correlates among cognitive beliefs, EBP implementation, organizational culture, cohesion and job satisfaction in evidence-based practice mentors from a community hospital system. *Nursing Outlook, 58*(6), 301–308.

Melnyk, B., Fineout-Overholt, E., & Mays, M. (2008). The evidence-based practice beliefs and implementation scales: Psychometric properties of two new instruments. *Worldviews on Evidence-Based Nursing, 5*(4), 208–216.

Role Model. (n.d.). *Dictionary.com Unabridged.* Retrieved June 21, 2011, from Dictionary.com website: http://dictionary.reference.com/browse/role model

Tobin, M. J. (2004). Mentoring: 7 roles and some specifics. *American Journal of Respiratory and Critical Care Medicine, 170,* 114–117.

Wallen, G. R., Mitchell, S. A., Melnyk, B. M., Fineout-Overholt, E., Miller-Davis, C., Yates, J. et al. (2010). Implementing evidence-based practice: Effectiveness of a structured multifaceted mentorship programme. *Journal of Advanced Nursing, 66*(12), 2761–71.

2

MENTORING CLINICAL CHAMPIONS

Fay Wright

Good timber does not grow with ease; the stronger the wind, the stronger the trees.

—J. WILLARD MARRIOTT FOUNDER OF MARRIOTT HOTELS

Implementing evidence-based practice (EBP) in the clinical setting is a challenging process. Here, the high-stress nature of the clinical environment, lack of organizational support, the nature of research information, and individual nurse characteristics all interact (Gale & Schaffer, 2009). Education about EBP process and benefits, however, is not enough to overcome the barriers that arise (Levin, Melnyk, Fineout-Overholt, Barnes, & Vetter, 2011). Direct care nurses, primarily responsible for providing patient care, need mentoring to translate their bedside skill beyond patient care. Certainly, engaging direct care nurses in the EBP process is essential to improve patient care. Also essential is a supportive infrastructure that includes education, practical experience, and mentorship as much to engage direct care nurses as to bridge the gap between EBP knowledge and EBP clinical practice.

As the most important part of a supportive infrastructure is a mentor, committed to nurturing and modeling the mentee (Davis, Little, & Thornton, 1977), this chapter illustrates a mentor–mentee relationship that supported the implementation of an EBP program at a community hospital. It also illustrates how the mentee and mentor helped direct care nurses to become clinical champions for EBP.

A MENTOR IS A GARDENER

Mentoring is a planned relationship between two individuals with mutually identified goals and outcomes (Davis et al., 1977; Dorsey & Baker, 2004). Mentorship can be described as a farmer planting and tending a garden. During the spring, a farmer will prepare the soil, adding fertilizer to provide a rich environment for growth, much as the mentor and mentee purposefully develop their relationship, setting goals, and identifying mutual learning needs. As a farmer plants seeds in the fertile ground, the mentor shares her expert knowledge with the mentee. Cultivating the garden during growing season, the farmer waters, fertilizes, and supports plant growth as the mentor teaches, guides, provides constructive feedback, and supports the mentee's growth. In the harvest, the mentee and mentor appreciate the fruits of their mutual learning and successful collaboration. Then, as the farmer prepares for another growing season, the mentee and mentor prepare to share their professional collegial relationship with others.

Preparing the Soil, Part 1: Collaboration

An innovative collaborative agreement for nursing student education and EBP education was the first step to prepare the environment for EBP. Northern Westchester Hospital (NWH) entered into partnership with Pace University, Lienhard School of Nursing (LSN) to mutually support each organization's strategic goals. NWH needed an expert mentor to implement an EBP initiative as part of the hospital's Magnet journey. LSN needed an expert nursing clinical instructor to support student enrollment goals. A master's-prepared, certified clinical nurse specialist was hired by NWH as a clinical instructor whose main responsibility was student clinical education. With a dedicated clinical faculty member at NWH, LSN was assured of a clinical instructor who met academic qualifications and who was oriented to the unit and institutional policies, facilitating a more coordinated clinical experience for the nursing students with guaranteed clinical placements and expert clinical instruction. The clinical instructor became the EBP mentee.

In return for NWH hiring the clinical instructor, LSN provided NWH with a doctorally prepared expert faculty who facilitated a series of education sessions for the nursing department about EBP. The faculty consultant was not only an expert in EBP but also an expert in practice improvement and mentoring. The mentor, who was experienced with education processes, nursing leadership, and EBP, joined with the on-site clinical expert, the mentee, and prepared a collaborative environment to begin to grow a robust EBP program that would be planted and tended by their mentor–mentee relationship.

Preparing the Soil, Part 2: Initiating the Mentoring Relationship

The hospital's EBP initiative needed an on-site facilitator, and the clinical educator was the obvious choice for the role (Dogherty, Harrison, & Graham, 2010). The mentee had participated in EBP workshops provided by the mentor as part of her LSN clinical instructor role. Experience with implementing and evaluating clinical EBP projects was not part of the mentee's skill set. As a master's-prepared nurse, the mentee was adept at project management, teaching, and clinical practice, but needed a mentor to help her support the hospital's EBP initiative.

The mentor and mentee initiated a relationship (Barker, 2006). The mentor would teach and support the mentee's understanding of how to implement EBP in the clinical setting; she would also facilitate the mentee's transition to becoming a mentor to the nursing staff at the hospital to support departmental EBP initiatives. The mentee would support the mentor's understanding of the NWH system to facilitate EBP program development and support the nursing staff in day-to-day project work, since she was on site and the mentor visited the hospital only one day a week.

As part of the initiation process, the mentor and mentee established norms of communication. The explicit discussion of methods of communication (phone or e-mail), time expectations for responses (within 48 hours), and how the partnership would evaluate progress and renegotiate the mentoring process (monthly discussions between mentee and mentor) established a true mentoring relationship focused on professional growth and outcomes (Barker, 2006).

The openness of the mentor to questions truly made a difference in the mentee's willingness to ask questions. As an expert clinician and clinical educator, the mentee was comfortable in her knowledge and abilities; however, she was a novice in her understanding of EBP. Knowing the mentor was sincerely engaged in the success of the mentee empowered her to ask questions that she sometimes felt she should know but did not. The mentee needed the mentor's EBP expertise and acceptance that as a mentee, the "clinical expert" was in a novice role. It is very difficult for a clinical expert to be placed in a situation in which she does not know where to find the answers and is not quite sure of all the questions. With active listening, openness, and understanding, the mentor created a safe space for the mentee to ask anything.

The mentee knew she could call or email with questions, and felt confident that the mentor's response would be learning focused. For example, the mentee was unsure of the quality and level of a specific piece of evidence. As a master's-prepared nurse, she felt she should know this. "I read journal articles all the time; how can I not know how to rate this one?" Without a supportive mentor, the mentee might not ask the question for fear of being negatively evaluated. In this relationship, the acceptance established during the initiation phase was essential, creating a safe haven for questions, and thus professional growth.

Planting EBP Seeds: Education

The mentor provided EBP workshops to build the knowledge base of all levels of nursing: the chief nursing officer, nursing executives/directors, nursing managers, nursing educators, and direct care nurses. The workshops were held at NWH with a representative from each clinical unit participating. During the workshops, the participants learned how to systematically search online databases such as CINAHL, PubMed, and the Cochrane Collaborative. The mentor led the group through the process of clinical question development using the PICO method, project planning, and the utilization of the plan, do, study, act (PDSA) method, which is based in practice or quality improvement models (Deming, 1986; Langley et al., 2009).

The workshops were interactive, engaging, and focused on skill acquisition. The mentor actively listened to the participants, supporting expert nurses' uncertainty and discomfort when learning new knowledge-based skills. The goal of the workshops was not only to learn the EBP process, but also to prepare the nurses at NWH to become leaders, disseminating EBP practice throughout the entire hospital. The mentor was committed to facilitate the learning of all the workshop participants, as they would be the clinical leaders, or "champions," for EBP.

Members of the workshops divided into teams to work on three projects: (1) fall risk prevention; (2) pain assessment; and (3) assessment of sedated, mechanically ventilated patients. Fall risk assessment and pain assessment were two institutional improvement priorities that participants of the EBP workshops agreed to champion, while the assessment of the mechanically ventilated sedation assessment was identified by an intensive care unit staff nurse as an important clinical question to examine. Each team met with the mentor to utilize the EBP knowledge learned during the workshops to develop and implement project plans. The teams worked to develop their skills, systematically searching and reading the evidence. In the weekly meetings with the mentor, questions were answered and each team's progress was discussed; however, forward movement was slow. The team members had basic knowledge from the EBP workshops and curiosity about ways to improve practice; however, the teams did not have system knowledge to move the projects forward.

Since the EBP initiative was the first major hospital initiative led by nursing, infrastructure was not in place to support the project work. The process of EBP implementation was being developed concurrently with the projects. The teams needed an internal advocate to smooth the bumps and to enable the nursing staff time to think and process. This was the critical role of the mentee: to be a hospital-based clinical "mentor" while her mentor continued to educate and support her. The mentee was needed on site to listen and to advise about internal process issues that were essential to successful EBP. The mentor could help with EBP educational needs, such as evidence discussion and identifying key internal data that was needed to clarify the clinical question; however, she could not help when a direct care nurse was unable to access the database search engines that were supposed to be accessible from unit computers but were not working, or when a nurse did not know how to print an article once it was found. The project teams needed to feel empowered and supported in their knowledge and to move forward toward implementation. The teams needed a clinical mentor to create a safe place for them to learn and grow in their EBP knowledge.

Cultivating the Mentoring Relationship

As the mentee moved into the role of clinical mentor, cultivation of the mentor–mentee relationship began (Barker, 2005). The mentee was gaining confidence in her knowledge of EBP and her ability to help facilitate the process from the weekly meetings with the mentor and project teams and from her individual mentoring sessions with the mentor. The mentor demonstrated successful mentoring and the mentee followed, applying her clinical and teaching expertise to a new knowledge area. The mentee was engaged in the mentoring process with clearly identified learning goals and motivation to succeed and support the EBP process, entrusting the mentor to show her the way (Anderson & Shannon, 1988). As the mentee worked with the mentor and the project teams, her confidence grew. The mentor respected the mentee's knowledge and growth, adapting her mentorship to the mentee's development (Allen, Eby, & Lentz, 2006; Barker, 2005). Mentoring does not produce an exact copy of the mentor; it empowers the mentee to grow into professional excellence (Barker, 2005). In this mentoring relationship, mutual respect, a love of nursing, and quality patient care were essential. Mutual respect is a hallmark of mentoring; without it, mentoring does not happen (Anderson & Shannon, 1988).

As the mentor's responsibilities at LSN changed, she could only meet with the project teams monthly; however, she continued to meet with the mentee weekly either in person or by phone. The mentee was the on-site support for the project teams and the mentor was the off-site support for the mentee. The weekly conversations cultivated the mentoring relationship maximizing learning and productivity (Barker, 2005).

During this time, the mentee and mentor regularly discussed what was working and, more importantly, what was not working. Two of the three projects were not progressing smoothly, the groups were not cohesive, and timeline goals were not being met. The mentee sought the mentor's counsel about possible barriers. The mentor would use clinical inquiry skills to peel back the layers of the barriers, working with the mentee to see all the issues and options. Discussing her assessment of the situation was a key method the mentee used to process issues. During the initiation phase, the mentee had identified that she needed time with the mentor to "think out loud" about what needed to be done to support the project teams. By establishing the mentee's need for verbal processing at the beginning of the relationship, a routine was in place for the mentee and mentor to discuss issues and concerns without having to identify how to address issues when problems arose.

The direct care nurse–led project was making great progress. While the project did not move forward without challenges, it made steady progress with the staff working on the project during which they were truly developing into a team. The mentor and mentee discussed the differences between the three groups. The major difference was the dedication of the direct care nurses to the clinical question that directly affected the quality of their patient care. The direct care nurse had identified the clinical question during the initial workshops, and was now leading the team of ICU nurses to follow the EBP process and to develop an EBP protocol to assess mechanically ventilated sedated patients. Direct care nurse ownership was shepherding the ICU project. An EBP clinical champion was born!

Coaching Clinical Champions

The EBP clinical champion was applying what she had learned in the workshops and regularly meeting with the mentor and mentee. She was asking questions and seeking help and support as needed. The mentor and mentee were coaching her, developing specific EBP skills to help her in her work (Homa et al., 2008). More direct care nurses from the ICU became members of this EBP project. The ICU team needed a coach to listen to what they knew and what they needed to know, to provide resources, and to provide system support for their EBP project. The mentor and mentee worked with the team—the mentor monthly and the mentee weekly, sharing their knowledge of EBP.

The mentee provided system knowledge to support the ICU team within the hospital (Homa et al., 2008). As a member of the nursing education department, the mentee could adapt her schedule to be available when team members were working. Making rounds to the clinical area, the mentee could coach the team for EBP skill application (Homa et al., 2008). The mentee's rounds enabled follow-up, provided informal time (not during a planned meeting) for questions, evidence discussion, and general team support. The mentee told the mentor that she felt her rounds were more cheerleading and support, encouraging the team to be confident in its work. Often during the mentee's rounds, a team member would share some concern about her knowledge or ability related to EBP. The mentee's ability to listen and support inspired the nurse to continue. As one of the nurse EBP champions stated, "The EBP mentor (mentee) guides me. She believes in me, even though I sometimes don't quite know where I am going. She takes it for granted that I am going to get it. And the funny thing is—I am getting it" (K. Peccoraro, personal communication, February 2, 2012).

The mentee's role as EBP coach was to advocate, troubleshoot, and inspire the project team (Homa et al., 2008). The mentee advocated for paid time for the direct care nurses to work on the project. A policy was developing that gave priority to EBP project work when there was unit downtime and staffing was sufficient. Troubleshooting took many forms, however, technology issues were foremost. The direct care nurses could complete literature searches on nursing unit computers, but were not able to download articles because a vital program was missing. The mentee worked within the system to have the program loaded to the computers. The most important role of the mentee was to provide inspiration and to acknowledge team progress. The mentee acknowledged and celebrated small steps of success to motivate and maintain the teams' energy for the projects. When the first evidence tables were completed, the coach provided coffee and chocolate to celebrate the "sweet success." Abstracts were submitted to the Pace LSN scholarly colloquium for the staff to receive recognition for their initial progress in identifying a new fall risk assessment tool, for example.

When the EBP teams were engaged in a project, they would seek out the mentee, wanting to learn more, not only to develop their skills, but also to "own" the project, with the clinical mentor passing on her knowledge, coaching the team, and developing their EBP skills. When EBP teams are enthusiastic and engaged in the clinical question, individual motivation blossoms, and staff blossomed into clinical champions.

When coaching, the old cliché that "there is no such thing as a stupid question" is essential to remember. A coach has specific skills and knowledge, but not all knowledge. The clinical champions needed to see that learning was ongoing and essential to professional development. When meeting with the mentor and clinical champions, the mentee would ask the mentor questions, role-modeling inquiry, comfortably acknowledging that she had more to learn. One quote from a member of the EBP team summarizes the value of this approach to coaching:

> Our mentor [coach] has shown us how to be professional even when we meet obstacles or are unsure of how to tackle the problem. The mentor [coach] will admit her mistakes and identifies when she doesn't know

> something. She'll say, "I don't know. Let's ask my mentor. Let's return to the article—I don't know what it says." Seeing someone who mentors others, teaches others, guides others, readily admitting that she is still learning and making mistakes, builds my confidence and the confidence of all the EBP teams. (K. Peccoraro, personal communication, February 2, 2012)

Challenges: Clearing the Weeds From the Garden

Fertile ground provides an environment for beautiful plants and weed growth. Weeds are barriers to the growth of the plantings. Weeds or barriers to progress are nothing more than opportunities for collaboration and partnership to develop infrastructure to support an environment for project growth.

At NWH, the Institutional Review Board (IRB) reviewed medical research. Before the EBP initiative, no nursing-led project had been reviewed by the IRB. While the EBP projects are designed to validate the application of evidence to the NWH clinical setting, all EBP projects are presented to the IRB chair for review to ensure the protection of human subjects and to maintain confidentiality of patient information. The IRB review proactively insures that the nurses involved have the potential to present and publish any findings from EBP projects. Utilizing the framework recommended by Newhouse, Pettit, Poe, and Rocco (2006), the mentor and mentee worked with the IRB chair and hospital lawyer to clarify the format for project review. The mentor and mentee worked with the clinical champions to complete the National Institute of Health Human Subjects Training (www.phrp.nihtraining.com/users/login.php) so they could be informed of human subject issues.

The hospital's electronic medical records (EMR) system, while streamlining bedside documentation, provided a challenge for EBP project implementation. Two of the projects involved new nursing assessment tools. The initial small tests of change for the tools were performed with written documentation to evaluate the tool's effectiveness. Without electronic versions of the tools built into the hospital's EMR, the bedside utility could not be evaluated with the written documentation forms. The informatics department collaborated with the mentee to develop a streamlined process to build the proposed tools in a "test EMR" format enabling the nursing staff to evaluate the tools in the EMR, thus maximizing the ability to evaluate the tools clinical utility.

Other infrastructures needed to be refined to support the EBP initiatives. The direct care nurses identified the need to regularly meet with the mentor, mentee, and each other to support the EBP project work. The hospital revised the model of shared governance and developed an

Evidence-Based Practice Nursing Research Council (EBP-NRC) to support the EBP initiatives (see Chapter 23).

Enjoying the Harvest: Redefining the Mentoring Relationship

As the mentor–mentee relationship evolves, the mentee grows in skills and knowledge and separation begins (Barker, 2006). The separation is an adjustment in the mentor–mentee relationship where the formal mentoring is replaced with a peer–collegial relationship (Barker, 2005). With the achievement of the mentoring goals that were established during the initiation phase, the mentoring relationship changes and is redefined. The fruits of the relationship are harvested and shared, enjoying the success as two colleagues. One of the prime fruits of the relationship was the development of the EBP-NRC council with 15 clinical champions who identify clinical questions and seek evidence to improve the quality of patient care at NWH. As the EBP-NRC evolved and the clinical champions grew in their knowledge, the mentee developed into the mentor for the EBP initiative at the hospital. The mentor evolved into the role of trusted advisor, ready to answer an e-mail or phone call but not with the regularity of the mentoring relationship.

The separation did not happen without planning. The mentor recognized the mentee's development and directly discussed the changes in the relationship, identifying that the mentee no longer needed formal mentoring, while offering collaboration in professional activities. The mentor guided the mentee on her journey toward doctoral education and other professional activities. The two colleagues presented the model of mentoring and coaching presented in this chapter in educational seminars and continue to collaborate on EBP initiatives in both the academic and clinical settings.

My mentor opened doors of knowledge and helped me build a team of dedicated professionals that are really making a difference for patient care and nursing! My ability to mentor others in the EBP process is directly related to the strong mentoring I experienced.

Planting a New Garden: Mentees as Mentors

Developing a successful mentoring relationship takes time and focus. Investing time in direct care nurses as EBP clinical champions provides professional development and extends the potential for EBP improvement. In mentoring and coaching, mutual goals and respect are essential for success. Developing professional caring relationships makes all the difference. The relationships established through mentoring continue to evolve. The clinical champions seek to move into a mentoring role, furthering their professional development. When asked about what EBP and mentoring means to her, one of the EBP clinical champions sums up the value of mentoring:

> I've had two EBP mentors [the mentor and mentee]. Their primary goal was not only to help our nursing staff to learn the EBP process, but also to prepare us to become leaders at disseminating the practice throughout the entire hospital. I worked closely with both mentors to provide support for my group, my unit, and my hospital. Luckily, I work with highly motivated and responsible nurses, both seasoned and young. Everybody is dedicated to the EBP process. When we started, most of us were new to EBP, and so our learning curve was large. The mentors taught and supported us. No question was ever ignored. We have completed many exciting projects, essentially changing practice and improving the care of many patients throughout the hospital. We did the work because we believed it would benefit our patients. This proved to be correct! But there was another byproduct of our efforts; nurses who were changing practice with EBP felt that their voices were heard. We were part of the decision-making process, and they were given an opportunity to learn and grow. Our mentors helped us find our voices. The nursing staff felt empowered and motivated. Suddenly, people were willing to move mountains. Lazy became active, shy were willing to speak in public, and followers became leaders. (K. Langer, January 25, 2012, personal communication)

REFERENCES

Allen, T. D., Eby, L. T., & Lentz, E. (2006). The relationship between mentoring characteristics and perceived program effectiveness. *Personnel Psychology, 59*, 125–153.

Anderson, E., & Shannon, A. (1988). Toward a conceptualization of mentoring. *Journal of Teacher Education, 39*(1), 38–42.

Barker, E. (2006). Mentoring—A complex relationship. *Journal of the American Academy of Nurse Practitioners, 18*(2), 56–61. doi:10.1111/j.1745-7599.2006.00102.x

Barker, E. (2006, February). Mentoring—A complex relationship. *Journal of the American Academy of Nurse Practitioners, 18*(2), 56–61.

Davis, L., Little, M., & Thornton, W. (1977). The art and angst of the mentoring relationship. *Academic Psychiatry, 21*, 61–67.

Deming, W. E. (1986). *Out of the crisis.* Cambridge, MA: MIT Center for Advanced Engineering Study.

Dogherty, E., Harrison, M., & Graham, I. (2010). Facilitation as a role and process in achieving evidence-based practice in nursing: A focused review of concept and meaning. *Worldviews on Evidence-Based Nursing, 7*(2), 76–89.

Dorsey, L., & Baker, C. (2004). Mentoring undergraduate nursing students: Assessing the state of the science. *Nurse Educator, 29*(6), 260–265.

Gale, B. P., & Schaffer, M. A. (2009). Organizational readiness for evidence-based practice. *JONA: The Journal of Nursing Administration, 39*(2), 91–97. doi: 10.1097/NNA.0b013e318195a48d

Homa, K., Regan-Smith, M., Foster, T., Nelson, E. C., Liu, S., Kirklan, K. et al. (2008). Coaching physicians in training to lead to improvement in clinical microsystems: A qualitative study on the role of the clinical coach. *The International Journal of Clinical Leadership, 16*, 37–48.

Langley, G. J., Moen, R. D., Nolan, K. M., Nolan, T. W., Norman, C. L., & Provost, L. P. (2009). *The improvement guide: A practical approach to enhancing organizational performance* (2nd ed.). San Francisco, CA: Jossey-Bass.

Levin, R. F., Melnyk, B. M., Fineout-Overholt, E., Barnes, M., & Vetter, M. (2011). Fostering evidence-based practice to improve nurse and cost outcomes in a community health setting: A pilot test of the ARCC model. *Nursing Administration Quarterly, 35*(1), 1–13.

Newhouse, R. P., Pettit, J. C., Poe, S., & Rocco, L. (2006). The slippery slope: Differentiating between quality improvement and research. *Journal of Nursing Administration, 36*(4), 211–219.

3

Mentoring Faculty for Evidence-Based Practice: Let Us Work Together

Rona F. Levin and Harriet R. Feldman

The greatest good you can do for another is not just to share your riches but to reveal to him his own.

—Benjamin Disraeli

This chapter builds on Chapters 1 and 2, and focuses on strategies to promote adoption of evidence-based teaching strategies with faculty in academic programs. We use the same definitions and framework presented in Chapter 1 to describe what mentoring vis-à-vis coaching is all about. Mentoring is a process between two people who are committed to growth of the mentee, whether the mentee is a student, practicing clinical nurse, educator, or administrator. That is one aspect of faculty development for evidence-based practice (EBP). Coaching, however, is a more accurate term to use when describing how to work with groups of faculty to facilitate their knowledge and integration of EBP into their teaching strategies. Also important to reiterate, as presented in Chapter 1, beginning research in this area, which Levin has conducted with colleagues (Levin, Melnyk, Fineout-Overholt, Barnes, & Vetter, 2011), supports the premise that didactic education or even an isolated workshop on EBP alone is insufficient to promote integration of EBP into clinical practice or teaching. This chapter focuses on strategies used with school of nursing faculties to help integrate EBP into curriculum development and teaching practices.

STRATEGY 1: FIND OUT WHERE FACULTY ARE

Levin has been asked to present many keynote addresses and/or lectures about EBP over the last 10 years, only some of which were followed by workshops or ongoing support for participants. The major assumption by program leaders was that we need to start at the beginning with definitions and introductory material about EBP. This may or may not have been an accurate assumption 10 years ago but is rarely accurate today. Depending on faculty's teaching and clinical experience, individuals are at different places when it comes to beliefs about EBP, knowledge of EBP, and ability to implement EBP strategies in their teaching and/or clinical practice. Most recently, Levin worked with a large group (over 70 individuals) of nursing faculty at a state university connected with a medical center to discuss integration of EBP teaching strategies into their courses and curricula. This particular program allocated one afternoon a month to faculty development that included an EBP workshop on one of those afternoons. For the first time offering one of these workshops, Levin decided to administer a few instruments for faculty to complete in order to have some data on where faculty were in relation to their knowledge of EBP and what they believed they needed to enhance that knowledge in order to make it functional. Among the tools administered prior to developing these workshops was the Learning Activity for Identifying Levels of Evidence (see Exhibit 3.1), a tool that Levin developed for this purpose. The result of this assessment was the basis for her decisions about content for faculty workshops.

STRATEGY 2: INCLUDE STUDENT LEARNING ACTIVITIES IN FACULTY DEVELOPMENT WORKSHOPS

One of the workshops Levin conducts on EBP for faculty focuses on teaching strategies that can be used in various clinical or didactic classes. In addition to discussing specific learning activities used with students, faculty is asked to engage in these same exercises. Some exercises are described in other chapters of this book. As an example, in order to fully understand how to level evidence, I use an exercise that was originally developed by Dr. Kathy Bowles from the University of Pennsylvania, where we provide students/faculty with several abstracts of studies and a specific scheme for leveling evidence (as there are many different ones). Learners are then asked to identify the level of evidence (LOE) of the study. Refer to Exhibit 3.1 for the actual exercise. Faculty finds this activity to be helpful in learning how to level evidence as well as providing a strategy for them to use with their students in helping them to understand that not all evidence is created equal.

After sharing a number of different learning activities that help a learner to better understand the model and processes of EBP, faculty begin to develop new, innovative learning activities of their own (see Exhibit 3.2). This type of exercise requires about an hour. First, faculty

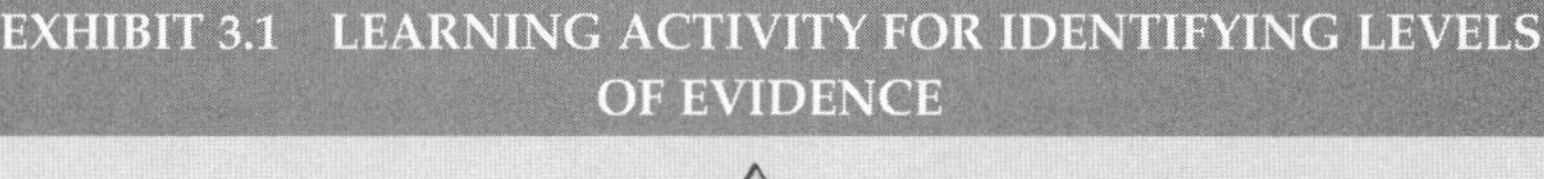

EXHIBIT 3.1 LEARNING ACTIVITY FOR IDENTIFYING LEVELS OF EVIDENCE

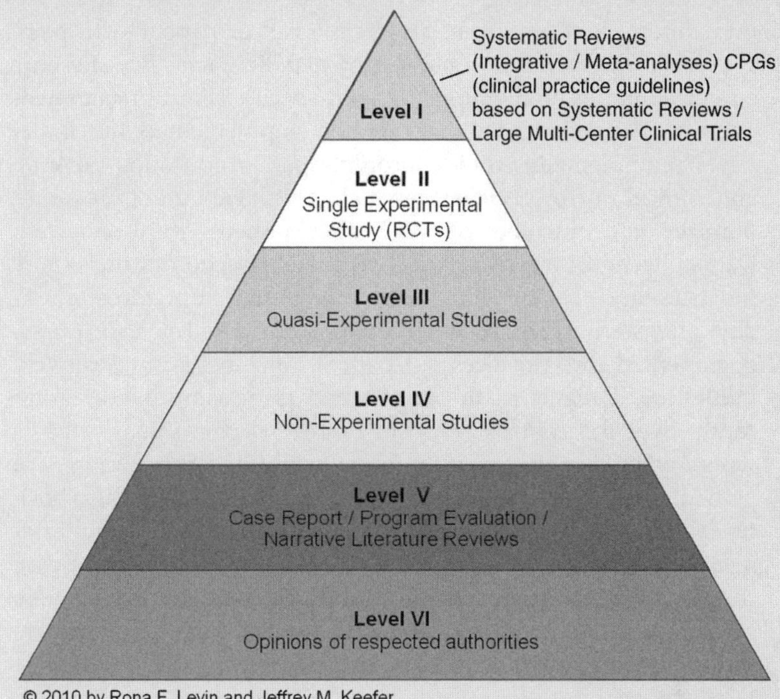

Adapted from the work of Stetler, Morsi, Rucki, Broughton, Corrigan, Fitzgerald, et al. (1998); Melnyk and Fineout-Overholt (2011); Levin (2008).

Using the "Levels of Evidence" pyramid above, read each abstract and then identify the level of evidence of the study.

1. McDonald, M. V., Pezzin, L. E., Feldman, P. H., Murtaugh, C. M., & Peng, T. R. (2005). Can just-in-time, evidence-based "reminders" improve pain management among home health care nurses and their patients. *Journal of Pain & Symptom Management, 25*(5), 474–488.
   Abstract: The purpose of this randomized, controlled, home care intervention was to test the effectiveness of two nurse-targeted, e-mail-based interventions to increase home care nurses' adherence to pain assessment and management guidelines, and to improve patient outcomes. Nurses from a large urban nonprofit home care

(*continued*)

EXHIBIT 3.1 (*continued*)

organization were assigned to usual care or one of two interventions upon identification of an eligible cancer patient with pain. The basic intervention consisted of a patient-specific, one-time e-mail reminder highlighting six pain-specific clinical recommendations. The augmented intervention supplemented the initial e-mail reminder with provider prompts, patient education material, and clinical nurse specialist outreach. Over 300 nurses were randomized and outcomes of 673 of their patients were reviewed. Data collection involved clinical record abstraction of nurse care practices and patient interviews completed approximately 45 days after start of care. The intervention had limited effect on nurse-documented care practices but patient outcomes were positively influenced. Patients in the augmented group improved significantly over the control group in ratings of pain intensity at its worst, whereas patients in the basic group had better ratings of pain intensity on average. Other outcome measures were also positively influenced but did not reach statistical significance. Our findings suggest that although reminders have some role in improving cancer pain management, a more intensive approach is needed for a generalized, nursing workforce with limited recent exposure to state-of-the-art pain management practices.

(a) Level I
(b) Level II
(c) Not applicable
(d) Level IV
(e) Level V/VI

2. Clark, L., Fink, R., Pennington, K., & Jones, K. (2006). Nurses' reflections on pain management in a nursing home setting. *Pain Management Nursing*, *7*(2), 71–77.

Abstract: Achieving optimal and safe pain-management practices in the nursing home setting continues to challenge administrators, nurses, physicians, and other health care providers. Several factors in nursing home settings complicate the conduct of clinical process improvement research. The purpose of this qualitative study was to explore the perceptions of a sample of Colorado nursing home staff who participated in a study to develop and evaluate a multifaceted pain-management intervention. Semi-structured interviews were conducted with 103 staff from treatment and control nursing homes, audiotaped, and content analyzed. Staff identified changes in their knowledge and attitudes about pain, and their pain assessment and management practices. Progressive solutions and suggestions for changing practice include establishing an internal pain team and incorporating nursing assistants into the care planning process. Quality improvement strategies can accommodate the special circumstances of nursing home care and build the capacity of the nursing homes to initiate and monitor their own process improvement programs using a participatory research approach.

(a) Level I
(b) Not applicable
(c) Level III
(d) Level IV
(e) Level V/VI

3. Dewar, A. (2006). Assessment and management of chronic pain in the older person living in the community. *Australian Journal of Advanced Nursing*, 24(1), 33–38.

Abstract: This paper reviews the nursing research literature on chronic pain in the older person living in the community and suggests areas for future research.

Background: Chronic pain is a pervasive and complex problem that is difficult to treat appropriately. Nurses managing chronic pain in older people in domiciliary/home/community nursing settings face many challenges. To provide care, the many parameters of chronic pain, which include the physical as well as the psychosocial impact and the effect of pain on patients and their families, must be carefully assessed. Beliefs of the older person about pain and pain management are also important.

Method: Relevant nursing studies were searched using CINAHL, Cochrane Database of Systematic Reviews, and Embase and PubMed databases using key words about pain and the older person that were appropriate to each database.

Results: Tools to assess pain intensity in the older person have been studied, but there has been less research on the other parameters of pain assessment or how the older person manages pain. An effective nurse–patient relationship is an important component of this process and one that needs more study. Few research studies have focused on how nurses can be assisted, or on the challenges nurses face when managing this vulnerable population.

(*continued*)

EXHIBIT 3.1 (*continued*)

Conclusion: A broad approach at the organizational level will assist nurses to manage this health care issue.
(a) Level I
(b) Level II
(c) Not applicable
(d) Level IV
(e) Level V/VI

4. Vallerand, A. H., Collins-Bohler, D., Templin, T., & Hasenau, S. M. (2007). Knowledge of and barriers to pain management in caregivers of cancer patients receiving homecare. *Cancer Nursing*. *30*(1), 31–37.
Abstract: Cancer treatment is increasingly being provided in outpatient settings, requiring many of the responsibilities for patient care to be undertaken by family caregivers. Pain is one of the most frequent and distressing symptoms experienced by cancer patients and is a primary concern for the family caregiver. Caregivers struggle with many issues that lead to inadequate management of cancer pain. The purpose of this study was to determine pain management knowledge and examine concerns about reporting pain and using analgesics in a sample of primary family caregivers of cancer patients receiving homecare. The Barriers Questionnaire and the Family Pain Questionnaire were administered to 46 primary caregivers. Between 46% and 94% of the caregivers reported having at least some agreement with the various concerns that are barriers to reporting pain and using analgesics, and up to 15% reported having strong agreement. The areas of greatest concern were about opioid-related side effects, fears of addiction, and the belief that pain meant disease progression. Results showed that caregivers with higher pain management knowledge had significantly fewer barriers to cancer pain management, supporting the importance of increasing caregivers' knowledge of management of cancer pain.
(a) Not applicable
(b) Level II
(c) Level III
(d) Level IV
(e) Level V/VI

5. Haynes, R. B., Yao, X., Degani, A., Kripalani, S., Garg, A., & McDonald, H. P. (2005). Interventions for enhancing medication

adherence (Article No. CD000011). *Cochrane Database of Systematic Reviews* Issue 4. DOI: 10.1002114651858.CD00001 1.pub2.

Background: People who are prescribed self-administered medications typically take less than half the prescribed doses. Efforts to assist patients with adherence to medications might improve the benefits of prescribed medications, but also might increase their adverse effects.

Objectives: To update a review summarizing the results of randomized controlled trials (RCTs) of interventions to help patients follow prescriptions for medications for medical problems, including mental disorders but not addictions.

Search strategy: Computerized searches were updated to September 2004 without language restriction in Medline, Embase, CINAHL, the Cochrane Library, International Pharmaceutical Abstracts (IPA), PsycINFO, and Sociofile. We also reviewed bibliographies in articles on patient adherence and articles in our personal collections, and contacted authors of original and review articles on the topic.

(a) Level I
(b) Level II
(c) Not applicable
(d) Level IV
(e) Level V/VI

6. Feng, C., Chu, H., Chen, C., Chang, Y., Chen, T., Chou, Y., ... Chou, K. (2012). The effect of cognitive behavioral group therapy for depression: A meta-analysis 2000 to 2010. *Worldviews of Evidence-Based of Nursing*, 9(11).

   The goals of the meta-analysis were to investigate the overall effectiveness of cognitive behavioral group therapy (CBGT) for depression and relapse prevention in depression from 2000 to 2010, and to investigate how certain variables (e.g., group size, therapist experience) could mediate the size of the treatment effect. The sample of studies was from the published literature during 2000 to 2010. The quality of the studies was assessed using the Cochrane Collaboration Guidelines. Thirty-two studies were included in the meta-analysis. CBGT showed an immediate and continuous effect over 6 months, but no continuous effect after 6 months. Also, the CBGT lowered relapse rate of depression. Researchers and clinicians should take note that CBGT had a moderate effect on level of depression and a small effect on relapse rate

(*continued*)

EXHIBIT 3.1 (*continued*)

of depression. The results of this study suggest that the patient should receive a course of therapy at least every 6 months.

(a) Level I
(b) Level II
(c) Not applicable
(d) Level IV
(e) Level V/VI

7. Marek, K. D., Popejoy, L., Petroski, G., & Rantz, M. (2006). Nurse care coordination in community-based long-term care. *Journal of Nursing Scholarship*, *38*(1), 80–86.

   Abstract: To evaluate the clinical outcomes of a nurse care coordination program for people receiving services from a state-funded home and community-based waiver program called Missouri Care Options (MCO).

   Design: A quasi-experimental design was used to compare 55 MCO clients who received nurse care coordination (NCC) and 30 clients who received MCO services but no nurse care coordination.

   Methods: Nurse care coordination consists of the assignment of a registered nurse who provides home care services for both the MCO program and Medicare home health services. Two standardized datasets, the Minimum Data Set (MDS) for resident care and planning and the Outcome and Assessment Information Set (OASIS) were collected at baseline, 6 months, and 12 months on both groups. Cognition was measured with the MDS Cognitive Performance Scale (CPS), activities of daily living (ADL) as the sum of five MDS ADL items, depression with the MDS-Depression Rating Scale, and incontinence and pressure ulcers with specific MDS items. Three OASIS items were used to measure pain, dyspnea, and medication management. The Cochran–Mantel–Haenszel (CMH) method was used to test the association between the NCC intervention and clinical outcomes.

   Findings: At 12 months the NCC group scored significantly better statistically in the clinical outcomes of pain, dyspnea, and ADL [activities of daily living]. No significant differences between groups were found in eight clinical outcome measures at 6 months.

   Conclusions: Use of nurse care coordination for acute and chronic home care warrants further evaluation as a treatment approach for chronically ill older adults.

   (a) Not applicable

(b) Level II
(c) Level III
(d) Level IV
(e) Level V/VI

EXHIBIT 3.2 LEARNING ACTIVITY: DEVELOPMENT OF AN EBP EDUCATIONAL EXERCISE

Purpose: To apply knowledge of the evidence-based practice (EBP) framework to the design of an educational exercise to promote student learning of EBP.
Desired Outcome: Draft of a brief proposal for an EBP learning activity to be more fully developed and refined at the faculty retreat in June 2012.
Directions: Work in groups of two to four to draft a proposal for an EBP learning activity, which will be presented to all workshop participants.
Timeframe: 30 minutes to draft proposal; 5 minutes to present draft.

Template for Proposal for an EBP Educational Exercise:

- **Title of Educational Exercise:**

- **Faculty Member(s):**

- **Student Audience/Course: (e.g., undergraduate students, medical-surgical course, clinical practicum):**

- **Purpose of Activity:**

- **Desired Outcome(s):**

(*continued*)

EXHIBIT 3.2 (*continued*)

- **Brief Description of Activity:**

Assessment of Learning Needs for Evidence-Based Practice*

In order to put together a workshop on evidence-based practice that meets your needs, I need to have an idea of the areas in which you would like to develop your knowledge and/or skills. Please rank the following topic in the order in which you would like a presentation using a one, "1," for your top priority.

______**Basics of EBP** (includes the definition of EBP, the rationale for why we need it, how to formulate a PICO question [with exercises], difference between background and foreground questions, levels of evidence)

______**How to conduct a systematic search of the literature**

______**How to appraise evidence (single studies, systematic reviews)**

______**How to access relevant clinical practice guidelines on www.guidelines.gov, use the new capabilities of that website for guideline comparison, and use the AGREE II tool to appraise clinical practice guidelines**

______**Models of EBP and providing exemplars of how they can be used to guide EBP initiatives**

______**Teaching strategies for integrating EBP into a nursing curriculum and into specific courses**

Please comment on any other type of EBP workshop that you would like if it is not listed above and give it a rank.

Thank you so much and I look forward to learning with you.

*Tool for Assessment of Faculty Learning Needs for Evidence-Based Practice reprinted with permission from the author.

members work together in collaborative groups for 20 to 30 minutes to complete the exercise. Then a spokesperson for each group shares with all workshop participants the work that was accomplished. Participants and the workshop facilitator then provide constructive feedback to each group about their proposed EBP learning activity. The time allotted for this interactive exercise depends on the number of participants involved in the workshop. My recommendation is to allow at least 10 minutes for each group to present their work and elicit collegial feedback. Consider that each group should have no more than five to six members.

One positive outcome of this approach was a clinical assignment devised by adjunct or clinical faculty in an undergraduate nursing program. The assignment entailed asking a focused clinical question about an issue that arose during the care of one of their patients and then accessing one or two primary sources to address the question. This was to take the place of one "nursing process paper." The clinical faculty convinced the tenured course coordinator to allow this change to course requirements. This was one small step for the involved clinical faculty yet it was one giant step for the integration of EBP into clinical course components.

STRATEGY 3: WORK WITH INDIVIDUAL FACULTY MEMBERS TO DEVELOP EBP LEARNING ACTIVITIES

Sometimes faculty members, just as students and clinical nurses, need individual support, whether it be mentoring or coaching, to help them devise and implement an EBP teaching strategy. Depending on faculty comfort with expressing their need for support, an individual may either come to you or you may need to go to them. I have had experience with both types of encounters as exemplified by the following:

Encounter One. A graduate faculty member who was teaching a clinical course for nurse practitioners approached Levin to work with her on developing a learning activity related to the use of the AGREE instrument to evaluate clinical practice guidelines. She asked Levin to co-teach a class with her on this. They developed the learning activity together and co-facilitated the class the first time she introduced it. Subsequently, the faculty member integrated this learning activity into her course and facilitated the class independently.

Encounter Two. In this example, a faculty member was encouraged to integrate the introduction of clinical practice guidelines into a sophomore clinical course in order to help students understand the evidence base for the material they were learning. The faculty member was eager to try this approach, yet lacked a thorough understanding of how to implement the learning activity. She wanted, however, to try this out on her own. She developed the learning activity yet did not ask for any review or comments prior to its introduction. During the semester in which she introduced the EBP learning activity, Levin had many of the faculty members' students in her undergraduate research/EBP course. Several of them approached to tell me of the assignment they had in their other course related to clinical guidelines. They also asked for Levin's help because they did not understand the assignment. After reviewing the directions, it was clear that the faculty member needed some assistance in providing clear direction and guidance for students. Levin asked to meet with her, shared the students' difficulty with the assignment, and then worked together to clarify any misunderstandings the faculty member had and revise the directions for the assignment.

STRATEGY 4: CO-TEACH A COURSE WITH YOUR MENTEE(S)

This strategy reflects mentoring. You are in constant contact with your mentee and are able to provide the continuous support needed for the mentee to successfully integrate new strategies into a course. For example, a number of years ago, Levin was asked to review a graduate research course usually taught by another faculty member at Pace University who was preparing to be on sabbatical, and to reframe the course to focus more on application. Levin first co-taught with the faculty member and slowly integrated an EBP approach into the course. During the sabbatical period, Levin solely taught the course, integrating additional strategies and content that used an EBP framework. At the conclusion of the sabbatical, the faculty member was able to move forward with the course, not only using some of the teaching strategies Levin developed, but by developing some of her own strategies as well as enhancing several of the strategies that had been used in the graduate course as learning activities and assignments.

Once the graduate research course was revised, Levin went on to teach the undergraduate research course. Levin used the same approach, first working with an undergraduate faculty member who had taught the course from a traditional perspective for many years. That was a beginning—we agreed to disagree. Yet a few new areas of content were integrated into the course. A few years later, the graduate faculty member mentioned in an earlier example for Strategy 4 began to teach the undergraduate course with this same faculty member. Slowly, "our" mentee began to move into the new paradigm but still did not fully understand or embrace it. It was not until the School of Nursing conducted a scholarly colloquium where a group of nurses from a partner hospital presented an EBP project that they developed and implemented successfully, did the faculty mentee finally exclaim: "Oh, now I understand what this is all about." This type of "ah ha" is not very different from the "ah ha" that students, clinical nurses, and health care agency administrators experience when they see what EBP can accomplish in actual practice. And so the bottom line is to begin by first bringing in frontline individuals who have improved practice using the EBP paradigm to share their methods and successes. This strategy has been used with students, faculty, and clinical nurses. When they see that EBP is real and does create positive change, buy-in is much easier. This approach is applicable at all levels of nursing education, and was used to initiate Strategy 6, which is described below.

STRATEGY 5: INCLUDE YOUR FACULTY MENTEE(S) IN PRESENTATIONS AND PUBLICATIONS

Even before we became interested in EBP, we used the venues of presentation and publication of our academic work as a strategy for facilitating faculty's growth in scholarly activity. This is all the more important now as we look for strategies to facilitate faculty's understanding of the value of EBP, and how to integrate it into curricula on a broad scale, and into individual courses on a smaller scale.

In devising the first edition of *Teaching Evidence-Based Practice in Nursing* (Levin & Feldman, 2006), faculty skeptical about EBP were recruited as chapter authors. In writing these chapters these authors began to understand and value the concept of EBP. Levin also engaged faculty in publications about the integration of the AGREE instrument in critical appraisal of guidelines, for example (Singleton & Levin, 2008), and in presentations about our work together (e.g., Londrigan, Shortridge-Baggett, Gordon, Levin, & Singleton, 2007).

STRATEGY 6: DEVISE A SERIES OF ADMINISTRATIVE SUPPORTED WORKSHOPS

In thinking about new ways to build nursing faculty scholarship at Pace University— a longstanding goal of Feldman— and knowing how important EBP was becoming in the practice setting, Feldman and Levin discussed a variety of approaches. A generous donor to the school had just made a commitment to supporting faculty development and details were being worked out as to how that funding could be used. In a brainstorming session with the donor, an alumnus of the school, we developed some tentative ideas that needed to be refined. The donor was very receptive to alternative approaches. Following this meeting, three approaches were identified: a faculty development program to expand faculty knowledge about EBP, funding individual faculty pilot initiatives in EBP, and holding a conference that would bring in national experts to share their work in EBP within the overall context of end-of-life care. The first initiative was implemented through a "Scholarship Development Series" (SDS) led by Levin and a School of Nursing graduate faculty member (Dr. Joanne Singleton—lead author of Chapter 22) who, in her role as family nurse practitioner, had been applying EBP in her clinical practice. The purpose of the SDS was to enhance EBP and research skills to facilitate faculty scholarship. Organized sessions were held, with mentoring arrangements of faculty with the two leaders. The end product for the series, accompanied by a well-established research peer support group, was to prepare a publishable manuscript based on their work.

The four sessions were organized as follows:

Session 1: **Focus**

- Participants were asked to identify the area of scholarship to which they wanted to contribute.
- Exercises for participants consisted of how to narrow the broad area of scholarship into a focused question for study, and how to clearly convey this idea in writing.

Anticipated Outcome: Participant will write a paragraph identifying one's focus area.

Session 2: **Search**

- Participants will identify their specific focus by applying efficient evidence search strategies to help answer their focused question and manage search results.
- Exercises for participants were to formulate searchable questions, construct and execute a search, and manage the search and search results.

Anticipated Outcome: Participants will write a paragraph about the search and results.

Session 3: **Synthesis of Evidence**

- Participants will learn how to construct an integrative review of the evidence that will be the foundation for their developing scholarship.

Anticipated Outcome: Participants will produce a bibliography of the articles they plan to include in their integrated reviews.

Session 4: **Critical Appraisal of Evidence**

- Participants will learn how to identify the level and quality of evidence on their selected topics.

Anticipated Outcome: Participants will develop a table rating the evidence and will write a summary of the evidence.

Combining the efforts of the SDS and the peer support group, which met monthly and focused on follow-up questions to the sessions and peer input on work in progress, we anticipated that participants would develop an abstract and publishable manuscript. Some participants were successful within the timeline; others required additional time and/or support.

In summary, faculty development initiatives, fostered by a strong mentoring plan, are essential to advancing faculty knowledge of and commitment to EBP. In order to implement these initiatives, administrative support in terms of providing released time or additional compensation to faculty and external funding are often essential ingredients for success.

REFERENCES

Levin, R. F., & Feldman, H. R. (2006). *Teaching evidence-based practice in nursing*. New York: Springer Publishing.

Levin, R. F., Melnyk, B. M., Fineout-Overholt, E., Barnes, M., & Vetter, M. (2011). Fostering evidence-based practice to improve nurse and cost outcomes in a community health setting: A pilot test of the ARCC model. *Nursing Administration Quarterly, 35*(1), 1–13.

Londrigan, M., Shortridge-Baggett, L., Gordon, S., Levin, R. F., & Singleton, J. K. (2007, April). R. F. Levin (Chair), *Integrating evidenced-based practice into nursing curricula: It takes a community*. Symposium conducted at the meeting of the Eastern Nursing Research Society, Providence, RI.

Singleton, J. K., & Levin, R. F. (2008). Strategies for learning evidence-based practice: Critically appraising clinical practice guidelines. *Journal of Nursing Education, 47*(8), 380–383.

4

Mentoring Preceptors in Evidence-Based Practice

Lucille Ferrara

One change makes way for the next, giving us the opportunity to grow.

—Vivian Buchen

Advanced practice nurses (APNs) are called upon time and again to act as preceptors to graduate APN students in clinical practice. Too often it is assumed that the APN, regardless of clinical experience and expertise, is willing and able to step into this role seamlessly without giving much thought to role development. Newer APNs are quite willing to serve in the preceptor role but are not always provided with the guidance and mentoring needed to help make this role exciting, interesting and, most importantly, sustainable. Seasoned preceptors frequently express frustrations in the role, which stem from a lack of preparation for and support in the role. Factors such as productivity quotas, limited space, and previous negative experiences with preceptors may discourage APNs from acting in this capacity, which in turn fuels the ever-growing shortage of preceptors and available clinical placement sites. A good approach to encourage busy APNs to act in this capacity is to ensure that preceptors, both new and seasoned, are mentored.

During the mentoring process, assisting the preceptor to learn and acquire strategies that will enhance the experience is vital. One very important strategy is the integration of evidence-based practice (EBP) into the mentor/mentee dyad and is an area that needs particular attention because it should not be assumed that all preceptors are familiar with EBP, have adapted its framework into their practice, or understand how to use the principles of EBP in clinical decision making.

Three common goals most preceptors share are to (a) have a solid knowledge base, (b) be confident in teaching students, and (c) keep a step ahead of the students they are mentoring. Much of the learning that takes place in clinical practice is "in the moment" learning. Preceptors need to be current with regard to prevention, diagnosis, and treatment and delivery of patient care, and be able to transfer and share this knowledge with students. I work with preceptors to achieve these goals by teaching them how to integrate EBP into their practice and to search for the best evidence that will support clinical decision making and at the same time build and expand on their knowledge base. By doing so, I can help them achieve the third goal, keeping a step ahead of their students. Once the preceptor becomes comfortable in searching for the best evidence, I can teach the preceptor how to navigate the data sites and interpret and translate the evidence into practice. Consider the following scenario.

> During a conversation with Lisa she explained to me that a student she was mentoring asked her for guidance in a school assignment that required the student to evaluate the quality of smoking cessation interventions in her placement site. Lisa explained to me that they were not offering smoking cessation interventions and that a formal program did not exist at that time. Lisa expressed, however, that she saw great value in instituting smoking cessation strategies in the clinic and that this type of student activity would certainly help her to realize the goal (Lisa's "what's in it for me" [WIIFM]. I showed Lisa the various databases available that address smoking cessation guidelines. Then Lisa searched those databases, that is, Cochrane Reviews, Joanna Briggs Institute, National Institute of Health, Agency for Healthcare Research and Quality, and the Centers for Disease Control, to familiarize herself with the content available on these sites as well as the nuances of navigating each one. Lisa was then able to work with her student and direct her toward sites that offered the best evidence. She also had the student perform a literature review of current research that looked at smoking cessation models. Based on the literature review, our collaboration, and the collaboration with her student, Lisa was able to develop a smoking cessation program in the clinic. The new knowledge acquired is empowering and ultimately builds the preceptor's level of self-confidence by equipping her with the tools and strategies she can use to not only incorporate EBP into her clinical practice, but to integrate EBP into her teaching.

Another example of how to mentor a preceptor about EBP integration is through debriefing. When mentoring new preceptors, it is beneficial to have them discuss and debrief their clinical day of mentoring.

> When we established our relationship Lisa and I agreed that we would meet every other week (either virtually or in person) to discuss her current students and debrief on how she was progressing with her mentoring experience. Keeping in mind the three goals (knowledgebase, self-confidence, and being a step ahead), the mentor provides guidance in the debriefing session to address these goals. For example, during a debriefing session, Lisa shared that her student learned in class about the United States Preventive Services Task Force (USPSTF) and had

> questions about navigating this site. Lisa was able to assist the student because this was one of the databases I reviewed with her, and her level of comfort with the material enabled her to easily assist her student. Lisa also shared that she used this site frequently for her patient teaching activities and found the evidence to be current and helpful in developing her patients' plan of care.

Through debriefing, Lisa was able to reflect on and appreciate the value of incorporating EBP into her practice.

NEED FOR ROLE DEVELOPMENT

As program director of a large and quite busy family nurse practitioner graduate program, my focus is on educating future nurse practitioners. Over the past few years the need for clinical placement sites has grown significantly, while the availability of these sights is becoming more competitive. The search for preceptors that are motivated, positive, student-focused, and current in the latest evidence is paramount! Because of these needs, it has become apparent that a major aspect of the director role includes spending time to develop and mentor clinical preceptors in order to ensure that students receive the best clinical experience as well as provide preceptors with clinical student experiences that are both satisfying and rewarding. Consider the following scenario.

> Lisa has been an APN for more than 5 years. She works in a federally qualifying health center (FQHC) where she sees approximately 20 to 30 patients per day. Her salary is supported by patient productivity numbers. On average, a full-time provider may be required to see as many as 3,000 patient visits per year to sustain his or her clinic position. Lisa has two exam rooms in which to see patients and, at times, due to internal factors such as resident training, may only have one exam room. This greatly limits space. Many of her patients are non-English speaking, requiring the use of translators, which increases the amount of time spent with patients. Lisa also specializes in chronic disease management (diabetes, hypertension, asthma, cardiac disease), where on specific days she devotes her time and practice to seeing this population, again requiring more time with each patient encounter. When approached with the request to be a preceptor, often the answer will be, "this will take up too much of my time," even though the APN may, in fact, want to be a preceptor (and is often required to do so for re-certification).

This scenario is all too common in today's clinical domain. A mentoring relationship with a preceptor can help to develop strategies for time management and other skills so that the APN can successfully take on the preceptor role that is so critical to the student's education. One important strategy that can be quite helpful is to show her the importance of incorporating the use of evidence into the clinical practice day, which can save her time, enhance her clinical practice, and increase positive patient outcomes.

Frequently, the assumption is made that all APNs working in clinical practice can be preceptors. A second assumption frequently made is that preceptors incorporate EBP into their clinical decision making. Both assumptions are false. Here's why. First, APNs need to have ongoing role development. Not every APN was born to mentor others, regardless of whether they are expert or novice clinicians. Much of the "I don't have time to be a preceptor" philosophy stems from a lack of preparation for the role. Second, many APNs, particularly those who completed programs over 10 years ago, may not be familiar with EBP, or, conversely, are familiar with EBP but may feel that they do not have time to incorporate it into the practice day, let alone include it in mentoring others. A major component of mentoring preceptors is assisting them in understanding the role of EBP in clinical practice, as well as helping them realize its utility. Perceived EBP usefulness is an important factor when entering into a mentoring relationship. If preceptors do not value EBP or identify its usefulness, then EBP will be considered extra work. How then does one begin to work with the very busy and overextended preceptor? The remainder of this chapter will help provide some insights and useful strategies for engaging in and developing mentoring relationships with preceptors.

MENTORING

Creating a Mentoring Culture

A mentoring culture needs to be created in the work environment in order for mentoring to be sustainable and successful (Fouche & Lunt, 2010; Zachary, 2005). APNs are not only preceptors to students with whom they work but often serve as role models, too (Henry, Bruland, & Sano-Franchini, 2011). With that point in mind, mentoring the preceptor accomplishes two important goals. First, mentoring provides support and guidance for the preceptor with regard to role definition and development. Second, effective mentors are also role models who can provide a mentoring experience in which preceptors can gain and acquire their own mentoring skill sets as well as maximize their own skills in this role. When creating a mentoring culture, it is important to assess the level of acceptance of mentoring and the philosophy of those with whom the mentoring will occur (Allan, 2010; Barker, 2006; Dorsey & Barker, 2004; Henry et al., 2011).

Both novice and expert preceptors can benefit from the mentoring experience, but will do so in different ways. Once established, the mentor and mentee can then enter into a relationship built upon the specific and unique needs of the mentee, taking into consideration the mentee's beliefs, assumptions, and values, as well as internal and external motivators (Allan, 2010). Because of my administrative role, I often discuss these elements with the preceptors as we begin to enter a mentoring relationship. I want to know what they expect and want to achieve during the process that will optimize their level of clinical practice and, at the same time, help develop them professionally and personally. As a mentor, I also need to understand and reflect upon my own values and beliefs so as to ensure that the mentee's goals, objectives, and agendas come first rather than imposing my own goals and agendas. Discussing the mentee's beliefs, values, goals, and objectives is vital to overall communication. The first step in the mentoring process is to establish clear lines of communication between the mentee and mentor.

Communication

Communication is a two-way conversation where listening is considered the most fundamental element. Effective listening can elevate communication from mediocre to exceptional because each person is heard and given a chance to be heard. Once the lines of communication are created, the mentor and mentee begin to develop trust. Trust is a powerful component in successful mentoring, especially for the mentee (Zachary, 2005), enabling both parties to embrace their vulnerability, foster freedom of expression, and allow for the flow of innovative and creative ideas. Effective communication is essential when setting goals for the mentoring process; also important is the mentee's desired outcomes.

Setting Goals and Evaluating Outcomes

Setting goals or desired outcomes is an essential step in the mentoring process (Caffarella, 2002; Merriam, Caffarella, & Baumgartner, 2007) for several reasons. First, each person's values, assumptions, and personal goals are unique and thus must be considered from both the mentee's and mentor's points of view at the outset of the relationship. Once these goals are on the table, the mentor has the responsibility of ensuring that the goals are realistic, measurable and, most importantly, achievable. Having goals at the beginning of the mentoring relationship also establishes a baseline for evaluating desired outcomes. For example, one goal the preceptor may have is to identify reliable sources when searching for specific clinical guidelines. Another goal may be to improve one's care delivery for specific patient populations based upon the current guidelines available. The population the preceptor has identified is patients with type 2 diabetes (DM2). By reviewing and implementing the recommended care options outlined by the American Diabetic Association and the National Institutes of Health (NIH) (reliable databases) the preceptor notices that her patients with DM2 have improved A1Cs and medication adherence (improved patient care delivery). These specific patient outcomes reflect her goal to improve the current care delivery of patients with DM2.

Established goals are the scaffold upon which outcome measures are set. Formal evaluations can be created in written form to provide an organized document to which both mentor and mentee (preceptor) can refer when looking toward future goal setting and changes to the initial plan. Incorporating an ongoing or formative evaluation is also essential. Reflection is one example of formative evaluation and is an important practice in the evaluation of mentoring activities. An example of how I employ ongoing evaluation of the mentoring experience involves setting up time with the preceptor for us to discuss our progress and work. We each take 15 minutes to highlight both the strengths of the partnership as well as the areas that need improvement. We then make changes and develop strategies for improvement as well as set new goals for continued success. Of particular interest to me is effective communication. During our session I ask the preceptor to reflect on how well he or she communicated with me, peers, patients, and colleagues throughout the week. We then look at what worked well and what needs improvement, followed by creation of a plan that will improve intra and inter-professional communication between us and with patients. Through reflection, both mentor and mentee are able to view the mentoring experience from different lenses in order to critically evaluate the overall experience.

STRATEGIES FOR MENTORING PRECEPTORS IN EBP

The need for formal mentoring of preceptors has been discussed broadly thus far. All of the principles, for example, creating a mentoring culture, opening lines of communication, establishing trust, setting goals, and evaluating outcomes are considered essential to mentoring preceptors in EBP. Besides general strategies, specific strategies are used to mentor preceptors in EBP. *Reflection, exploring attitudes and beliefs* of EBP, and *identifying perceived usefulness* of EBP are crucial to successful integration of EBP into the preceptor's clinical practice and preceptor role.

Integrating EPB Into Clinical Practice: What's in It for Me?

Integrating EBP into clinical practice will be the biggest challenge for the preceptor, but with proper mentoring and guidance, can be achieved successfully. One way to facilitate integration is to have the preceptor identify and define the utility of EBP as it relates to his or her practice. This is what is often referred to as the "what's in it for me" (WIIFM) phenomenon (Author, 1988–2008). One's personal WIIFM is central to any change, transformation, or definition of self, practice, or learning. The WIIFM represents internal drivers and forces for motivation. Thus, it is a key objective for the mentor to identify and understand the mentee/preceptor's WIIFM. Being a preceptor for over 35 years has taught me to understand how I make the role work for me. As a mentor, I can appreciate the importance of acknowledging the mentee's internal drivers and forces in order to help one to operationalize and integrate specific elements into clinical practice. Once the preceptor understands how integrating EBP will meet one's needs and WIIFM, the utility and usefulness of EBP becomes apparent. This "ah-ha" moment for the preceptor should be harnessed in order to assist in defining how EBP is going to work, and then help to own it. If we return to the challenges described earlier for Lisa, her main WIIFM is to be able to mentor, meet the demands of a busy practice, provide excellent care that she can be proud of, and be able to teach and guide APN students in a meaningful way. Integrating EBP into practice can become a useful tool here. The mentor can now help Lisa identify what she needs to know about EBP and understand ways to incorporate EBP into the practice day and in different roles, for example, provider, preceptor, and patient educator. How can this be accomplished?

Reflection

Reflection provides preceptors with an opportunity to look at the what, how, and why of their clinical practice. At the end of the day a reflective preceptor asks, "What worked best?," "What did I do well?," "What could have been done better?," "What do I need to do to change?," "Where does the change need to take place?," and "What strategies can I incorporate into my practice to help make these changes?" Through reflection, the preceptor can also ask "Did I use the best evidence to care for this patient (population, community)?," "How could the current evidence inform my practice (my colleagues, my preceptees)?," "How much do I know about EBP?," and "What are the best resources for finding the best evidence?" Reflective practice can be established by employing various methods to assist preceptors to reflect in a meaningful and effective way (Schon, 1983). Methods include journaling or writing down one's thoughts, dialoging with other preceptors, and establishing a time each day to reflect and debrief with the mentor. Part of the debriefing process includes helping the preceptor appreciate the value of the information gleaned from the reflection. Another interesting aspect of reflection, especially when exploring the use of and defining a place for EBP in clinical practice, is assisting the preceptor in exploring his or her attitudes and beliefs with regard to EBP.

I also evaluate the preceptor's learning of EBP through reflection. Consider the following. Fred had been mentoring a nurse practitioner graduate student at his clinical practice site for 3 weeks. Fred shared with me that he had made several observations with regard to the student's use of unacceptable websites for retrieving patient education materials. He also shared that although he knew these were not the best sites, he was not sure what would be the best approach in addressing this student's current practice. We discussed the various sites the student was using and why these were unacceptable. We then developed a script that the preceptor could use to confront the student in positive and strategic ways—a teachable moment! Through reflection, we were able to view Fred's experience as a preceptor from different lenses in order to enhance the effectiveness of his teaching.

Exploring Attitudes and Beliefs

It should not be assumed that every preceptor will be willing to integrate EBP into clinical practice. To assess willingness, an exercise for the mentee could focus on attitudes and beliefs toward EBP (Allan, 2010; Berger, 2010). With well-established, open lines of communication and a trusting mentoring relationship, the mentor can assist the mentee in exploring attitudes, beliefs, and thoughts about integrating EBP in the clinical practice day as well as learning activities. It is here that reflection, sharing stories, clarification of misconceptions of EBP, and other discourse will arise. Through discourse, the preceptor begins to make meaning of EBP and to internalize the practice (Berger, 2010). An important goal for preceptors to achieve is transforming their attitudes toward and understanding of the utility of EBP in both clinical and mentor practice. It is here that the mentor will spend the most time with the preceptor, because without the preceptor's understanding of one's perceived usefulness of EBP, successful integration of EBP into clinical practice will most likely not occur (Allen, Eby, & Lentz, 2006). Seeing the use of EBP as a skill set can further frame its utility. Preceptors can incorporate EBP into practice if they view this as a skill to enhance and build upon their clinical experience. I often share my experiences as a preceptor with other preceptors to give examples of how I incorporate EBP into my clinical practice as well as my activities in the mentoring role. I do this by discussing experiences when using EBP was successful, informed my practice, and assisted preceptees to achieve their clinical practical goals.

SUMMARY

Providing excellent clinical experiences for APN graduate nursing students is central to our work as graduate faculty. Theoretical frameworks are tested in the clinical arena, which shape and define APN students' clinical practice and voice, as well as overall professionalism. Preceptors serve as the bridge that links theory with practice. Developing, refining, and cultivating the preceptor role is the cornerstone for building the strength and sustainability of the theory to practice bridge.

Too often, well-spent time is dedicated to optimizing the student's clinical experience, and less in developing clinical preceptors. Establishing well-defined mentoring relationships with preceptors creates a scaffold upon which the preceptor role is supported and fortified. Assuming that every APN is "born" to the preceptor role is erroneous. Although novice APNs may recognize the need for role development, many experienced and expert APNs also need mentoring for preceptor role development. As demonstrated in Lisa's case scenario, excellent APNs may be deterred from serving as preceptors. Developing the preceptor with the proper guidance and direction through mentoring can provide the tools, skills, and strategies for preceptors to create meaningful learning environments and experiences for students and themselves. Establishing a mentoring relationship that incorporates trust, communication, reflection, and mutual respect will be most effective in developing and educating preceptors.

Through mentoring, the preceptor (mentee) acquires many strategies and tools, one of which is the integration of EBP into clinical practice and teaching. Respecting and understanding the beliefs and attitudes of the preceptor toward EBP and assisting the preceptor (mentee) to embrace integration of EBP into his or her role are crucial. Once the preceptor understands one's WIIFM in how EBP relates and translates to clinical practice, then the practice can be internalized.

The work of the mentor is to guide and facilitate these best practices through the integration of EBP. The most important aspect of mentoring preceptors is developing role models and mentors for APN students, colleagues, and peers. The true success of the mentoring experience is measured by the mentee's incorporation of all that is learned and the application of this learning to his or her clinical and professional lives. In the case of EBP, the preceptor's effective use of the best evidence that informs and guides best practices is a powerful exemplar to those who he or she interact with, teach, and mentor.

REFERENCES

Allan, H. (2010). Mentoring overseas nurses: Barriers to effective and non-discriminatory mentoring practices. *Nursing Ethics, 17*(5), 603–613.

Allen, T. D., Eby, L. T., & Lentz, E. (2006). The relationship between mentoring characteristics and perceived program effectiveness. *Personnel Psychology, 59*, 125–153.

Author. (1988–2008). AcronymFinder.com, *The free dictionary*. Retrieved March 25, 2012, from http://acronyms.thefreedictionary.com

Barker, E. (2006, February). Mentoring—A complex relationship. *Journal of the American Academy of Nurse Practitioners, 18*(2), 56–61.

Berger, R. (2010). EBP: Practitioners in search of evidence. *Journal of Social Work, 10*(2), 175–191.

Caffarella, R. (2002). *Planning programs for adult learners* (2nd ed.). San Francisco: Jossey-Bass Company.

Dorsey, L., & Baker, C. (2004). The art and angst of the mentoring relationship. *Academic Psychiatry, 21*, 61–67.

Fouche, C., & Lunt, N. (2010). Nested mentoring relationships: Reflections on a practice project for mentoring research capacity amongst social work practitioners. *Journal of Social Work, 10*(4), 391–406.

Henry, J., Bruland, H., & Sano-Franchini, J. (2011). Course embedded mentoring for first-year students: Melding academic subject support with role modeling, psychosocial support, and goal setting. *International Journal for the Scholarship of Teaching and Learning, 5*(2), 1–22.

Merriam, S. B., Caffarella, R. S., & Baumgartner, L. M. (2007). *Learning in adulthood* (3rd ed.). San Francisco: Jossey-Bass Company.

Schon, D. (1983). *The reflective practitioner: How professionals think in action*. NewYork: Basic Books.

Zachary, L. J. (2005). *Creating a mentoring culture*. San Francisco: Jossey-Bass Company.

Part II

Evidence-Based Teaching Practices: Let Us Practice What We Preach

Part II describes strategies for teaching specific, and often difficult, concepts related to evidence-based practice. These include formulating clinical questions, searching for evidence, understanding complex statistical concepts, teaching treatment effectiveness formulas, using assessment tools, and more. Various aspects of implementing evidence-based practice are also described, for example, involving stakeholders or conducting a gap analysis. We want to equip faculty and practitioners with the tools they will need to be effective in these areas.

5

Describing the Practice Area for Improvement

Rona F. Levin

The first edition of this book identified problem identification, problem clarification, and problem focus as important steps in forming a focused clinical question (see Chapter 7). Those steps are still extremely relevant. An increasingly widespread, new emphasis on aspects of problem identification and refinement or clarification now informs and enhances our approach to clinical practice improvement. In brief, while the pure evidence-based practice (EBP) paradigm begins with a focused clinical question, clinicians and administrators still find clarifying that question a challenge. Not only do we need to start with identifying a clinical problem, clarifying that problem, and then focusing the problem into a searchable clinical question, but we also need to pay attention to whether or not the problem that an individual clinician, administrator, or educator may consider important is also important in an organizational and societal context. This chapter and the chapter that follows address how to assess whether or not to expend resources in studying a problem or attempting to improve a practice. Important to that decision is the identification of key stakeholders, and using methods to involve them in determining whether to pursue a clinical practice improvement effort.

According to Levin, Keefer, Marren, Vetter, Lauder, and Sobolewski (2010), what the individual clinician may identify as a clinical problem may be only the first step in describing a practice area for improvement. The larger agency/organization and societal context must also be considered. The former may be gleaned from internal agency data and the latter from external literature or other evidence, which supports the problem's significance beyond the specific health care setting in which the problem was identified.

INTERNAL DATA

Thus once a problem or area for improvement is identified, the project team needs to access internal data to "more fully describe the problem in quantitative terms in order to place the problem within the larger context significance" (Worral, Levin, & Coté Arsenault, 2009–2010, p. 13). Such information may be gleaned from: (1) quality data that an organization regularly collects; (2) patient record audits, which the project team may request permission to access from the agency's Institutional Review Board (IRB); or (3) prospective data that nurses and other health care providers may collect during the routine care of patients. The following are some examples of each of these types of data.

Routine Quality Data

Every organization must keep statistics on certain aspects of care. Some are mandated by the Joint Commission on Hospital Accreditation and others are developed at the behest of each agency. For example, if you find that the patient fall rate at your agency is higher than the intended benchmark, you should contact the quality management department or individual in charge of compiling such data to find out the current fall rate, how that rate may differ on each type of inpatient unit, and whether or not the statistics actually support a problem. That is, an individual clinician may identify a problem with patient falls based on one incident on a particular hospital unit. That incident, however, may not be indicative of a larger hospital-wide issue. Only by accessing the quality or patient safety data is a project team able to judge the wider significance of the problem to the institution.

Patient Record Audits/Nurse Focus Groups

Often internal agency data does not supply us with all the quantitative information we need to develop a focused clinical question. In such circumstances, we may need to audit patient records to glean additional quantitative data to support the notion that a problem exists and to aid in its description. On another level we may need to interview patients and/or nurses to find out more about the possible problem (qualitative data). Two examples follow, of which the first deals with patient record audit results.

During an actual evidence-based practice improvement (EBPI) project regarding pain management in a community health agency, nurses involved on the project team had to access patient records in order to determine how home health nurses were documenting patients' pain. Initially, each nurse on the project team reviewed the same patients' records using

Visiting Nurse Service Of New York
We Bring The Caring Home

Renfield Project: Pain Management Team Audit Tool			
Reviewer's Name: ______ **Diagnoses:** ______ COC____ Other____ **Period of Time** **Reviewed: 10/1/-11/30/2007** **Region:** %Brooklyn % Bronx **Team#:** ____ **Time Frame**-October 1, 2007–November 30, 2007 (at least 4weeks) **Total # of visits in time frame including last and prior OASIS** ______ **Case#:** ______ **SOC:** ______ **Case is:** % Active % Discharged			
			Instructions Comments
OASIS Assessment/Clinical Findings/Pain Management Problem			
1. Presence of pain is assessed on each visit (VNS0337). Include "None" as an assessment.	___**Of**___	**NA**	Answer as %. For example "4 of 8" (meaning total number of notes reviewed 4 assessed pain out of 8 charts)
2. Pain was rated 4 or greater. (**Include pain rating in the pain management problem-example,** SN rated pain as 2 under clinical findings but rated pain under "pain management problem as 5 as "worst " since last visit.)	___**Of**___	**NA**	Answer as %. **If no notes have pain 4 or greater then STOP review at this point**. If "5 of 8" had 4 or greater pain rating then **continue review of the 5 charts only.**
3. If Pain is scored as 4 or greater, were the following additional items completed? a. (VNS0338) Type	___**Of**___	**NA**	Answer as %. for each category. For example, of the 5 charts reviewed (with pain 4 or more) "2 of 5" completed the "type" of pain.
b. (VNS0339) Location	___**Of**___	**NA**	
c. (VNS0340) Characteristics	___**Of**___	**NA**	
d. (VNS0341) Relieved by	___**Of**___	**NA**	
e. (VNS0342) Effectiveness	___**Of**___	**NA**	
Pain Management Problem			
1. If pain score is 4 or more is there documentation in the Pain Management Problem? **(IF NO DOCUMENTATION ON PAIN MANAGEMENT PROBLEM SKIP TO QUESTION 3)**	___**Of**___	NA	Answer as %. For example, of the 5 charts reviewed (with pain 4 or more) **"4 of 5"**"documented in the pain management problem."
2. Interventions documented against. a. Assessed	___**Of**___	NA	Answer as % **only** charts that documented in pain problem. For example, of the 4 charts that document in pain problem 3 documented under assessment. "3 of 4"
Pain Status: Pain symptom rating: worst pain/least pain Frequency of symptoms reported: Pain interferes with: ______ Aggravating factors: ______ Alleviating factors: ______	**Check (✓) what was "assessed" during the time period of review.** (For example, If in all 5 charts reviewed with a pain level of 4 or greater assessed aggravating factors –5 checks should be in front of that assessment.		

FIGURE 5.1 Sample audit tool for pain management EBPI project.

b. Taught	___Of ___	NA	Answer as %. For example, of the 5 charts reviewed 3 documented under teaching.
Reason for pain **Medication management** Rationale for around the clock dosing Filling prescriptions in a timely manner Initially causes drowsiness Manage constipation Difference between drug tolerance/drug addiction **Behaviors/ techniques to manage pain:** Engage in activities that distract from pain Exercise, as tolerated Repositioning Immobilization Rest/exercise schedule Imagery Meditation Breathing exercises Develop structured routines Expression of feelings Avoid stressors Manage nausea and vomiting **Symptom/complications to report to care provider:** Increase in pain New pain Constipation Stupor Confusion			**Check (✓) what was "taught" during the time period of review.**
c. Managed	___Of ___	NA	Answer as %. For example, of the 5 charts reviewed 3 documented under managed.
Contact MD for medical consultation, pain regimen ineffective (See Coordination of Care) Referred to other VNS programs: Acute Care, Hospice, LTHHCP, Choice, Infusion Care Referred for additional VNS services: Nursing, SW, PT, OT, SLP, Paraprofessional, Nutritionist Referred to outside healthcare services			**Ch eck (✓) what was "managed" during the time period of review.**
d. Supported	___Of ___	NA	Answer as %. For example, of the 5 charts reviewed 3 documented under supported.
Participation in support groups Acknowledged response to pain			**Check (✓) what was "assessed" during the time period of review.**
e. Evaluated	___Of ___	NA	Answer as %. For example, of the 5 charts reviewed 3 documented under evaluated.
Check (✓) what was "evaluated" during the time period of review. (TURN PAGE OVER)			

FIGURE 5.1 Sample audit tool for pain management EBPI project (*continued*).

Patient response to care: Treatment tolerated ✏ Treatment tolerated poorly Clinical Actions: ______ ✏ Patient experienced pain related to treatment Clinical Actions: ______ Treatment observed to be effective ✏ Treatment observed to be ineffective Unable to determine effectiveness -Condition/symptoms unchanged since last visit Condition/symptoms improved since last visit ✏ Condition/symptoms declined/worsened since last visit Clinical Actions:______	Patient/Caregiver learning/return demonstration: **Has adequate knowledge** Can perform treatment /care without supervision Knowledge inadequate, requires further supervision -✏ Unable to recall information and/or follow detailed instruction Clinical Actions: ______ ✏ Unable to perform Clinical Actions:______ Requires further supervision		**Patient /Caregiver–Follows suggested Plan:** As often as necessary -✏More often than necessary Clinical Action Taken______ -✏Less than necessary Clinical Action Taken______ -✏Rarely or Never Clinical Action Taken______ **Primary symptom management since last visit** Managed independently Managed with assistance (caregiver, family, HHA) Required intervention of skilled professional Required unplanned /emergent care
Other "Problems" and "Outcomes"			
3. Did the note include documentation on a Pain **<u>Medication</u>** Management Problem (Only pain medications or adjuvant therapy)	____**Of** ___	**NA**	
4. Did any other "problems" documented on the note include **specific instruction** in "pain"? *	____**Of** ___	**NA**	*Example, in "OA or HIV Problem check if instructed in pain management, S/S of pain to report etc.
5. Did the note include documentation of "outcomes" related to pain? **Include only if documented under outcomes**	____**Of** ___	(Found after evaluation under care plan problem" pain management".	
Coordination of Care (COC): Check under "Problems"-"Managed", "Evaluated" & in "Narrative" (last part of visit note) & in COC Notes			
6. Based on **<u>patient assessment</u>** was F/U indicated?	**Yes or No**	This is reviewer's conclusion, i.e., pt had pain greater than 6 for 6 week period and nothing was done.	
7. Did the note document F/U was needed? (Check Managed, Evaluated, Narrative or COC.)	____**Of** ___	**NA**	If needed, briefly explain.
8. **If f/u was needed** was it done? (Check "Managed, Evaluated, Narrative or COC.)	____**Of** ___	**NA**	If needed, briefly explain
9. If documented, where? Managed Evaluated	Narrative		COC
10. If follow up, what was the follow up? **Check ALL that apply.** Contacted MD to change POC related to pain regime Referral to pain clinic F/U tests Change in pain/adjuvant meds Referral PT other, explain notes			
11. During the review time period, did the pain rating improve (Interventions were effective)?	**Yes or No**	**NA**	(Evidence can be - improvement in pain rating and/ or Improvement 420) If needed explain
12. List all pain medications including adjuvant therapy (Check POC):			
13. Was there a change in pain medications or adjuvant therapy during the time period? (Check POC and dates medications ordered)	**Yes or No**		If yes, briefly explain change
14. Was Rehab involved? (Check POC)	**Yes or No**	**NA**	
(TURN PAGE)			

FIGURE 5.1 Sample audit tool for pain management EBPI project (*continued*).

Episode Outcome		
Frequency of pain interfering w/ activity (M0420)	Score on **Last OASIS** = Date_______________	Score on **Prior to Last OASIS** = **Date**_______________
NOTES:		
Pain and Adjuvant Medications		
Opioid-Codeine, Codeine and Acetaminophen (Tylenol #3 or #4), Oxycodone (Roxicodone, Percolone), Oxycodone and Acetaminophen (Percocet), Hydrocodone and Acetaminophen (Vicoden, Lorcet, Lortab), Morphine (MS Contin, Oramorph)) , Hydromorphone (Dilaudid), Methadone (Dolohine), Ketobemidone, Fentanyl Transdermal System (Duragesic), Propoxiphene(Darvon), Propoxiphene and acetaminophen (Darvocet)		
Non-Opioid/NSAIDS-Acetaminophen, Aspirin, Ibuprofen,Choline Magnesium Trisalicylate (Trilisate), Naproxenl (Naprosyn), Nabumetone (Relfan), Ketorolac (toradol), Celecoxib (Celebrex), Tramadol (Ultram)		
Antidepressants-Amitriptyline (Elavil), Nortriptyline (Pamelor), Desipramine (Norpramin), Duloxetine (Cymbalta)		
Anticonvulsants-Gabapentin (Neurontin), Carbamazepine (Tegretol), Lamotrigine (Lamictal)		
Corticosteroids-Dexamethasone (decadron), Prednisone		
Other -Baclofen (Lioresal), Lidoderm Patch (Topical Lidocaine)		

FIGURE 5.1 Sample audit tool for pain management EBPI project (*continued*).

the same audit tool (see Figure 5.1) in order to determine how each nurse was interpreting the documentation. After discussion of differences, all agreed to a single interpretation of data for each item on the tool (see Chapter 10 for additional information on interrater reliability).

Project team leaders also arranged to conduct a focus group with nurses who were visiting patients in chronic pain. They interviewed these nurses to find out where the visiting nurses believed they needed additional education so as to more fully address their patients' pain needs. Based on the data accumulated from both the patient record audits and the focus group with visiting nurses, the project team was able to better understand the challenges involved and where to focus the improvement effort (see Chapters 25 and 26 for a more detailed description of this project).

Prospective Patient Data

At times retrospective data on patients specific to a clinical question is not readily available through patient record audits or quality data. Thus it becomes necessary to accumulate data related to a clinical problem prospectively. An example of this type of data collection is surveying or interviewing patients about their hospital experience after discharge. More specifically, one institution wanted to find out more about why some patients were not 100% satisfied with their postoperative pain management. This institution used the Press Ganey Hospital Quality Performance Survey (2011) as the only parameter of patient satisfaction with pain control. These data showed that overall patient satisfaction with pain control was high, but not perfect. In order to find out specifically about patients' satisfaction with postoperative pain management, and where improvement was needed, one of the hospital's patient advocates conducted telephone interviews on surgical patients post discharge to find out firsthand how they experienced pain management postoperatively. Depending on whether such information collection is considered an aspect of quality improvement by the organization, those wishing to obtain such information may need to receive IRB approval. Checking with the IRB administrator about the procedures and processes at your organization is always advised.

EXTERNAL DATA OR SUPPORTING LITERATURE

According to Worral and colleagues (2010), "... external data ... [puts] the problem in a larger context of importance to the population in question ..." (p. 13). This information is usually not part of the systematic search for evidence on a focused clinical problem, but provides background on the problem or issue that may be appropriate for an EBPI initiative. For example, during one EBPI project at a community hospital, nurses observed that patients who were on assisted ventilation in an intensive care unit (ICU) and receiving propofol for sedation had a difficult time waking up when sedation was discontinued. They also experienced profound muscle weakness among other adverse effects (Misiano, Levin, Wright, Comiskey, & D'Arcy, 2011). The nurses involved in the project started accessing related literature to determine if their observations were supported by other health care providers and whether a guideline existed to monitor and evaluate patients receiving propofol in an ICU setting.

Once you have described the clinical practice problem and are able to focus in on exactly what concerns you, you must ask yourself whether the question you are asking is a *background* or a *foreground* question. A *background* question usually asks for a fact, a statement on which most authorities or experts would agree. For example, what is the etiology of congestive heart failure? What are the most frequently prescribed analgesics for the management of postoperative pain? What are the adverse effects of treatment X? The answers to these types of questions can usually be found in a textbook and are not controversial. A *foreground* question requires an extended search for evidence to answer a specific clinical question (Straus, Richardson, Glasziou, & Haynes, 2005).

Figure 5.2 provides an abbreviated example of how an EBP project team in one organization developed its proposal for change based on both internal and external data.

TEACHING STRATEGIES

I have used several strategies to teach the above content to learners. First, it is important to "tell" learners that this content alone is not sufficient for learning. They must engage in experiential learning in order to internalize this content, and feel at least a beginning comfort with applying these approaches to their own practice. Regarding patient record audits, I ask advanced practice students to interview a quality management or performance improvement staff members in the organization to find out if they use or have used any specific tools to conduct patient audits in the agencies in which they practice. I also ask them to request copies of these tools to either bring to class (if conducting traditional classroom courses), or post on a course online platform for discussion (for virtual courses). In both instances, I ask students to address specific

Description of the Problem

The most recent Cochrane meta-analysis (Gillespie, Gillespie, Robertson, Lamb, Cumming, & Rowe, 2003) and a later systematic review (Oliver, Daly, Martin, & McMurdo, 2004) identify falls as a significant factor associated with morbidity in older people. Gillespie et al. cite several sources to support that 30% to 50% of people over the age of 65 fall each year. These authors, however, do not parcel out the rates for falls in hospitalized elderly. The Oliver et al. review focuses on hospitalized patients and cites literature that indicates rates from 2.9 to 12 falls per year per 1,000 bed days (Morse, 1995), and that approximately 30% of such falls may result in injury (Rhymes & Jaeger, 1988).

At Northern Westchester Hospital (NWH) the 2006 Patient Falls Statistics indicate that there were 163 falls during the year. This was an increase in our fall rate from a 2005 fall rate of .32 per 100 patient days to .39 per 100 patient days in 2006, not meeting our goal fall rate of .28 to .35 per patient days. The percentage of fall injuries, however, decreased from 42% in 2005 to 24% in 2006. The 6th and 7th floors had the highest number of falls with Behavioral Health having the third highest. The percentage of falls per shift was only slightly higher on the night shift. Also noted was that:

- 7% of patients had been identified as high fall risk
- 17% had bed alarms in place
- 22% had had sleep meds within 4 hours
- 15% had footwear as a factor in the fall

During 2005 to 2006, NWH interventions and/or factors to decrease the fall rate were put in place. These included:

- Hiring and training an increased number of nursing techs (2005–2006)
- Purchasing and implementing the use of bed alarms
- Increasing the number of "sitters" used for high-risk fall, confused and difficult to manage patients

All these interventions were costly. For example, $25,000 was budgeted in 2006 for sitters. Yet, the actual cost of sitters was $75,000. Despite these interventions, we were still not able to reach our benchmark figure for number of falls.

Source: Worral, P.S., Levin, R.F., & Coté Arsenault, D. (2009–2010). Documenting and EBP project: Guidelines for what to include and why. *Journal of the New York State Nurses Association, 40*(2), 14. Reprinted with permission.

FIGURE 5.2 The background section of a problem description document's internal and external evidence.

questions in an in-person class or a discussion board online. Some of these questions are:

1. What is the purpose of the tool you have accessed? What does it measure?
2. Who is responsible for conducting audits in your agency?
3. Who receives the results of these audits?

4. How has the validity and reliability (with a focus on interrater reliability) been evaluated? Has it been evaluated?
5. What are critical comments about this tool? How would you improve the tool or the process by which it is used?

Another focus group strategy is to have students simulate this type of data collection with groups of classmates and/or colleagues in their work environment. In person or with online groups data collection is also appropriate. For example, suppose the student thinks there is an issue with how nurses and technicians are approaching falls prevention strategies on the unit in which they are a staff nurse or a manager. The student might ask one or two nurses and one or two technicians to meet for an hour one day prior to or after their usual work shift for a focus group on the topic. There are many references available on how to conduct focus groups should you need assistance. Additional readings are also provided at the end of this chapter.

In summary, this chapter emphasizes the importance of describing a clinical problem with supporting internal and external data prior to making a decision about its importance within an organizational context and its wider societal significance. This and the following chapter on stakeholder involvement also contain perspectives that should engage users prior to any decision about whether to go forward with studying a focused clinical question within a specific organizational system. Several examples and strategies for teaching how to access and/or develop internal data are discussed.

REFERENCES

Levin, R. F., Keefer, J. M., Marren, J., Vetter, M., Lauder, B., & Sobolewski, S. (2010). Evidence-based practice: Merging 2 paradigms. *Journal of Nursing Care Quality*, *25*(2), 117–126.

Levin, R. F., & Wright, F. (2011). Introduction to evidence-based practice. In D. Ignatavicious, & M. L. Workman (Eds.), *Medical-surgical nursing: Patient centered collaborative care*. St. Louis, MO: Saunders/Elsevier.

Misiano, B. M., Levin, R. F., Wright, F., Comiskey, M., & D'Arcy, A. (in press). *An evidence-based protocol for propofol administration in mechanically ventilated ICU patients: Improving patient outcomes and decreasing hospital costs*. Manuscript submitted for publication.

Press Ganey Associates . (2011). *Quality performer SM: Reporting and analysis for hospital performance improvement*. Press Ganey Associates, Inc. http://www.pressganey.com/ourSolutions/hospitalSettings/clinicalSuite/qualityPerformer.aspx

Straus, S. E., Richardson, W. S., Glasziou, P., & Haynes, R. B. (2005). *Evidence-based medicine: How to practice and teach EBM* (3rd ed.). Edinburgh, Scotland: Elsevier.

Worral, P. S., Levin, R. F., & Coté Arsenault, D. Fall/Winter (2009–2010). Documenting an EBP project: Guidelines for what to include, why. *Journal of the New York State Nurses Association, 40*(2), 12–19.

ADDITIONAL READINGS

Clinical Audits

Borbasi, S., Jackson, D., & Lockwood, C. (2010). Undertaking a clinical audit. In M. Courtney, & H. McCucheon (Eds.), *Using evidence to guide nursing practice* (pp. 113–130). Sydney, Australia: Churchill Livingstone.

Focus Groups

Krueger, R. A. (1998). *Moderating focus groups.* Thousand Oaks, CA: Sage.

Morais, R. J. (2010). *Refocusing focus groups: A practical guide.* Ithaca, NY: Paramount Marketing Publishing.

Morgan, D. L. (1998). *The focus group guidebook.* Thousand Oaks, CA: Sage.

6

Involving Stakeholders in Determining the Clinical Problem: A Learning Activity

Rona F. Levin

Stakeholders are the people that build the community . . . that inspire the community . . . that serve the community.

—Gianni Longo

Since the first edition of this book, I have had the privilege of working consistently with two health care agencies (a community hospital and a prominent, home health care agency) to facilitate the evolution and integration of an evidence-based practice (EBP) culture. This chapter and its companion chapter, "Describing the Practice Area for Improvement" (Chapter 5), thus provide important information and perspectives on how to initiate any performance or practice improvement effort. This chapter focuses on stakeholder involvement and a learning activity/assignment I conceived to help doctor of nursing practice (DNP) students develop skills in obtaining stakeholder input to define a clinical problem for improvement in their agencies.

In a column that one of my DNP students and I wrote for *Research and Theory in Nursing Practice* (Burke & Levin, 2010), we noted that although several authors coming from performance improvement or evaluation perspectives (Holden & Zimmerman, 2009; Langley et al., 2009; Patton, 2008; Preskill & Catsambas, 2006) emphasize the importance of stakeholder involvement, the EBP paradigm has not explicitly included this important activity in any of the phases or components of the EBP process as it has been described historically (e.g., DiCenso, Guyatt, & Ciliska, 2005; Melnyk & Fineout-Overholt, 2005; Sackett, Straus, Richardson, Rosenber, & Haynes, 2000; Straus, Richardson, Glasziou, & Haynes, 2005).

THE IMPORTANCE OF OBTAINING STAKEHOLDER INVOLVEMENT

While Patton (2008), Holden and Zimmerman (2009), and Preskill and Catsambas (2006) define stakeholders in a project evaluation context as those who "... can affect or be affected by an evaluation process or its findings" (Patton, 2008, p. 63), this definition can easily be refined for an evidence-based practice improvement (EBPI) project (Levin et al., 2010). Most important to realize is that stakeholders must be included at the initiation of a project, not brought in only at the implementation or evaluation phase. According to Burke and Levin (2010), "... [e]ngaging stakeholders serves two major functions in the EBPI [evidence-based performance improvement] process: (1) It provides a better understanding of an agency's culture, expectation, and perspectives; and (2) it engenders buy-in throughout the EBPI process" (p. 156). Ownership of any project or change initiative is the first key to its success. Often, however, a group of individuals who believe in a project work through the planning and beginning implementation stages without including those responsible for actually implementing a new practice or those whom the implementation may affect. Then, when implementation raises issues, the initiators wonder why it was not more successful. The answer is clear: project initiators did not obtain "buy-in" from key stakeholders.

A Case in Point

Several nurses from a variety of inpatient units in a community hospital were concerned about the incidence of patient falls and embarked on an EBPI project (Levin et al., 2010) with the goal of achieving a benchmark rate for falls. They followed the initial steps of the EBP process in a systematic way; that is, they developed their focused clinical question, systematically reviewed and critiqued the relevant evidence on falls prevention, and developed an implementation plan, which the hospital approved for testing the improvement innovation. After an initial small test of change, the nurses with the assistance of their EBP mentor, realized that there were process issues related to the implementation, which had not been dealt with. Those issues were about patient care assistants' (PCAs) resistance to implementation of a toileting schedule for patients on their units. Once this issue was realized, the nurse educators in the hospital conducted interviews with the PCAs and the nurses on the test units to determine their perceptions of the problem. The PCAs shared that they felt that all the work of toileting was being "dumped" on them and that the nurses were not helping with this intervention when they were busy with other patient care responsibilities.

After meetings between the nurses and PCAs, as much to openly share issues as to educate both groups about the new intervention (from its importance in preventing patient falls and the ramifications of positive patient outcomes, to how to engage in collaborative practice), the intervention was implemented more successfully. Had the PCAs been included as major stakeholders from the beginning of the project, many of the process issues and challenges that arose could have been avoided. The beauty, however, of starting the project with a small test of change allowed the project implementers to uncover this process issue before dissemination of the new innovation to the entire hospital. Being open to learning from key stakeholders and allowing small tests of change to uncover process issues are key ingredients in any successful EBPI project.

APPROACHES TO INTERVIEWING STAKEHOLDERS

There are several frameworks that may guide the interview process. Burke and Levin (2010) wrote:

> . . . [W]henever you begin the stakeholder interview process, it is important to identify a systematic method that your project team is comfortable with and that works for them. There are several effective approaches identified in the literature, including appreciative inquiry (Preskill & Catsambas, 2006), Multimethod Assessment Process (Kairys et al., 2002), and positive deviance (Bradley et al., 2009; Walker, Sterling, Hoke, & Dearden, 2007). The take-home message is that the approach you use is not as important as the commitment to involve stakeholders in the process of EBPI from day one. (p. 157)

The multimethod assessment process (MAP) is touted as an "innovative quality improvement methodology" that combines both quantitative and qualitative techniques to gather data in order to understand organizations at a systems level and guide quality improvement initiatives (Kairys et al.). The positive deviance approach begins to focus on the positive aspects of organizational work but emphasizes nonnormative positive or "honorable" behavior, behavior that is unexpected but derives from the individual's good intentions, in order to understand where improvement needs to begin (Spreitzer & Sonenshein, 2004). Taking the positive approach to a new level and integrating it into how one goes about interviewing organizational stakeholders, Preskill and Catsambas (2006) not only provide the framework of appreciative inquiry (AI) to guide one's approach to organizational improvement, but provide the "how to" of conducting an interview to determine where an organization is doing well and how to build on that good work to achieve excellence.

Because all students in two classes I have taught chose the AI approach (Preskill & Catsambas, 2006) to guide their interviews, I will elaborate on that interview framework. Important to using this framework is a positive attitude toward improvement. What that means is that you approach the interview situation attempting first to find what people think is their most important contribution to the organization and where both the organization and the individual excel. This approach is often difficult for students to master as the organizational culture in which they have been working has tended to focus on what is wrong and what needs improvement rather than what is good and how both the organization and individual can get better.

According to Preskill and Catsambas (2006), the AI interview focuses on what interviewees value about their personal experiences within an organization and/or about the organization itself. The AI interview framework provides the context in which to develop interview questions that elicit information about:

- The interviewee's perceived moments of excellence
- Successful initiatives (processes and outcomes) in relation to the focus of the interview, for example, quality improvement
- How both processes and outcomes can be improved to increase excellence (Preskill & Catsambas, 2006)

Sample AI interview questions include:

- What do you believe has been the greatest accomplishment of your organization/agency?
- What has been your most positive contribution to the organization/agency?
- What about your work gives you the greatest pleasure?
- Can you tell me the three things that your organization/agency does best?
- If you could have one wish for organizational enhancement, what would that be?

THE LEARNING ACTIVITY

The learning activity in Exhibits 6.1 and 6.2 is the first paper that students were required to submit in the second EBP course in their DNP program, a course that focused on the reality aspects of the process, getting them ready to work with an agency on an EBP clinical improvement project. This first paper combines two important exercises for students to develop skills for

EXHIBIT 6.1 GAP ANALYSIS OF A PRACTICE AND STAKEHOLDER ASSESSMENT: PAPER I

Purposes

To gain experience and beginning skill in:

1. Conducting a gap analysis of a specific clinical practice within your organization, and
2. Identifying the stakeholders whom you would involve in an EBPI project to address the gap, specifically focusing on the project evaluation component.

Guidance

Identify individuals in your setting who you believe are stakeholders in determining best clinical practices. Then,

1. Identify all individuals in your setting who you believe are stakeholders in any EBPI effort.
2. Interview at least three of these individuals in your setting to assess what they consider current best practices, and practices that they believe could be improved or enhanced.
3. Use one of the models or approaches to stakeholder assessment from your readings to guide your interviews.
4. From these interviews, in collaboration with your stakeholders, determine the clinical practice for which you will perform a gap analysis.
5. Conduct the gap analysis.
6. Write a report in a form that you would use to present your findings to the stakeholders who you interviewed. (Of course, this report would be in APA format.)

Method of Evaluation (see Exhibit 6.2)

EBPI. One is conducting a gap analysis, the focus of Chapter 16; the second is identifying and interviewing key stakeholders for a practice improvement effort within the agency in which the DNP student is employed. Exhibit 6.3 provides the purposes of the assignment and directions or guidance for how to carry them out. Exhibit 6.2 provides the rubric for evaluating students' papers. Refer to Chapter 16 to learn more about the gap analysis portion of this assignment.

EXHIBIT 6.2 GRADING RUBRIC FOR ASSIGNMENT

Rubric for Grading Paper I

Components for Evaluation of Paper I	Outstanding (100–90)	Acceptable (89–83)	Not Acceptable (below 83)	Score
Identification of stakeholders (15%)	You clearly identify stakeholders, including a description of their position and job title in the organization; their particular informal role in practice improvement and the organization. Your rationale for including them in your interviews is presented.	One of the criteria for an "outstanding" grade is not addressed.	More than one criterion is not addressed.	
Interview with stakeholders (40%)	You present the parameters of the interview: 1. Time and length 2. Place 3. Who You present a short (150) word summary of each interview. You present your synthesis of the common themes, and support the identification of a practice that needs improvement or enhancement.	A gap exists in the discussion of how the stakeholders view the practice change that might occur and your interpretation of their thinking. One of the parameters of the interview is not addressed.	Two or more gaps exist in discussion of how stakeholders view the practice change in question, and/or the summary of the interviews do not connect the synthesis or common themes that you glean from the interviews to the practice change. The practice change you identify is not connected to stakeholder concerns.	

(continued)

EXHIBIT 6.2 *(continued)*

Components for Evaluation of Paper I	Outstanding (100–90)	Acceptable (89–83)	Not Acceptable (below 83)	Score
Driver diagram or flow chart (20%)	The diagram/flow chart of the practice you identify above contains all aspects of the current practice in need of improvement and clearly identifies aspects of the practice.	The diagram/flow chart omits up to two aspects of the practice or does not clearly identify aspects of the practice.	The diagram/flow chart omits more than two aspects of the practice and/or does not describe the practice.	
Clarity of discussion (15%)	Discussion is directed to the practice audience in "user-friendly" language, understandable to stakeholder groups within the organization.	Discussion occasionally includes terms and phrases which are more appropriate for an audience of researchers than for an audience of organizational stakeholders.	Most or all of the discussion consists of terms and phrases that an educated layperson or professional not conversant with EBP or evaluation is not likely to understand.	
Grammar and referencing (10%)	Correct use of grammar, spelling, and punctuation is evident throughout the paper. All sources are cited correctly in the text and on the reference list using APA style (2009).	There are isolated instances of incorrect use of grammar, spelling, and punctuation that limit understanding of the content. There are isolated instances of sources cited incorrectly in the text and/or on the reference list.	There is repeated incorrect use of grammar, spelling, and punctuation that limits understanding of the content and/or demonstrates limited knowledge of written English. Sources are repeatedly cited incorrectly in the text and on the reference list.	

EXHIBIT 6.3 DISCUSSION BOARD ACTIVITY—GRADED DISCUSSION

For the first week (September 17 through September 24) in order to get some experience with interviewing stakeholders for EBPI initiatives, each person in the class is to conduct one AI interview in one's practice setting. This interview should be in real time and so you should consider setting up a 1-hour appointment with the interviewee. Using the framework and approach in Preskill and Catsambas (2006), develop your own interview questions to guide your interaction. Record your interview and do not forget to ask permission of the interviewee to do so. Besides the recording keep detailed notes on the responses to your questions. **Post the questions you posed to the interviewee and summarize the interviewee's responses to each of your questions (limit to no more than four questions) in one paragraph of no more than 75 words.** Be sure to include one question that asks the interviewee about a practice that one believes could be enhanced in your setting. Provide a one-paragraph synthesis of your interview findings and describe your personal experience in conducting this interview.

Each student is to respond to one other peer's posting during the third week of the semester **(by Wednesday, September 29 at 9 a.m.)**. Please critically appraise your chosen peer's questions and presentation, and offer at least one constructive collegial criticism to facilitate your classmate's learning.

Discussion will be graded!

STUDENT FEEDBACK

There are several ways to evaluate the impact of these assignments (the discussion board learning activity and the paper). The following are excerpts from their discussion board assignment regarding their experience with an AI interview:

Student 1:

I think you [writing to another student] hit the nail right on the head. It seems to me that the value of AI is to help the interviewee push past any existing negativity by reframing the concern and becoming empowered. When we come to the interview relationship with the sole purpose of facilitating the inner awakening/empowerment of the individual with whom we speak, I think we are able to achieve the purest form of AI. Once the barriers of frustration and feelings of lack of control are reframed as opportunity, helping the interviewee to tap into inner strength, vision, and power, [and] progress replaces stagnation.

Student 2:

My personal experience, during this appreciative interview, helped me recognize a human connection to a person I thought of as administrator. The challenge I had with appreciative inquiry was not to lead the answers and to allow for pregnant pauses. It is much more fulfilling to ask questions that will evoke positive answers then to complete typical root cause analysis questions that all too often lead to blame, judgment and negativity. I reflected on why I chose this stakeholder to ask the questions of and came up with three answers. First, I thought she would be the most receptive to my inexperienced questioning, second, because I believe she is looking for someone to share growth and unit cohesiveness with, and lastly, I think she is interested in facilitating real change in the unit. I was honored and fulfilled with her last comment that I had evoked the need for further reflection in her. I was humbled, honored, and empowered after conducting this interview. "... appreciative inquiry is about conversations that matter ...." (Preskill & Catsambas, 2006, p. 11)

Student 3:

What came out of this process was the fact that we identified the need for a unified, interdisciplinary-team approach to achieve our goals. Next week the program director is planning a meeting with the nurse practitioners from both the medical and surgical cardiology services to discuss workflow and ways to improve program practices and meet patient needs. We discussed using an AI perspective, starting out by creating a list of what each service thinks works best and to try to build off of commonalities from these lists to meet our goals.

Several students mentioned during in-person class discussion that they were initially very uncomfortable with conducting an interview from an AI perspective, as it was foreign to them. When, however, they received consistently positive feedback from the interviewees and left the interview feeling that they had accomplished a small step toward practice improvement, they grasped this approach and found it extremely satisfying. In fact, all students (~40) in two different classes chose the AI framework for interviewing stakeholders rather any other framework proposed in their readings. Two students, one from each of two different classes, shared that this learning activity, particularly the use of an AI interview to determine area in the organization that need enhancement, led immediately to the development of practice improvement initiatives in their agencies.

Engaging students in realistic as well as conceptual/theoretical learning, and facilitating their application of that learning to improving practice in their own agencies and the agencies in which they are assigned for a mentorship experience in EBP, is key to helping students the confidence and skill they will need to lead evidence-based clinical practice improvement projects as doctorally prepared clinical leaders.

REFERENCES

Bradley, E. H., Curry, L. A., Ramanadhan, S., Rowe, L., Nembhard, I. M., & Krumholz, H. M. (2009). Research in action: Using positive deviance to improve quality of health care. *Implementation Science, 4*(25). doi: 10.1186/1748-5908-4-25.

Burke, R., & Levin, R. F. (2010). Describing the problem for an evidence-based practice Improvement Project: A missing ingredient. *Research and Theory Nursing Practice, 24*(3), 155–158.

DiCenso, A., Guyatt, G., & Ciliska, D. (2005). *Evidence-based practice: A guide to clinical practice.* St. Louis, MO: Elsevier/Mosby.

Holden, D. J., & Zimmerman, M. A. (2009). *A practical guide to program evaluation.* CA: Sage.

Kairys, J. A., Orzano, J., Gregory, P., Stroebel, C., DiCicco-Bloom, B., Roemheld-Hamm, B. et al. (2002). Assessing diversity and quality in primary care through the multimethod assessment process (MAP). *Quality Management in Health Care, 10,* 1–14.

Langley, G., Moen, R., Nolan, K., Nolan, T., Norman, C., & Provost, L. (2009). *The improvement guide: A practical approach to enhancing organizational performance* (2nd ed.). Philadelphia, PA: Jossey-Bass.

Levin, R. F., Keefer, J. M., Marren, J., Vetter, M., Lauder, B., & Sobolewski, S. (2010). Evidence-based practice: Merging 2 paradigms. *Journal of Nursing Care Quality, 25*(2), 117–126.

Melnyk, B. M., & Fineout-Overholt, E. (Eds.). (2005). *Evidence-based practice in nursing and Healthcare: A guide to best practice.* Philadelphia: Lippincott Williams & Wilkins.

Patton, M. Q. (2008). *Utilization-focused evaluation* (4th ed.). Los Angeles, CA: Sage Publications.

Preskill, H., & Catsambas, T. (2006). *Reframing evaluation through appreciative inquiry.* CA: Sage.

Sackett, D., Straus, S. E., Richardson, W. S., Rosenberg, W., & Haynes, R. B. (2000). *Evidence-based medicine: How to practice and teach EBM* (2nd ed.). UK: Churchill Livingstone.

Spreitzer, G. M., & Sonenshein, S. (2004). Toward the definition of positive deviance. *American Behavioral Scientist, 47*(6), 828–847.

Straus, S. E., Richardson, W. S., Glasziou, P., & Haynes, R. B. (2005). *Evidence-based medicine: How to practice and teach EBM* (3rd ed.). UK: Churchill Livingstone.

Walker, L. O., Sterling, B. S., Hoke, M. M., & Dearden, K. A. (2007). Applying the concept of positive deviance to public health data: A tool for reducing health disparities. *Public Health Nursing, 24,* 571–576.

7

Formulating Clinical Questions: Follow My Lips

Rona F. Levin

Instruction begins when you the teacher learn from the learner; put yourself in his place so that you may understand ... what he learns and the way he understands it.

—Soren Kierkegaard

Faculty and students both struggle with identifying a focused clinical question, whether it is for a dissertation, evidence-based project, or simply for a course paper. After 6 years, I still use the same approach to facilitate focusing the clinical question. What I do want to share, however, is another approach to writing such a question that has been more recently advocated by Melnyk and Fineout-Overholt (2011). They recommend adding a "T" for time frame to the PICO (population, intervention, comparison, and outcome) question thus making it a PICOT question. What this does is detail the outcome to a greater degree. For example, a PICO question might be: Does guided imagery decrease the pain of labor in primiparous women? Thus, based on the theory and evidence about the cognitive state of women during the different phases of labor, might there not be a specific phase in which guided imagery is more effective than in others? An appropriate PICOT question based on this idea might be, Does guided imagery decrease the pain of labor during the second phase of labor in primiparous women? Of course, in order to narrow the question with a time frame, there would need to be sufficient evidence (at least theoretical) to identify a specific time during which an intervention might be most effective.

The literature on EBP does a wonderful job of helping students and clinicians to formulate focused clinical questions (e.g., Nollan, Fineout-Overholt, & Stephenson, 2004; Sackett, Straus, Richardson, Rosenberg, & Haynes, 2000). When teaching the novice about clinical problems, however, we need to meet the students where they are at the moment, that is, in their practice settings, at a point where they might not yet know how to identify the problems that exist. We also need to keep in mind as teachers that although it may be easy for us to put clinical problems in the format of a focused, searchable question, this is a skill that takes nurturing and practice. Therefore, I believe there are at least two steps of cognitive activities that need to occur prior to asking students to formulate focused, searchable clinical questions: identification and clarification. We can form a teaching trajectory or process to approach this material, which leads eventually to the focused, searchable question. The steps are:

- Problem identification
- Problem clarification
- Problem focus

PROBLEM IDENTIFICATION

Somewhere along the path of my teaching career, I came across a principle that I am sure we have all happened upon: Start where you find the student! I cannot remember where or when I heard or read it or who authored the saying, but I have always put it to good use. In terms of helping students to identify clinical problems, it means letting them tell you what is on their minds about their clinical experience in their own words as a first step in formulating a focused, searchable question.

Engaging students in a discussion of problems they are encountering in practice creates the practical link between the content you are teaching and how that content relates to students' daily clinical experience. Thus, this is where we begin. As part of an introductory class or as an out-of-class assignment, depending on the length of class, have students describe in a paragraph a clinical problem they are experiencing in their setting. (The exercise may also be done as an online teaching strategy using a discussion board with students and instructor or via e-mail with the instructor.) This activity allows students to first describe their clinical problem in their own words, an easy first step in the identification–clarification–focus format. Such an exercise also helps you as the instructor to assess students' current thinking about clinical problems and how much time needs to be devoted to helping them clarify their clinical problems, which is the next step.

Several years ago, one of my service colleagues attended the class I taught on identifying clinical problems. Each student had written a paragraph describing a problematic situation in their practice for homework and was now reading it aloud to the rest of the class. My service colleague was quite impressed with the students' ability to describe practice problems "in their own words." While the students themselves had thought about what they wrote in the past, they never took pen to paper to articulate their thinking—a first and necessary step preceding clarification and focus.

PROBLEM CLARIFICATION

When students are able to describe a clinical problem, the next step is to clarify their thinking about it. One of the ways to approach the clarification task is through Socratic dialogue between student and teacher. An abbreviated example of the use of this approach is as follows:

> I recently had the opportunity of introducing EBP to nurses in a hospital setting as part of a pilot study to test the success of EBP educational interventions. Using the Socratic method, I asked the nurses to describe what they considered to be a problem on their unit. One of the nurses replied, "Patient satisfaction." I then asked, "How is patient satisfaction a problem?" The nurse went on to say that patients complained about noise on the unit. "Ah," I said, "are they having a problem with noise on the unit?" "Yes," she responded, "noise is the problem." Once noise was identified as the problem, we could proceed to looking at patient outcomes that noise was affecting, patient satisfaction being one. Other outcomes we discussed were sleep/rest patterns and pain. The focused, searchable question was evolving.

Another way to approach the task of clarifying the clinical problem is through group discussion, whether face-to-face or electronically through interactive dialogue. An electronic interactive assignment might include students providing a transcript of the dialogue they have had with at least one other classmate or colleague about their identified clinical problem, providing the focused question that results from that dialogue.

PROBLEM FOCUS

Now it is time to help students formulate the focused, clinical question that will guide the search for evidence. In a chapter by Nollan, Fineout-Overholt, and Stephenson (2004), "Asking Compelling Clinical Questions" (see Exhibit 7.1), they do a wonderful job providing question templates for asking PICO questions; that is, population, intervention, comparison, and outcome (see chapter 1 of Nollan et al., 2004) related to therapy, etiology diagnostic tools, prevention, prognosis, and harm. Their chapter also

EXHIBIT 7.1 QUESTION TEMPLATES FOR ASKING PICO QUESTIONS

Therapy
In _____, what is the effect of _____ on _____ compared with _____ ?

Etiology
Are _____ who have_________at _____ risk for/of_________com-pared with _____ ?

Diagnosis or Diagnostic Test
Are (Is) _____ more accurate in diagnosing _____ compared with _____ ?

Prevention
For_________does the use of_________reduce the future risk of _____ compared with _____ ?

Prognosis
Does_________influence_________in patients who have _____ ?

Meaning
How do _____ diagnosed with _____ perceive _____ ?

Source: Nollan, Fineout-Overholt, & Stephenson, 2004, p. 31.

includes clinical scenarios, which may be used as an exercise to give students practice in formulating focused questions before they tackle their own. Of course, depending on the students' clinical focus or nurses' current practice specialties, you may wish to develop your own clinical scenarios so that they are relevant for your particular audience. Once students have clarified their clinical problem and are able to articulate the intervention or diagnosis of interest, the outcome or outcomes in which they are interested, and the population in which the problem exists, I then challenge them to put all this information in the appropriate PICO or PCD (see Exhibits 7.1 and 7.2) format.

To review, the PICO format includes the client *population* of interest; the *intervention,* which can be a treatment, exposure to disease or risk behavior, or prognostic variable; a *comparison,* which may include an alternate or standard therapy, absence of risk or prognostic factor, or alternate prognostic variable; and the *outcome* of interest. The PCD format stands for *population* of interest, the observed *cues* or *cue cluster,* and the *differential*

EXHIBIT 7.2 QUESTION TEMPLATE FOR PCD QUESTIONS

In ______________ who exhibit ______________, what are the possible nursing diagnoses to consider?

Source: Levin, Lunney & Miller, 2004.

diagnoses (see Chapters 1 and 2 for an explanation of these terms). Exhibits 7.3 and 7.4 provide sample exercises for developing questions in a PICO format in an acute care setting and a home-care setting, respectively. To view a sample clinical scenario, for developing a PCD question, refer to Chapter 15.

As I introduce the question templates to students, I say, "Read my lips!" At one time, I thought that by using this approach students would simply be able to fill in the blanks and immediately have a beautifully focused, searchable question. I have learned, however, that not everyone is able to lip-read; apparently that is also a skill to be learned. Sometimes it takes several in-person or electronic conversations before students have the appropriate question to guide their evidence search. Therefore, I have students submit their focused clinical question by e-mail or on a discussion board to obtain instructor and peer feedback prior to the next class or before beginning an evidence search. As you can see, another of the principles on which I base my teaching is that students need to master the foundation before they can build the house. Using this approach, students should be able to have a focused clinical question in 1 or 2 weeks that will lead them to the next step in the EBP process.

The teaching trajectory and strategies for helping students learn how to identify, clarify, and focus clinical questions is especially important if their work on formulating questions is a prelude to a term paper or assignment, which includes synthesizing evidence on a clinical question and

EXHIBIT 7.3 EVIDENCE-BASED PRACTICE EXERCISE: FORMULATING SEARCHABLE, ANSWERABLE CLINICAL QUESTIONS (ACUTE CARE)

Scenarios and Question Templates for Asking PICO Questions

Purpose: To practice formulating various types of clinical questions in order to locate evidence that will provide answers.

(*continued*)

EXHIBIT 7.3 (*continued*)

Questions of Therapy

"Urinary tract infection is the most common hospital acquired infection" (Brosnahan, Jull, & Tracy, 2004). You note that the number of UTIs in patients who have had urethral catheters for short-term voiding problems on your unit is 20% over the benchmark. The protocol for catheter insertion and care includes use of sterile technique for catheter insertion and hygienic procedures. You have read that there is a variety of catheters available and wonder if one kind is better than another for reducing the incidence of infection. You decide to search the literature to find the best evidence to answer this question.

In _____, what is the effect of _____ on _____ compared with _____?

Questions of Secondary Prevention

Recent quality assurance studies show that the percentage of falls in your hospital has increased steadily over the passed year. You know that falls are particularly prevalent in patients over the age of 65. The protocol for fall prevention in your agency includes such precautions as keeping side rails up at specific times with specific clients, referral to physical therapy (PT) by a physician when indicated, and explaining to patients when and how to use the call button when necessary. You wonder if there are other preventative nursing measures you can provide to your patients that would decrease falls, especially among elderly patients. You decide to search the literature to determine if there is evidence to support the effectiveness of a program of risk assessment and intervention and what that might include.

For _____, does the introduction of _____ reduce the risk of _____ compared with _____?

Questions of Prognosis

One of your patients is a 55-year-old woman who recently had a myocardial infarction. She smokes at least one pack of cigarettes a day. Although she has been admonished by her primary care physician to stop smoking, she has not stopped. You know you have an obligation to discuss smoking cessation with your patient and its effects on her health status and want to provide the best evidence to her of the relationship between smoking and heart disease.

Does_________influence_________in clients who _____ ?

Adapted from Nollan, Fineout-Overholt, & Stephenson, 2005. (Prepared by Rona F. Levin, PhD, RN, for a presentation to nursing staff in an acute care setting, December 8, 2004.)

EXHIBIT 7.4 EVIDENCE-BASED PRACTICE EXERCISE: FORMULATING SEARCHABLE, ANSWERABLE CLINICAL QUESTIONS (HOME CARE)

Scenarios and Question Templates for Asking PICO Questions

Purpose: To practice formulating various types of clinical questions in order to locate evidence that will provide answers.

Questions of Therapy

You pay a home visit to a 75-year-old woman who has an in-dwelling catheter. A home health aide comes in every week day to assist this woman with her activities of daily living (ADL). Her daughter, who is a practical nurse, visits at least every 3 days, at which time she changes the catheter. Over the past month this woman has had two urinary tract infections, which have been treated with courses of antibiotics. You wonder whether frequent catheter change may be responsible for the infections and decide to search the literature to find the best evidence to answer this question.
In _____, what is the effect of _____ on _____ compared with _____ ?

Questions of Secondary Prevention

Recent OASIS (Outcome Assessment and Information Set) reports show that the percentage of falls in your region of the long-term-care division has increased steadily over the past year. You have read that at least 30% of people over 65 who live independently in the community fall each year (Gillespie, Gillespie, Robertson, Lamb, Cumming, & Rowe, 2004).You know there is a protocol for fall prevention in your agency, which mainly involves referral to physical therapy (PT) by a physician. You wonder if there are preventative nursing measures you can provide to your clients other than referral to PT.

(*continued*)

EXHIBIT 7.4 (*continued*)

You decide to search the literature to determine if there is evidence to support the effectiveness of a program of home hazard assessment and modification and what that might include.
For _____, does the introduction of _____ reduce the risk of _____ compared with _____ ?

Questions of Prognosis

One of your clients is a 55-year-old woman who recently had a myocardial infarction. She smokes at least one pack of cigarettes a day. Although she has been admonished by her primary care physician to stop smoking, she has not stopped. You know that you have an obligation to discuss smoking cessation with your client and its effects on her health status and want to provide the best evidence to her of the relationship between smoking and heart disease.
Does _____ influence _____ in clients who _____ ?

Adapted from R. Nollan, E. Fineout-Overholt, & P. Stephenson, 2005. (Prepared by Rona F. Levin", PhD, RN, for presentation to nursing staff at the Visiting Nurse Service of New York, October 25, 2004.)

coming to a conclusion about its application in practice. In my experience, unless students have the appropriate and guiding question, they may get lost along the way. More often than I would like to admit, students have retrieved studies that do not belong in the same evidence base or are irrelevant. Therefore, before students proceed with the next steps of EBP, they must have developed the focused, searchable question, the foundation from which to build their house of answers.

REFERENCES

Brosnahan, J., Jull, A., & Tracy, C. (2004). Types of urethral catheters for management of short-term voiding problems in hospitalized adults. *The Cochrane database of systematic reviews 2004*, Issue 1, Art. No. CD004013.pub2. DOI: 10.1002/14651858.CD004013.pub.2.

Fineout-Overholt, E., & Stillwell, S. (2011). Asking compelling, clinical questions. In B. M. Melnyk, & E. Fineout-Overholt (Eds.), *Evidence-based practice: A guide to best practice* (2nd ed., pp. 25–39). Philadelphia: Wolters Kluwer Health/Lippincott Williams & Wilkins.

Gillespie, L. D., Gillespie, W. J., Robertson, M. C., Lamb, S. E., Cumming, R. G., & Rowe, B. H. (2004). Interventions for preventing falls in elderly people (Cochrane Review). *Cochrane library*, Issue 3. Chichester, UK: Wiley.

Levin, R. F., Lunney, M., & Krainovich-Miller, B. (2004, October–December). Improving diagnostic accuracy using an evidence-based nursing model. *International Journal of Nursing Terminologies and Classification, 15*(4), 114–122.

Nollan, R., Fineout-Overholt, E., & Stephenson, P. (2004). Asking compelling clinical questions. In B. M. Melnyk, & E. Fineout-Overholt (Eds.), *Evidence-based practice: A guide to best practice* (pp. 25–37). Philadelphia: Lippincott Williams & Wilkins.

Sackett, D. L., Straus, S. E., Richardson, W. S., Rosenberg, W., & Haynes, R. B. (2000). *Evidence-based medicine* (2nd ed.). Edinburgh, Scotland: Churchill Livingstone.

8

INTEGRATION OF CRITICAL THINKING AND EBP INTO "ROUTINE" PRACTICE

Jeffrey M. Keefer and Rona F. Levin

Tell me and I'll listen. Show me and I'll understand. Involve me and I'll learn.

—TETON LAKOTA INDIANS

Working together in an internship program for newly graduated baccalaureate-prepared nurses in a large urban home health agency, we developed a program to link critical thinking and evidence-based practice (EBP)—to explicitly marry these two paradigms. We want nursing students and novice nurses to learn to use both critical thinking skills and an evidence-based approach in their practice. The knowledge and skills gleaned from these paradigms are essential for enhancing current nursing practice with the goal of improving patient outcomes in a cost-conscious environment. The challenges both students and new graduate nurses face in their first year seem overwhelming. Yet this is an extremely formative time and educators have the opportunity to shape their practice for the rest of their careers.

The focus of the program was clinical decision making. Students in academic programs are often taught critical thinking as a separate course or this content may be integrated into a beginning course that covers many introductory concepts. Key is the explicit experience of understanding how the theoretical concepts and propositions of critical thinking theory are of practical use in clinical decision making, and are specifically related to the application of the most current and best scientific evidence in their own discipline. The program we developed (see Exhibit 8.1) included several teaching strategies that are designed to engage learners and promote critical thinking. These included Socratic teaching methods, case studies, and collaborative group work. Socratic methods were used to encourage new nurses to think about how they think, and to understand how they form their care decisions. Case studies provided an opportunity to think through and understand how nurses formulate nursing diagnoses

EXHIBIT 8.1

Outline of the Initial Workshop

This chapter presents some of the work done on the first day of a 2-day workshop. This is an approximate outline for what we did so you can see our scheduling.

Outline of Day 1

1. Introduction to the day and us (what are our roles, and what are our backgrounds that qualifies us to be here)
2. Case scenario exercise 1
3. Discuss and debrief scenario exercise

Break

4. Introduction to critical thinking principles

    - What are assumptions and why do we make them?
    - Inferences and conclusions
    - Questions
    - What is critical thinking?
    - Why engage in critical thinking?
    - Steps in critical thinking
    - Inferences

Lunch

A critical thinking approach to clinical decision making = evidence-based practice (EBP)

5. Case scenario exercise 2 + debrief
6. Introduction to EBP
7. Asking clinical questions
8. Exercise on formulating clinical questions from case scenarios

Break

9. Begin speaking about searching for evidence (use computers and small groups to search for evidence together)

using previously learned critical thinking skills. Collaborative group work was intended to provide a nonthreatening venue for sharing ideas and coming to consensus on diagnoses, an important skill to learn for practice.

While this program was developed specifically to meet an identified need, namely assist with the orientation of bachelor of science in nursing (BSN) interns in home care, we repurposed what we learned for other audiences. After we presented this program twice with the interns and then refined it, we adapted it into a well-attended and well-received interactive presentation at the 2007 New York State Nurses Association (NYSNA) Convention, Integration of Critical Thinking and EBP into Novice Nurse Practice (Levin & Keefer, 2007). Further, we incorporated many of the teaching strategies we developed while working together at the home care agency into our teaching practices at the academic institutions where we teach. The programs emphasized identifying and uncovering assumptions, asking clinical questions, understanding that not all evidence is created equal, critically appraising evidence for use in practice, and learning how to create change. We have found that students and nurses alike are eager to learn these strategies and skills to improve their practice and patient outcomes.

EXHIBIT 8.2 CLINICAL DECISION-MAKING LEARNING ACTIVITY I

Case Scenario 1

You are making the first home visit in Manhattan to Mrs. Bridges, an 80-year-old, Hispanic woman who was discharged from the hospital 2 days ago. She had been hospitalized for chest pain. When you arrive, she opens the door for you after you wait several minutes. You note that she is using a rolling walker. She then returns to her recliner and sits down, as she says, "*Venga, enferma. No tengo ninguna energia.*" The hospital referral indicates that Mrs. Bridges was discharged with Hgb. of 10 and vital signs as follow, BP = 102/60, pulse = 88, respirations = 16, and temperature = 100.2. The note also indicates that Mrs. Bridges has a daughter who lives in Queens and her phone number is included. Upon physical examination, you note that Mrs. Bridges is pale, her vital signs are similar to those on the hospital referral note, and her lungs are clear bilaterally. To your surprise you observe a stage II pressure ulcer on her sacrum. The referral made no mention of this.

Directions for Group Work

I. *Individually*, write the answers to the following questions.

(*continued*)

EXHIBIT 8.2 (*continued*)

1. Explain the purpose of your visit to Mrs. Bridges.
2. By the end of your time with her, what do you hope to accomplish?
3. What is your initial assessment?
4. What do you think are the patient's primary health problem(s)?

II. *In a small group*, discuss what you wrote. Did you all come up with the same assessment? If not, what were the different assessments?

A CASE STUDY IN CRITICAL THINKING

Before we begin discussing the content of critical thinking in earnest, let us have a little warm-up with a brief case study activity similar to the one we presented in our program. Imagine how you might respond to the questions in Exhibit 8.2.

While each program participant initially read and jotted down responses individually, we found it very valuable to debrief the experience together in a group using a flip-chart. So, how did you do? Did you identify some of your own assumptions? Did you identify some when you discussed this with your small group? Did you check their accuracy and validity? How about considering alternate perspectives, for example, things that may be possible but which you initially shied away from? What were some of the assumptions you made? What did you *assume* about Mrs. Bridges? That her husband was still alive? That her daughter lives near or is even on talking terms with her? That she does not speak English or speaks fluent Spanish? That the hospital was careless? These and many other factors lead to assumptions, all of which, if unchecked, can result in taking uninformed action that may result in not achieving your (or your organization's, or even the patient's) care goals.

We then take the exercise a step further, and ask nurses to respond to the following questions:

- As a result of your assumptions, and based on the evidence provided in the case, what inferences did you draw?
- Did you perhaps *assume* that a hemoglobin of 10 indicates anemia?
- What sort of differential diagnosis did you make, perhaps involving anemia versus dehydration?
- Do you see how different assumptions, even those without evidence in the case, can lead to the potential for different outcomes?

All of this is a result of asking yourself different questions about what assumptions lurk quietly behind your decisions.

Finally, to debrief we ask: What did you learn? Have you ever seen assumptions lead to less-than-optimum patient outcomes? How can you bring this learning into your clinical practice and/or your teaching?

CRITICAL THINKING

Critical thinking is a term that is used frequently in learning environments, and while most would agree it is a valuable concept and process in which to engage, ironically it can mean different things to instructors and students alike. Thus, there is no better place to begin than by stating how we have chosen to use "critical thinking" in this chapter and why we took this position. The framework developed by Stephen Brookfield, the adult learning and critical theory researcher, serves as a way to understand how critical thinking describes the process used to uncover and check assumptions so we can consider alternative perspectives and take informed action (Brookfield, 2006). While there are many definitions that focus on internal logical thinking (Ennis, 1996; Paul & Elder, 2002), we chose to root our work in the common and easily overlooked concept of assumptions, as they are so pervasive in thinking patterns, occur often, and lead us into mischief without our even realizing it! Brookfield's steps in critical thinking are:

1. Identify assumptions
2. Check accuracy and validity
3. Consider alternative perspectives
4. Take informed action

Assumptions are unstated entities that are nevertheless perceived as being true and taken for granted. They are almost never directly acknowledged or discussed, as it is easy to *assume* that other people who are like us believe in ways similar to us; likewise, those people not like us may believe something differently. Assumptions such as these are all based on models in our mind that we often do not discuss or confirm with others. People tend to believe that others behave or think as they do. For example, people who engage in health behaviors may think that everyone should engage in those behaviors just as people who do not engage in healthy behaviors probably think that most others do not engage in them either.

If we *assume* we know the reasons for people's behavior without trying to better understand them, then we put our patients into a box (*these* people are like *this*) without really understanding them as individuals. These assumptions are alive and well in the minds of instructors and learners alike, and without giving voice to and acknowledging them, critical thinking work can be diverted by focusing solely on internal ways of processing that information.

So pervasive are assumptions that you, the reader, are probably holding many of them right now! Consider that assumptions may be divided into three categories to more easily be able to organize them—paradigmatic, prescriptive, and causal (Brookfield, 2006).

Paradigmatic assumptions structure how we see the world, and comprise our worldview of what exists and is real. "Students really want to learn how to do the best work" or "families will care for one another when they are sick" are examples of paradigmatic assumptions. People who believe that either of these assumptions is true often believe that *all* people see things in this way. Paradigms are often considered to be common sense, especially if there is a group or community that so firmly shares this same perspective that they cease to realize that not everybody sees the world in the same way. These paradigmatic assumptions are especially difficult to uncover, as we *assume* how people will think, act, or believe about a certain phenomenon, not to mention what we perceive the phenomenon to mean itself.

Prescriptive assumptions are value-based and are exemplified by the fact that people believe certain things should happen. These are the assumptions behind mission statements or moral codes. "All people should do this," or "think this," or "believe this" are examples of prescriptive assumptions. We prescribe, or abide by prescribed thought processes or beliefs, often insisting upon them or *assuming* that others around us hold these same thoughts. Even when we say we believe the same things, such as we believe increasing patient self-management is beneficial, we are often still assuming we all mean the same thing when we use the same terms.

Causal assumptions are all about believing we can see and understand simple cause and effect relationships. In this way, single causes are at times perceived to lead to direct effects. This is often an overly simplified view of very complex human and social interactions, and may lead to mental isolationism. Examples like "poor people are that way because they refuse to work," or "this patient's lung cancer must have been caused by smoking." While it is easier to think that single causes lead to their natural effects, there are many exceptions in life, so many in fact that some theories, such as chaos theory (Hodge & Coronado, 2007) or actor-network theory (Latour, 2005), posit that clear cause and effect is difficult, perhaps impossible to clearly explain. Left unchallenged, causal assumptions can result in implementing programs, initiatives, and education in ways that do not get to the root problem or problems. This is a key concept in using an EBP approach to practice.

While it is not imperative that we determine what sort of assumptions we are confronting, it is valuable to determine that an assumption is being made. Once we have identified assumptions that cloud our thinking, it is time to check their accuracy and validity. Is what we are assuming accurate? Is it valid in our situation for anybody who may be involved with it? Accounting for these assumptions and their applicability to some decision or thinking process, it is then time to begin reasoning toward inferences.

Inferences are the thoughts that we form as we reason toward conclusions. This presumes that we have clear, logical, justifiable, and reasonable thoughts or evidence to support the development of these inferences. When we have the best available evidence to support our inferences, we can then engage in reasoning, take our inferences, and begin to draw conclusions from developed observations, facts, or hypotheses. The patient assessment process is an example of reasoning. A hypothesis is the result of what happens when we make inferences from the evidence. Making a differential diagnosis for a patient condition would be an example of developing a hypothesis or alternate hypotheses.

Once we have considered alternate perspectives, we are able to draw a reasoned conclusion that is not built on unexamined assumptions. This will allow us to take informed action, such as making a diagnosis. Without following these steps, our reasoning is to our own conclusions that may not match the reality around us.

A SECOND CASE STUDY IN CRITICAL THINKING

While critical thinking principles may seem relatively straightforward in isolation, their value comes alive when they are explored in real context. One way of doing this is through creating a simple case study (see Exhibit 8.3 to continue to illustrate the steps, followed by several questions about action-oriented next steps. After reading the case, participants individually answered the questions, after which they worked in small groups to discuss their responses. How do you think you did with this one? Were you able to recognize some of your assumptions, check their accuracy and validity, and consider alternative perspectives to take informed action?

EVIDENCE-BASED PRACTICE

EBP is a concept that during the past decade has become a common term, almost a "buzz word," in the health care professions. Others may discount the term as a trend that will disappear. Whatever you call a scientific and systematic approach to finding the best evidence to answer your clinical

EXHIBIT 8.3 CLINICAL DECISION-MAKING LEARNING ACTIVITY II

Case Scenario 2

While doing chores at home one summer afternoon, ... [Nicole] noticed that the sky had become overcast and dark and looked particularly threatening. She turned the radio on to a news weather station and heard a forecast for a severe thunderstorm. The wind started to blow fiercely, so she began to close the windows. While closing the bedroom window, she looked out and saw a huge black wind tunnel full of debris and dirt heading toward her home. The sound was deafening and the air pressure changes made her feel that her head would explode. She ran to an inside bathroom and knelt on the floor on the inside corner of the room. Within 20 to 30 seconds, her home, garage, and large storage barn were flattened with portions falling in on themselves. Other walls and sections of roof were totally swept away. The afternoon was now dark. Golf ball–size hail was falling. Rain and wind battered the demolished home. She cowered in the corner of the bathroom; heart pounding, pupils dilated, wary of another impending assault. She later stated that she had been terrified and had remained extremely apprehensive for the duration of the storm.

Adapted from Whitley (1992, p. 158).

Directions for Group Work

I. *Individually*, write the answers to the following questions:
   What is your assessment of this person's emotional state?
   What would be your diagnostic hypothesis?
II. *In a small group*, discuss what you wrote. Did you all come up with the same assessment? If not, what were the different assessments?

questions is not as important as the meaning behind the term and how we as nurses carry out this approach in practice (Levin, 2008). Evidence-based practice has been referred to as "evidence-based medicine" (Straus, Richardson, Glasziou, & Haynes, 2005), "evidence-based nursing" (DiCenso, Guyatt, & Ciliska, 2005), and "evidence-based practice" (Levin & Feldman, 2006; Melnyk & Fineout-Overholt, 2011), among others. The EBP process is cross-disciplinary and we believe it has useful terminology that is not discipline specific. Our definition combines the approaches of several authors and is as follows:

EBP is a framework for clinical decision making that uses . . .

1. The best available evidence
2. The clinician's expertise
3. And a patient's values and preferences

. . . to guide judgments about a patient's personal health condition (Levin & Feldman, 2006; Melnyk & Fineout-Overholt, 2011; Straus et al., 2005).

With this fundamental understanding of EBP, following the discussion of critical thinking, by the end of the 2 days interns are expected to:

1. Define EBP
2. Identify the processes of EBP
3. Discuss the rationale for using an evidence-based approach to practice
4. Identify a problem that comes from their clinical practice
5. Formulate a focused, searchable clinical question in PICO format
6. Identify search strategies for finding evidence
7. Appraise a clinical trial

Thus, the EBP content we included focused on answering the following questions:

- What is EBP?
- Who needs EBP?
- Why engage in EBP?
- What are levels of evidence?
- What are quality ratings?
- What are clinical questions?
- Kinds of clinical questions?
- How do you formulate clinical questions?
- How do you focus clinical questions?

Content for each of these objectives can be found elsewhere in this book. Here the emphasis is on how integrating critical thinking concepts and an EBP approach enhanced the program for the interns at the Visiting Nurse Service of New York (VNSNY), and the teaching strategies used to do so.

MARRYING THE CONCEPTS

Critical thinking and EBP are theoretical approaches that are integral to providing quality care. Marrying them seemed a natural process, as critical thinking without a goal for its use was a process without an end, while using evidence without thinking critically about it or how it is used does not lead to best practice and desired outcomes. Once we linked these two concepts and decided we could meet the learning needs of the interns using a combination approach, we set about designing a teaching and learning strategy that would engage adult learners. We spent some time discussing our own pedagogical approaches and found we agreed with two fundamental premises that guided our design:

1. Teaching and learning are active, interactive, and collaborative processes between learner and teacher.
2. Students create their own knowledge rather than use someone else's knowledge.

A purely didactic lecture presentation does not facilitate critical thinking, since lecture as a strategy focuses on the individual as a receptacle for someone else's knowledge.

TEACHING STRATEGIES THAT FOSTER CRITICAL THINKING

The illustrations that follow are not intended to be a comprehensive list. Rather, these suggestions are to help you get started with educating adults as to marry critical thinking and EBP work. As with all marriages, success depends on looking at the merger as a collaborative endeavor.

CASE SCENARIO/CASE STUDY

You have already seen two examples of case studies we used in our teaching. You may find it helpful to develop your own, too. If you do, the case study should be broad enough to avoid having a single correct answer, as the point of a case scenario is to help people to think through processes with limited evidence. Case studies are meant to foster critical thinking and can often support diverse perspectives that benefit from discussion and debriefing (Brickman, Glynn, & Graybeal, 2008; Hodge & Coronado, 2007; Krauss, Salame, & Goodwyn, 2010; Utterback, Davenport, Gallegos, & Boyd, 2012).

Case scenarios are meant to benefit learner processing of some content, often in a real-world manner. As they are not intended to have objective right or wrong answers, they often invite deep introspection and navigation of things that may or may not be explicit. In this way, case studies are an excellent vehicle to promote critical thinking and personal reflection. Important to note is that cases should be written or otherwise presented in ways that are open-ended enough that learners can develop whatever knowledge, skill, or attitude the instructor seeks to develop; length can vary as needed. It is not necessary that the instructor has the "correct answer," but rather that the exercise allows for the process of evidence-based, critical thinking to develop something that is often easier in a collaborative conversation.

SOCRATIC METHOD

According to Paul (1995), the Socratic method of teaching leads students to content or subject matter understanding by providing students with guiding questions, leading them down a teacher-led path to find the "correct" answer. This method uses an interactive dialogue between student and teacher. The questions the teacher asks are intended to:

- Stimulate thinking
- Clarify thinking
- Hold students accountable for their thinking

As an example related to EBP, nurses have often expressed a clinical problem as one word as in "pain," "falls," or "infection." Over the years, Levin has had the opportunity of introducing EBP to nurses in both hospital and home care settings. Using the Socratic method, she has asked nurses to describe what they considered a problem on their unit or in their practice (Levin & Feldman, 2006, chapter 3). In the hospital setting, one group of nurses indicated that monitoring of postoperative vital signs was a problem. She then asked, "How is monitoring of postoperative vital signs a problem?" In response, the nurses began to elaborate on two aspects of monitoring: (1) the frequency of monitoring vital signs according to the current hospital protocol and (2) the accuracy of measuring vital signs according to whether a nurse or assistive personnel (e.g., "nurse's" aide) was taking the readings. The next question might be, "Are these the same questions?," or "Are you having a problem with the frequency of vital sign monitoring or with the category of health care worker who is assigned to monitor vital signs?" Note here that the interaction started out with questions, not answers. The questions helped the nurses clarify their thinking, and as a first step in their EBP project, led to their decision to search the literature for evidence on the comparative accuracy of vital sign readings by registered professional nurses versus patient care assistive personnel.

BEYOND THE SOCRATIC METHOD

Golding (2011) takes us a step beyond the Socratic method into a teaching realm that he calls "using thought-encouraging questions in a community of critical thinking" (p. 357). He refers to Paul (1995) but differentiates his method from Paul's in that he believes the Socratic method leads students to a teacher-desired outcome, whereas his method may lead students to a different answer—not necessarily the one "correct" answer. To use this method, however, a teacher has to be totally comfortable with the subject matter of the course and the ability to be flexible. According to Golding, important premises in his strategy rest on basic skills that students need to develop in order to become critical thinkers. Included in these basic skills are

1. Skills and abilities such as knowing how, or being able, to evaluate or analyze
2. The tendency or disposition to engage in critical thinking
3. Ability to engage in contextual thinking; that is, there is no one right answer for every situation
4. Understanding of the disciplinary subject matter

As an example, in critiquing a research report, there may be different opinions as to whether a particular aspect of the study may be considered a strength or weakness. While some researchers may consider tight controls as strength to avoid threats to internal validity, others may consider tight controls a compromise to external validity. This is important to clinicians who wish to translate the research into clinical practice in a setting where tight controls are nonexistent. The teacher in this scenario needs to understand the relationships between research and clinical practice, and how to help students learn to apply research findings to practice. This is not black and white, but instead takes knowledge of the intricacies of translating evidence into clinical practice.

COLLABORATIVE LEARNING

Another strategy that informs our approach to teaching is collaborative or cooperative learning. Some authors (e.g., Abrami et al., 1993; Johnson, Johnson, & Smith, 1991)[1] differentiate these two approaches by indicating that they are at either end of a continuum. That is, cooperative learning is more structured than collaborative learning. Others use the terms interchangeably. In either case these approaches share common assumptions:

- Learning is active
- Learning requires challenge

- Learning is illuminated by multiple perspectives
- Learning is a social activity
- Learning is a shared experience between students and teacher

Learning Is Active

Learning is a process. Therefore, our primary goal is to help students learn how to learn in a world of constantly changing knowledge. To accomplish this goal, we must engage students in intellectual activity—activity that goes beyond taking in new information. Carl Rogers, in his classic 1969 book *Freedom to Learn*, aptly addresses this assumption:

> We are, in my view, faced with an entirely new situation in education where the goal of education, if we are to survive, is the facilitation of change and learning. The only ... [person] who is educated is the ... [person] who has learned how to learn; ... [the person] who has learned how to adapt to change; ... [the person] who has realized that no knowledge is secure, that only the process of seeking knowledge gives a basis for security. Changingness, a reliance on process rather than upon static knowledge, is the only thing that makes any sense as a goal for education in the modern world. (p. 104) [We have taken the liberty of editing his sexist language. We're sure if he were writing today he would have done the same.]

Learning Requires Challenge

As teachers, we need to challenge the intellect of our students. We need to ask them to think about the content, issues, and premises we share with them and to reach their own conclusions about this knowledge. This principle/assumption is in direct contrast to simply passing on our knowledge to students.

Learning Illuminated by Multiple Perspectives

A principle of collaborative/cooperative learning is that there is never one correct answer to a question or issue. Our job as teachers is to encourage students to keep an open mind to all perspectives on an issue—to listen to others and question the rationale for the comments that emanate from these different perspectives. Then after hearing and processing all views on a question or issue, come to an independent conclusion with supporting rationale.

Learning Is a Social Activity

We have all heard of the intellectual genius who is a hermit and develops ideas and creations in isolation. Still, even one who isolates oneself from social interaction interacts with the ideas of others by reading and thinking, and these days perhaps from virtual interaction with others who hold similar interests. In a class of students, however, interaction (preferably collaborative interaction) fosters learning, hence the recent emphasis on collaborative group projects. This type of social interaction (whether it be for professional or personal growth goals) is essential for success.

Learning Is a Shared Experience

Learning is about sharing an experience that brings both students and teacher to a new level of understanding. As an example, several colleagues developed a model for merging the EBP and practice improvement paradigms (Levin et al., 2010). When discussing this model with a class of doctoral students, one student offered that he thought something was missing from the model. Levin (second author) was open to his thoughts. As a result, a co-published article was written to include what Burke thought was the missing ingredient (Burke & Levin, 2010).

COLLABORATIVE LEARNING APPROACH

Regardless of whether one is more comfortable with greater or lesser structure for a class of students, there are major learning objectives to which each school of thought adheres. These are that students work together (and, we might add, with the teacher) to:

- Achieve understanding of course content
- Search for new meaning
- Solve related problems
- Create a product

There is no argument that the collaborative/cooperative approach to learning is:

- A student-centered approach
- Student (or shared teacher/student) responsibility for governance and evaluation
- Encouraging diversity of thought
- A group/team experience (process as well as content)

One final experience we want to share is the way we end each class. Following again from the work of Stephen Brookfield, we adapted and use an ongoing, formative assessment instrument, the Critical Incident

EXHIBIT 8.4 CRITICAL INCIDENT QUESTIONNAIRE

Date: _________

Please take a few minutes to respond to any of the questions below about today's class. Do not put your name on this paper, as your responses are anonymous. If you do not have a response for any question, feel free to leave it blank. Responses will be shared with the class the next time we meet. This is intended to help make the class more responsive to your needs and concerns.

1. At what *moment* in today's class did you feel *most engaged* and/or *least engaged?*
2. What *action* (if any) did anybody take that you found *most affirming/helpful*?
3. What *action* (if any) did anybody take that you found *most puzzling/confusing*?
4. What was the most *important information* you *learned* during today's class?
5. Do you have any *questions or suggestions* about today's class?

Critical_Incident_Questionnaire_v7

Adapted by Jeffrey Keefer from Brookfield, S. (1995). *Becoming a critically reflective teacher*. San Francisco, CA: Jossey-Bass.

Questionnaire (see Exhibit 8.4) to allow learners to give anonymous feedback about their experiences in class. This instrument allows learners to process what and how they learned, and to share it with the instructor, and ultimately with each other. Whether as a reflective activity or a collaborative exercise that cuts across everybody in the learning event, it is better to help learners process when more closely rooted in the experience than if it were completed at the end of a course or omitted (Keefer, 2009).

SUMMARY AND CONCLUSION

We hope we were able to show you how and why we married critical thinking and EBP together as linked strategies for teaching integration of both into clinical practice. While we initially did this as a natural approach to teaching and learning in our internship program, we never dreamed it would snowball into something much larger.

We took this same approach and integrated into our own teaching practices in different academic programs, further helping to influence teaching and learning strategies in ways to hopefully improve clinical practice. We hope that this approach will contribute positively to care satisfaction and patient outcomes.

NOTE

1. Note that the references here are "dated" because the topics of cooperative and collaborative learning were a major focus of educational study and writing during the 1990s. This is when the second author started to integrate principles of this approach into her teaching. The Johnson et al. reference is well-worth reading today.

REFERENCES

Abrami, P. C., Chambers, B., Poulsen, C., Howden, J., d'Apollonia, S. et al. (1993). *Using cooperative learning*. Dubuque, IA: Brown & Benchmark.

Brickman, P., Glynn, S., & Graybeal, G. (2008). Introducing students to cases. *Journal of College Science Teaching, 37*(3), 12–16.

Brookfield, S. (2006). *Developing critical thinkers. (11/22/11)*. Retrieved from http://www.stephenbrookfield.com/Dr._Stephen_D._Brookfield/Workshop_ Materials_files/Critical_Thinking_materials.pdf

Burke, R. E., & Levin, R. F. (2010). Evidence-based practice: Describing the problem for an evidence-based practice improvement project: A missing ingredient. *Research and Theory for Nursing Practice, 24*(3), 155–158.

DiCenso, A., Guyatt, G., & Ciliska, D. (2005). *Evidence-based nursing: A guide to clinical practice*. St. Louis, MO: Mosby, Inc.

Ennis, R. H. (1996) *Critical thinking*. Upper Saddle River, NJ: Prentice-Hall.

Golding, C. (2011). Educating for critical thinking: Thought encouraging questions in a community of inquiry. *Higher Education Research & Development, 30*(2), 357–370.

Hodge, B., & Coronado, G. (2007). Understanding change in organizations in a far-from-equilibrium world*. *Emergence: Complexity and Organization, 9*(3), 3–15.

Johnson, D. W., Johnson, R. T., & Smith, K. A. (1991). *Cooperative learning: Increasing college faculty instructional productivity. ASHE-ERIC Higher Education Report No. 4*. Washington, DC: George Washington University, School of Education and Human Development.

Keefer, J. M. (2009, May). The Critical Incident Questionnaire (CIQ): From research to practice and back again. *Adult Education Research Conference*. Chicago, IL.

Krauss, D. A., Salame, I. I., & Goodwyn, L. N. (2010). Using photographs as case studies to promote active learning in biology. *Journal of College Science Teaching, 40*(1), 72–76.

Latour, B. (2005). *Reassembling the social: An introduction to actor-network-theory.* Oxford: Oxford University Press.

Levin, R. F. (2008). Evidence-based practice: EBP by any other name is still a rose. *Research and Theory in Nursing Practice, 22*(1), 5–7.

Levin, R. F., & Feldman, H. R. (Eds.). (2006). *Teaching evidence-based practice in nursing: A guide for educators.* New York: Springer Publishing.

Levin, R. F., & Keefer, J. M. (2007). *Integrating critical thinking and evidence-based practice in novice nurses.* Paper presented at the New York State Nurses Association Convention, Atlantic City, NJ.

Levin, R. F., Keefer, J. M., Marren, J., Vetter, M., Lauder, B., & Sobolewski, S. (2010). Evidence-based practice: Merging two paradigms. *Journal of Nursing Care Quality, 25*(2), 117–126.

Melnyk, B. M., & Fineout-Overholt, E. (2011). *Evidence-based practice in nursing & healthcare: A guide to best practice* (2nd ed.). Philadelphia: Wolters Kluwer Health.

Paul, R. W. (1995). *Socratic questioning and role playing.* Santa Rosa, CA: Foundation for Critical Thinking.

Paul, R., & Elder, L. (2002). *Critical thinking: Tools for taking charge of your professional and personal life.* Upper Saddle River, NJ: Prentice-Hall.

Rogers, C. (1969). *Freedom to learn.* Columbus, OH: C. E., Merrill.

Straus, S. E., Richardson, W. S., Glasziou, P., & Haynes, R. B. (2005). *Evidence-based medicine: How to practice and teach EBM* (3rd ed.) . Edinburgh, Scotland: Elsevier Churchill Livingstone.

Utterback, V. A., Davenport, D., Gallegos, B., & Boyd, E. (2012). The critical difference assignment: An innovative instructional method. *Journal of Nursing Education, 51*(1), 42–45.

Whitley, G. G. (1992). Concept analysis of fear. *International Journal of Nursing Terminologies and Classifications, 3*(4), 155–161.

9

SEARCHING THE SEA OF EVIDENCE: IT TAKES A LIBRARY

*Rona F. Levin**

It has been said that man is a rational animal. All my life I have been searching for evidence which could support this.

—BERTRAND RUSSELL

This chapter is based on four columns published in the *World Council of Enterostomal Therapists* (*WCET*) *Journal* that were designed to assist in the search for evidence. The emphasis is on how to search for the best evidence. This first column in the series will provide you with an algorithm for how to structure a search. Subsequent columns will provide guidance on how to use appropriate search terminology, keep track of the evidence you find, and how to summarize individual studies that are relevant to your question into a table of evidence (TOE).

PART I

The first step you need to take is to formulate a focused clinical question to help guide your search. The algorithm in Figure 9.1 depicts the next step as identifying search terms. If you are a novice or expert at literature searches, it behooves you at this point in your search to "befriend a librarian," preferably a health sciences or medical librarian, who is an expert in searching for the best evidence on a topic. As a seasoned evidence searcher, I still enlist the assistance of my instructional services librarian at my university to make sure that I am using the most appropriate search terminology.

*Levin, R. F. (2009). Translating research evidence for WCET Practice: Clinical effectiveness formulas. Part II. *WCET Journal, 29*(3), 38–39; Levin, R. F. (2010). Translating research evidence for WCET Practice: Clinical effectiveness formulas. Part III *30*(1), 25; Levin, R. F. (2010). Translating research evidence for WCET Practice: Clinical effectiveness formulas. Part IV. *30*(2), 17. Permission to reproduce these articles for this book is granted by WCET (www.wcetn.org) who continues to own the copyright for this content.

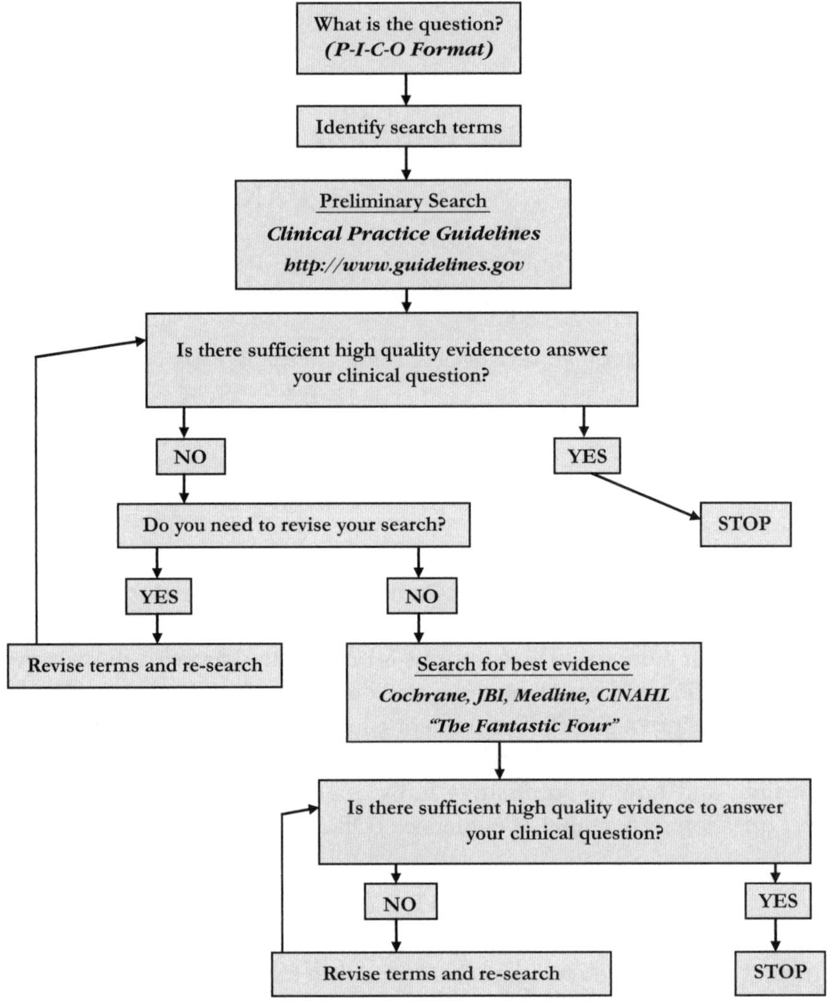

Source: © Burke & Levin, 2010. Reprinted with permission of the authors.

FIGURE 9.1 Algorithm for systematic review of the published evidence.

The extra time and effort you spend meeting with a librarian at the beginning of an evidence search will save you many more hours than you can imagine.

Levels of evidence (LOE) are addressed. The top level of evidence consists of clinical practice guidelines (CPGs) supported by high-level, quality evidence and systematic reviews. I have come to believe that large, multicenter trials should also be considered top-level evidence. I propose this because sometimes a quantitative systematic review or meta-analysis of evidence, for example, may only include two or three randomized controlled trials (RCTs) and the sample size can vary significantly. Three RCTs may only have a combined sample size of a few hundred. On the other hand, a multicenter clinical trial usually has a large sample size across geographic and treatment settings.

To begin your search for evidence to answer your clinical question, you start with looking for the top level of evidence, that is, systematic reviews, clinical practice guidelines based on top-level evidence, and/or multicenter randomized clinical trials in the case of quantitative questions. I am emphasizing this here because that is, I believe, the focus of your work; that is, assessing wounds, preventing wound development, and promoting wound healing. The beauty of the systematic approach to evidence searching is that you do not have to "reinvent the wheel." That is, if evidence syntheses of reasonable quality already exist on your topic of interest and/or burning clinical question, then you do not need to delve into finding, summarizing, and critiquing single primary studies. That is a difficult task if you do not have the appropriate research background or education to be able to do this. Thus, one of the purposes of providing systematic reviews of evidence on a topic is that busy clinicians would not have to spend many hours finding original research and then synthesizing primary studies in order to answer a clinical question. If, however, published guidelines and/or systematic reviews on your topic do not exist or are of low quality, then you are obligated to search further. Subsequent searching would consider single studies of a nature appropriate to the question; that is, if you are trying to answer a question about treatment effectiveness, the next level of search would be for single RCTs, the next level search would be for quasi-experimental studies, and so on down the evidence hierarchy.

The algorithm in Figure 9.1 is intended to help you with the systematic steps you need to take to find the evidence (if it exists) to answer your clinical question. This column focuses on the overall approach to searching. The next two columns will provide you with practical hints for identifying search terms, documenting your search for evidence, and summarizing and synthesizing the evidence that you find.

PART II

Rona F. Levin, Robert E. Burke, and Shannon B. Kealey

The second part addresses searching for the best evidence to answer a focused clinical question. Once you have identified your focused clinical question, and accessed and evaluated clinical practice guidelines, the next step is to locate relevant systematic reviews related to your PICO question. The two best databases for locating relevant reviews are the Cochrane Library and the Joanna Briggs Institute. This column will focus on how to search the Cochrane Library. As I stated in my first column in this series, I still befriend a librarian to be sure I am searching in the correct sea with the most updated sonar equipment. Thus, I enlisted the help of Ms. Shannon Kealey, an instructional services librarian at Pace University, to develop the search strategy outlined below. In addition, Mr. Robert Burke, a doctor of nursing practice student from Pace University, worked on these columns.

We will now take you on a sail into the Cochrane Library and help you to navigate your way through the Cochrane Sea of Systematic Reviews. Come aboard! We begin with a clinical question in PICO format, for which a team of clinicians is looking for an answer. Our sample PICO question for this learning experience is: In patients with venous ulcers, how do compression garments compare with traditional interventions for promoting healing and preventing recurrence?

When identifying your initial search terms, we recommended that you match keywords to the population (P) and intervention (I) terms first. (From our sample PICO questions above, the population is "patients with venous ulcers" and the intervention is "compression garments"). Including the comparison (C) and outcome(s) (O) terms too early in your search may narrow your findings and omit retrieval of important studies. When searching a database as circumscribed as the Cochrane Library, you do not want to be too demanding. Remember that every keyword you enter is a term you are requiring to appear in each result, so try to be as flexible as possible with certain related or synonymous terms.

You may begin with a simple search of the Cochrane Library. For example, try starting with venous ulcers and compression garments. This approach will yield results from all seven databases included in the library for your keywords. You will notice that a search of venous ulcers AND compression garments will not find articles that use other terms for compression garments, such as compression stockings or compression bandages. To let the search engine know that you are flexible with the terms garments, stockings, and bandages, link these terms together in a separate single "search box" using the connector OR and putting the entire string in parentheses (Figure 9.2).

For the purpose of this chapter, we suggest using the Advanced Search mode to navigate the Cochrane Database of Systematic Reviews. Choosing the advanced search function does not imply that you have to have advanced skills to utilize it. This function actually gives you more control over your search and simplifies the process. The advanced search allows you to limit the search to the Cochrane Database of Systematic Reviews (e.g., Figure 9.2).

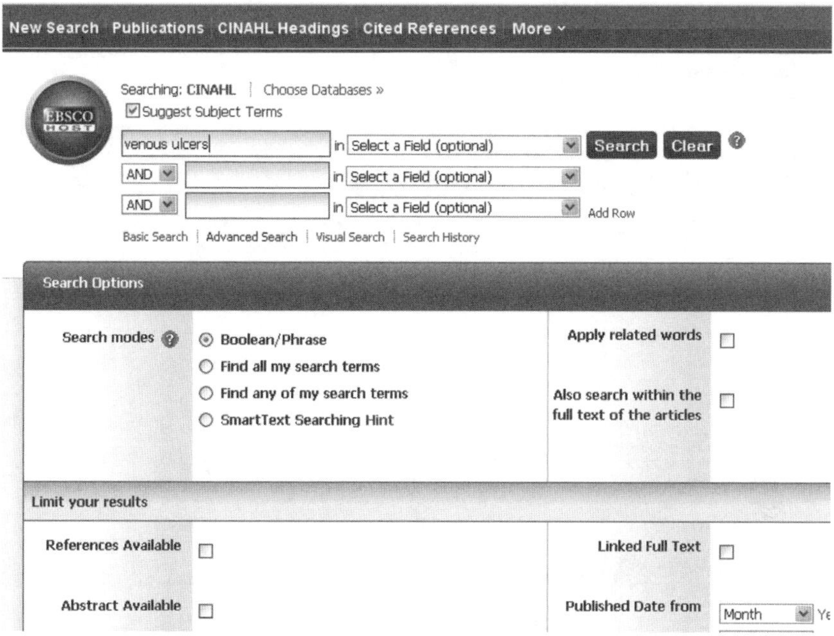

FIGURE 9.2 Enter primary topic term, venous ulcers.

We recommend that you search for your keywords in the Abstract section, since a search of the text of the documents is too broad, and a search of "Titles" is too narrow. We believe that this is a good way to ensure relevant results. In addition, you may find using Medical Subject Heading (MeSH) terms, which allow you to browse and search, using the official subject headings of the database. This is something you might want to try if you are not sure what keywords are most appropriate for your search, or if your keyword search is returning irrelevant results.

Figure 9.3 shows the results page that materialized using the keywords search depicted in Figure 9.1. To open any of the resulting systematic reviews, click on the article title. Figure 9.4 demonstrates that the abstract of the review appears after you click on the review title. You may now open the full review in HTML or PDF format, save it to a file, and/or print the document. Clicking on the review title takes you into the HTML version, which will contain hyperlinks to the different parts of the article, including illustrations and graphs. It also may contain links to other related articles in the Cochrane Library.

The PDF version of the article will be an exact replica (scanned version) of the original review as it appears in print form. If you would like to see the PDF version, click on the PDF link on the left-hand side of the page.

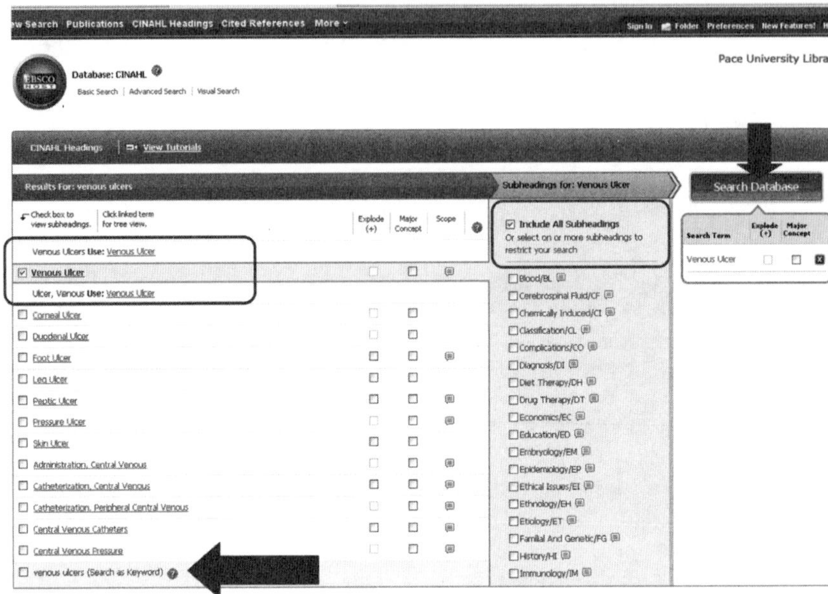

FIGURE 9.3 Search terms.

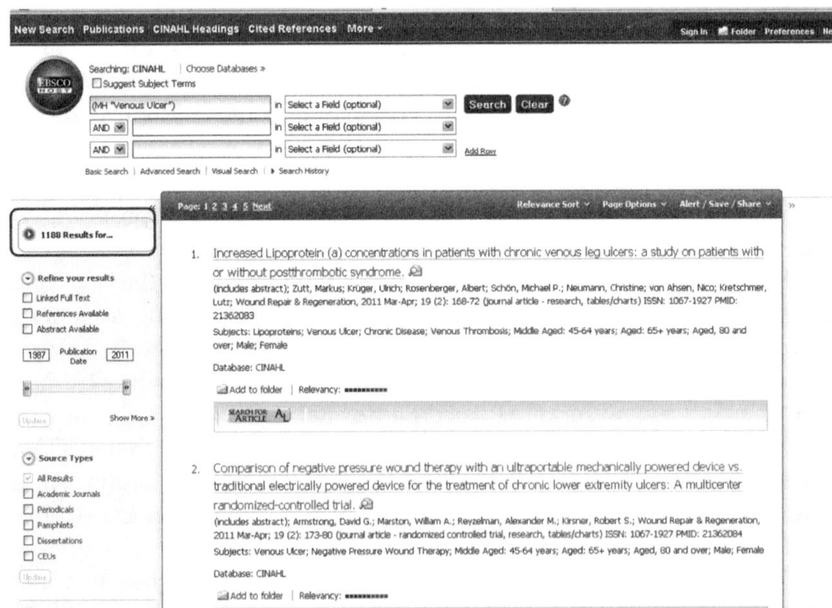

FIGURE 9.4 Number of citations retrieved by using the CINAHL subject heading *venous ulcer*.

You have now completed your sail through the sea of the Cochrane Database of Systematic Reviews, the #1 tool for locating full-text meta-analyses, and arrived safely at shore with your treasure (the full review). Please keep in mind that your organization or a library with which you are partnering needs to subscribe to this database in order for you to have access to the full text of a review. Systematic reviews also can be found with other databases and search engines, such as CINAHL, PubMed or Medline, and Sum Search, but the Cochrane Database of Systematic Reviews is guaranteed to give you access to the actual article, not just a citation or abstract. In the next column we will be discussing how to search CINAHL and PubMed (or Medline).

PART III

Rona F. Levin, Robert E. Burke, and Shannon B. Kealey

The third part addresses searching for the best evidence to answer a focused clinical question. While the second part gave you a map for negotiating the *Cochrane Library of Systematic Reviews*, what happens if you cannot find evidence-based guidelines or systematic reviews in either the Cochrane Library or the Joanna Briggs Institute (JBI) Library of Systematic Reviews? The answer is that you need to then focus on finding systematic reviews or individual studies in the extant literature that are not supported by Cochrane or JBI. This column will focus on how to search the CINAHL* database on EBSCOhost in order to uncover evidence pertinent to your clinical question, using a step-by-step approach that we have found successful. As you recall, the *WCET Journal* is indexed in CINAHL.

First, enter your primary topic term and make sure that "suggest subject terms" is checked. Then click search (Figure 9.2). Next, select the most appropriate subject heading. In this case, it is our entry term without the "S"—*venous ulcer*. If you cannot find an appropriate subject heading, you can click the keyword search for your entry term (in this case, not necessary). Then click search database (Figure 9.3). As a result, we retrieve 1,188 articles tagged with the subject heading *venous ulcer* (Figure 9.4). If you replicate this search, you will likely retrieve different numbers of results because additional articles on the topic may have

*A note to the reader: Just as the sea changes, so too do the results of a literature search. The following search and its examples were run on a specific date. If you practice this search at a later date, it may yield different results.

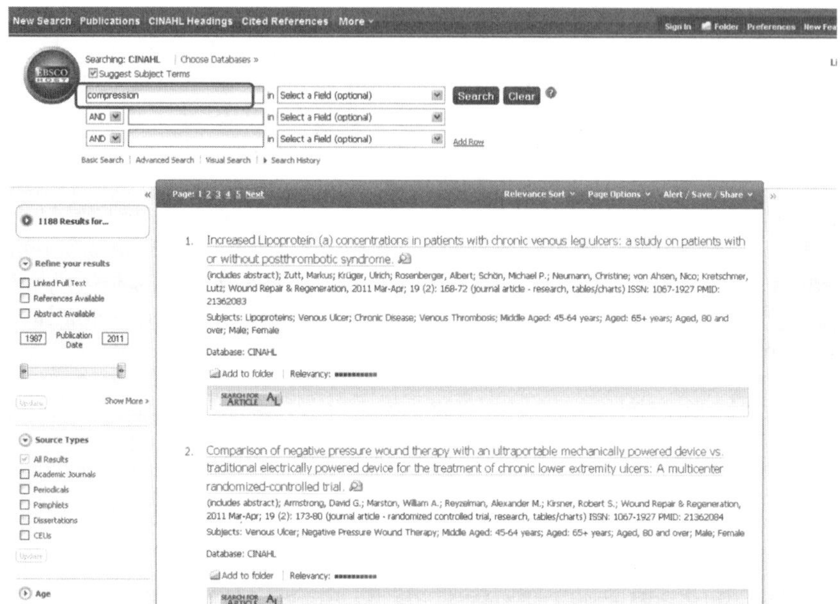

FIGURE 9.5 Intervention keyword, compression.

been added to the CINAHL database between the time of publication and when you run your search.

Now we must combine the topic of venous ulcers with our Intervention, compression (Figure 9.5). Select "Compression Garments" (Figure 9.6). This should include articles that call compression garments by other names, such as stockings and bandages, but to be safe we can add a keyword, *Element*. For now, select compression garments and click Search Database (Figure 9.6). This search results in 1,007 articles in CINAHL that are tagged with the subject heading "Compression Garments" (Figure 9.7). To make sure we do not miss articles, we can search again with keywords (Figure 9.8). The 294 results of the keyword search may or may not be included in the 1,007 tagged with the subject heading "Compression Garments"—let us now see if this search uncovered evidence that our previous search did not find.

The next step would be to clear the search field, click on Search History, select S2 and S3, and click "Search with OR." As a result, we have 1,157 hits—150 additional articles are in the search for compression garments (Figure 9.9). Now, combine S1 and S4 with AND. The result is 185 citations (Figure 9.10). To narrow the search even further, hide the history and then on the left sidebar click "Show More." To limit citations to the highest level of evidence, use the "Publication Type" limiter to

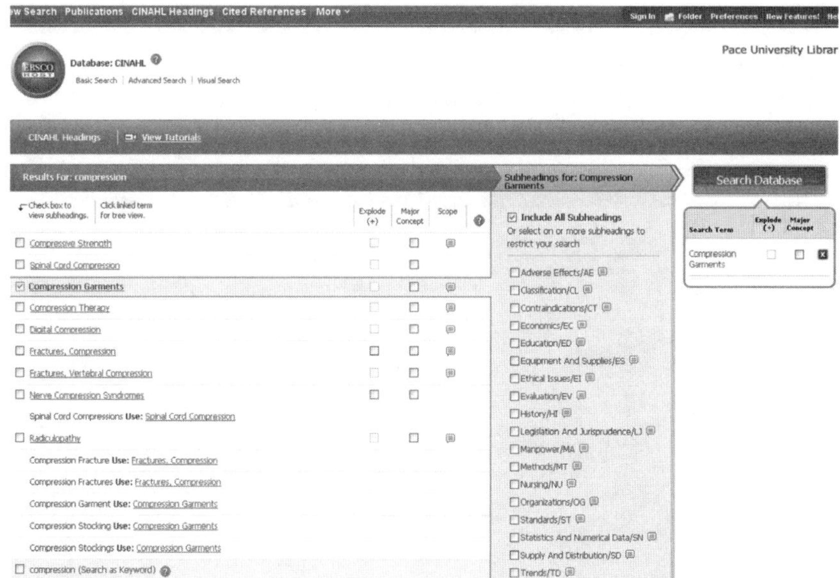

FIGURE 9.6 Select "Compression Garments" and click on Search Database.

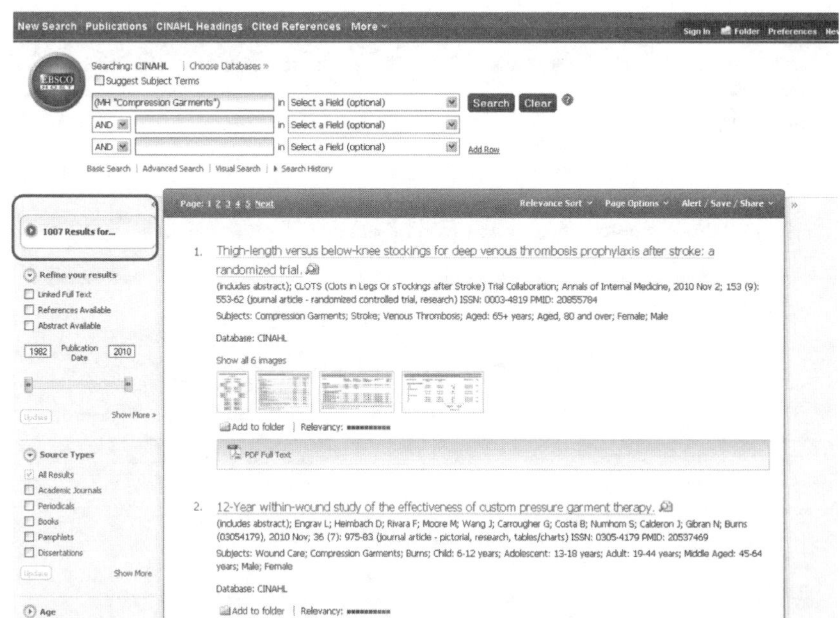

FIGURE 9.7 Number of results for CINAHL subject heading "Compression Garments."

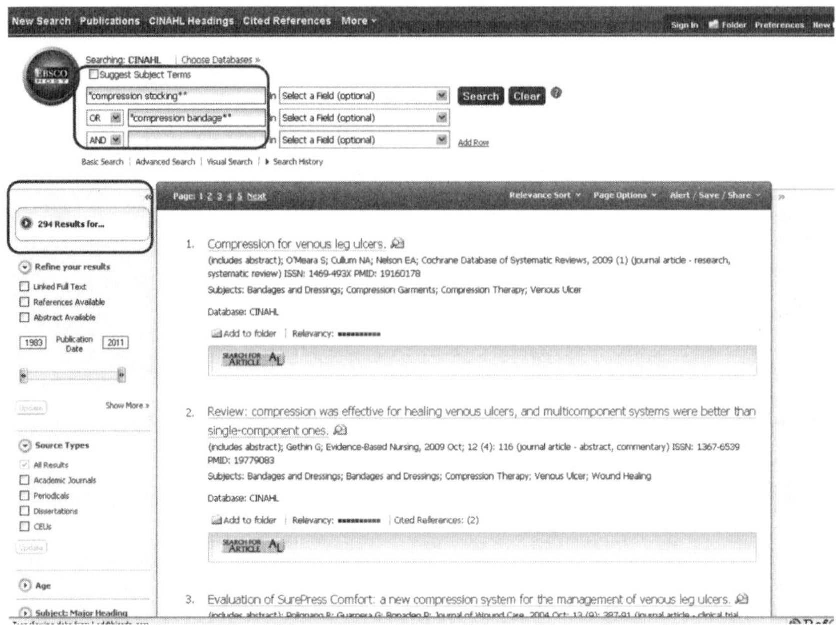

FIGURE 9.8 Results for search of keywords for compression garments.

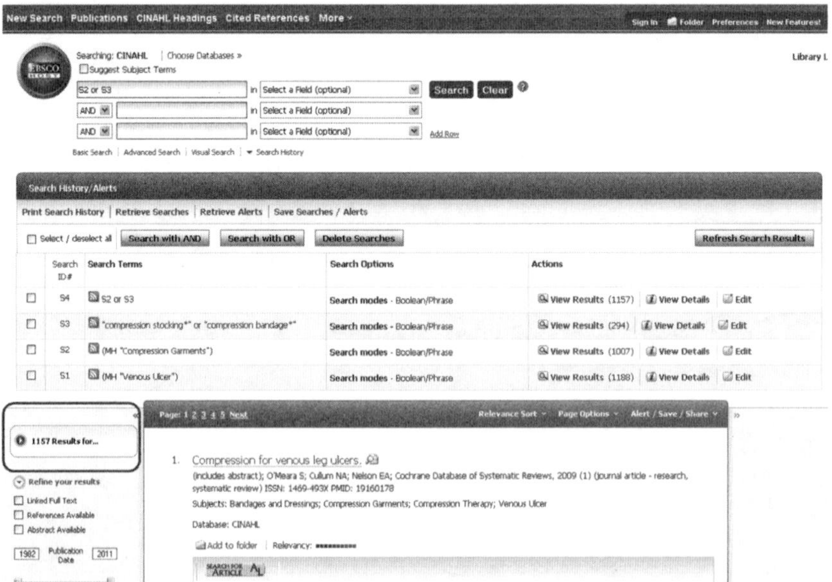

FIGURE 9.9 Results of combining CINAHL subject heading and keyword searches for "Compression Garments."

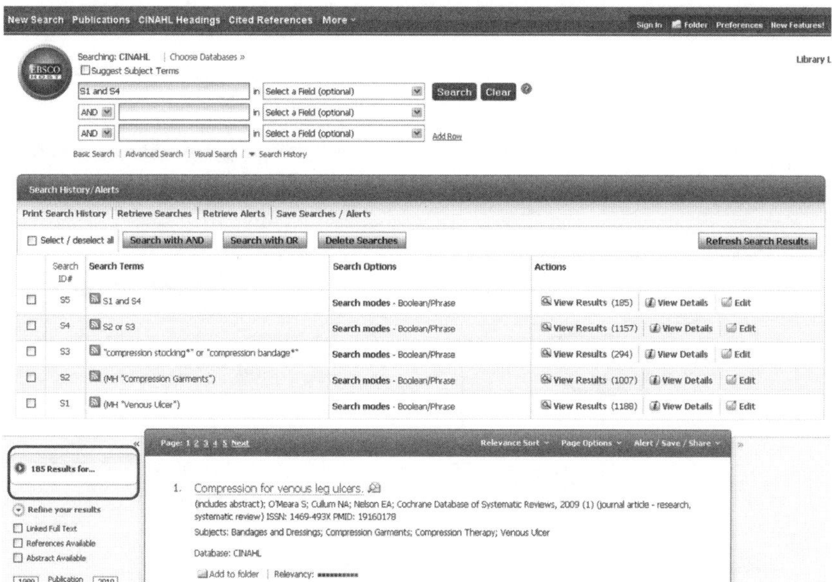

FIGURE 9.10 Results of combining searches for *venous ulcer* and "Compression Garments."

target the level of evidence you need, for example, systematic reviews or clinical trials.

Use this limit option to narrow your search (Figure 9.11). If you only read English, you may also want to limit to the English language. If you read languages other than English, you might want to extend your search to include those languages. Age group is another limit to use if relevant to your clinical question. Of the 185 articles initially retrieved, we are now down to 11 systematic reviews in the English Language (Figures 9.12 to 9.15).

Depending on your institution, you may have direct access to the full text for one or more of these articles. For example, in Figure 9.13, the fourth article was immediately available for a "PDF Full Text" download (see circle around this in Figure 9.13). When this is available, you can easily save the article as an electronic file and/or print it out for immediate use. However, if your institution does not have access to the desired article, you will have to order it through interlibrary loan or purchase it.

This entire process can take less than an hour once you become conversant with how to navigate the CINAHL Sea of Evidence. In the next column, Robert Burke will give you some "Tips of the Trade" that he learned while a student in a doctor of nursing practice program. Stay tuned!

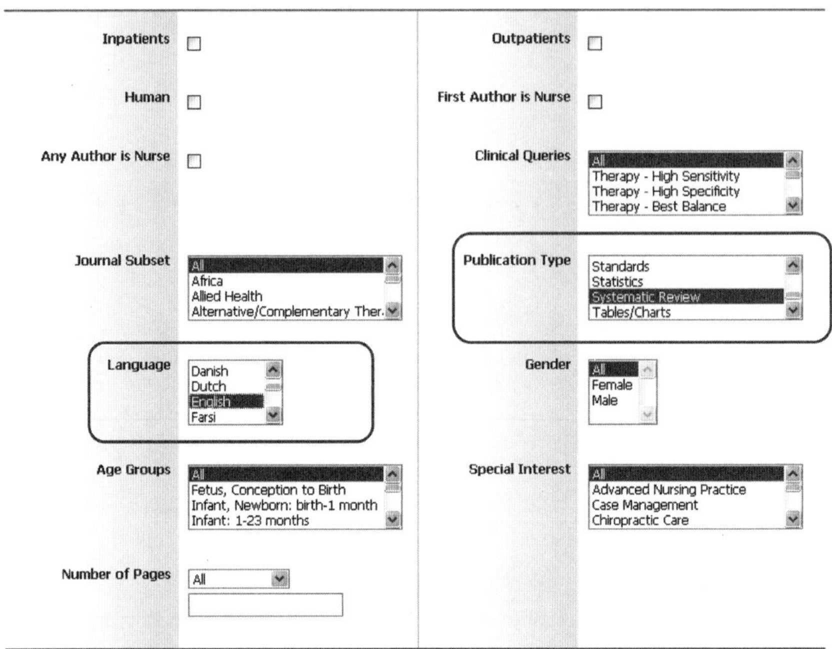

FIGURE 9.11 Limiters for targeting specific criteria for search.

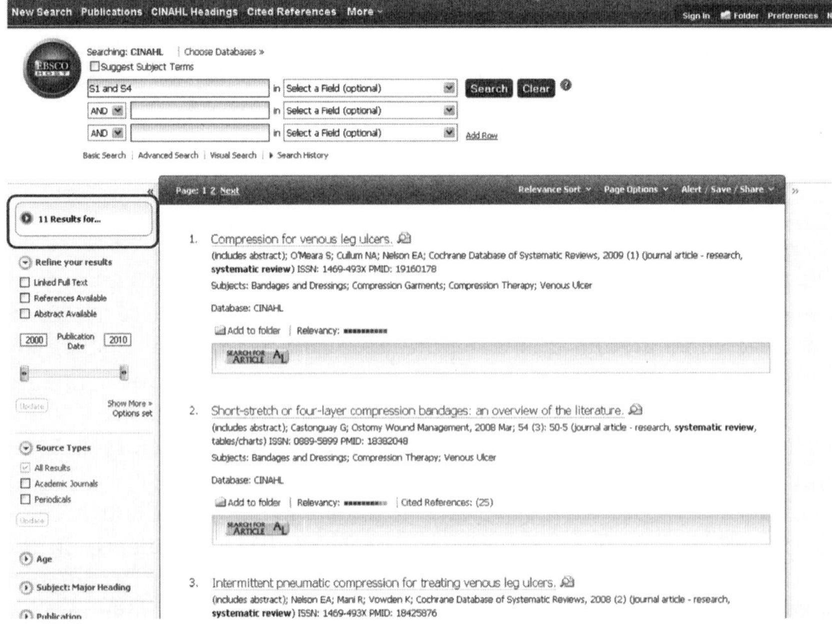

FIGURE 9.12 Results of search and display function for reference availability.

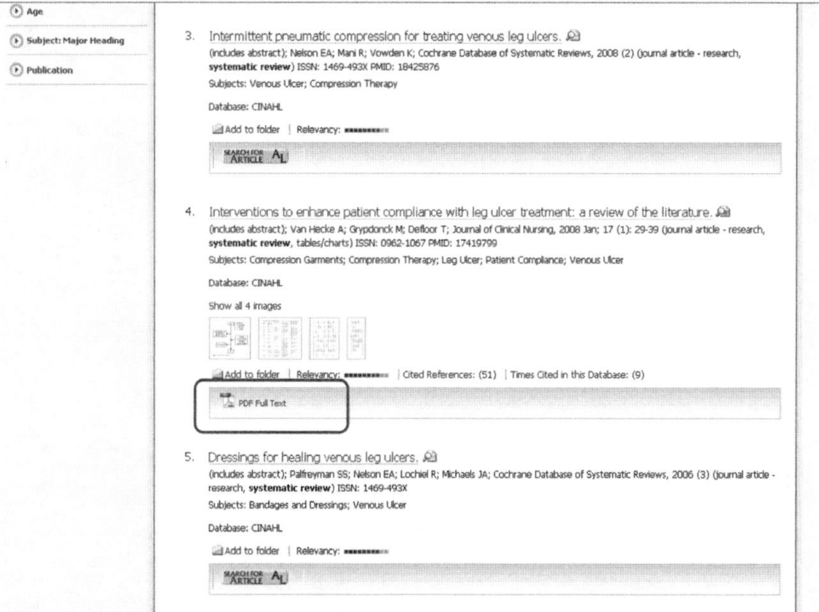

FIGURE 9.13 PDF full text available.

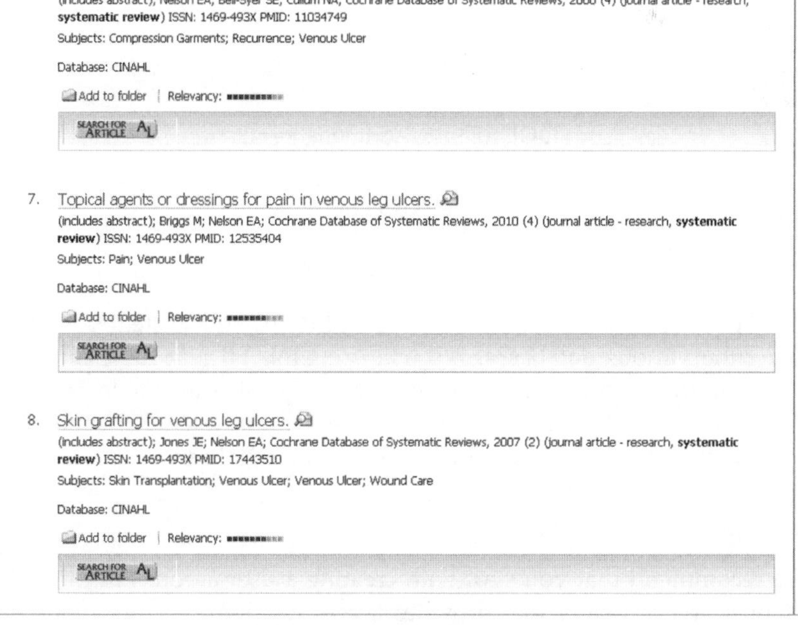

FIGURE 9.14 Additional results.

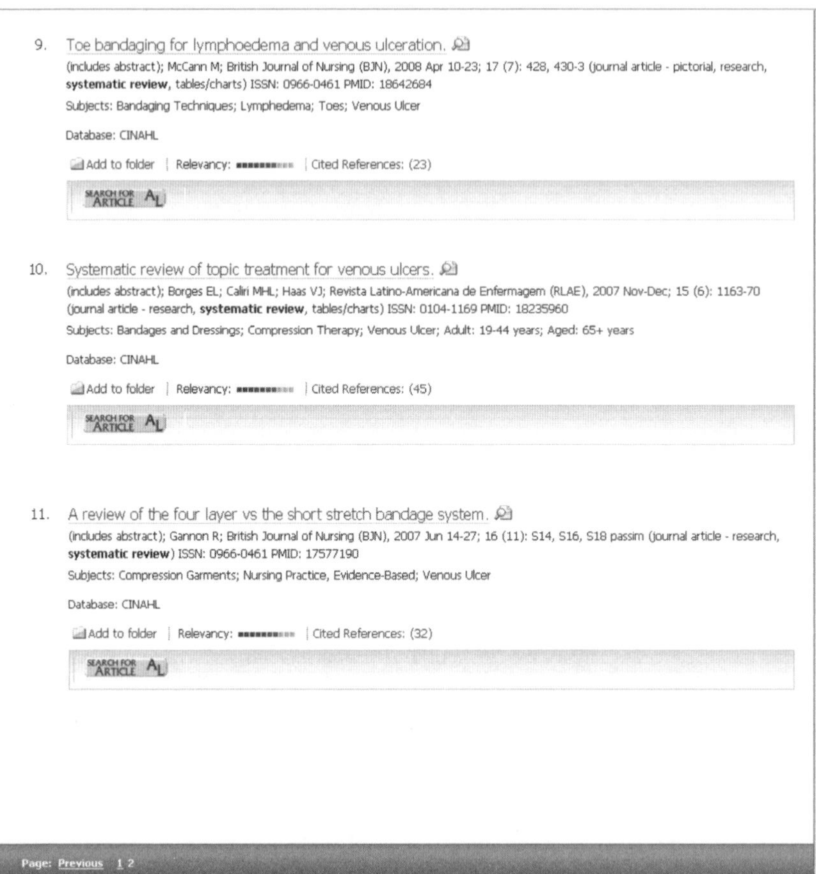

FIGURE 9.15 Additional results.

PART IV

Robert E. Burke, Rona F. Levin, and Shannon B. Kealey

The fourth part focuses on some helpful tips and strategies when utilizing the various databases. We will use CINAHL via EBSCOhost as a guide. Many of these tips and strategies are also available on OVID, PubMed, and the Cochrane Library; however, each system has slight differences that you can explore using the lessons that follow.

Registering for an Account

We recommend that you start with creating a user account through EBSCOhost, the company that provides access to CINAHL and a variety of other databases. This first step is essential for you to access the myriad features associated with this service. Creating an account will enable you to save preferences, organize your research within folders, save and retrieve your search histories, create e-mail alerts, and access your saved research remotely.

Setting Preferences

Once you create an account and log-in, you can set your preferences. This simple step allows EBSCOhost to remember how you like to arrange your research and prevents you from having to manually do it each time you use the system. For example, one of the authors prefers to maximize the number of hit results per page and view all articles in the detailed format, allowing him to view the article information along with the abstract 50 at a time. You can also present your page layout to display one, two, or three columns at a time. In general, the central column has information relating to the identified article. The left column contains advanced options to refine your search, while the right column displays articles you have previously saved in your folder. Another helpful option is presetting your preferred e-mail address so you do not have to continually enter it each time.

Saving Searches

Saving your research at the end of each session will allow you to pick up exactly where you left off and prevent you from needlessly reentering your search strategy each time. When saving a search, you will be asked to define your search and the duration of the save. Choosing the "Permanent" option is recommended as you can delete it later if needed. Once this is done, your search is saved and ready to be opened the next time you log-in. This is done by opening up your Folder, clicking on the Saved searches tab, and retrieving the saved search. Following this approach, the search engine will import your search back into the search history section and allow you to refresh your search and begin anew.

Creating Alerts

Using alerts is another helpful tip that allows EBSCOhost to work for you behind the scenes. Alerts are tools that enable EBSCOhost to continually run your search strategy and look for new evidence even when you are not logged in. Alerts are flexible in their structure and allow you to define the frequency, duration, format, and recipients for the alert. For example, you may be developing a protocol for best practices over the course of

3 months. You can set your alert to search for new evidence twice weekly during this period and create your alert to send you and the entire team new abstracts in the detailed format. Thus, if new evidence is published during this time, you will have immediate access to it.

Tools

The last tip is maximizing the use of the "Tools" tab. This function allows you to add individual articles to your folder and e-mail them to colleagues, along with a few other useful functions. Saved articles are stored in your EBSCOhost folder and easily retrievable when you log in. E-mailing individual articles to your colleagues circumvents the previous need to cut and paste them into a separate e-mail.

The main theme throughout all of these tips is that appropriate use of technology can assist you to stay organized, remain efficient by reducing redundancies, and share work easily with colleagues. These tips and strategies are simple in nature, but will significantly help you maximize your limited time as you conduct searches to find the best evidence for a focused clinical question.

RESOURCES

Levin, R. F. (2009a). Translating research evidence for WCET practice—Clinical effectiveness formulas: What do they mean? *WCET Journal, 29*(3), 38–39.

Levin, R. F. (2009b). Translating research evidence for WCET practice—Clinical effectiveness formulas: Part II. *WCET Journal, 29*(4), 34–35.

Levin, R. F. (2009c). Translating research evidence for WCET practice—Evidence levels and quality ratings: What do they mean? *WCET Journal, 28*(1), 30–31.

Levin, R. F. (2010a). Translating research evidence for WCET practice—Searching the sea of evidence: Part I. *WCET Journal, 30*(4), 18–19.

Levin, R. F. (2010b). Translating research for WCET practice—Clinical effectiveness formulas: Part III. *WCET Journal, 30*(1), 25–26.

Levin, R. F., Burke, R. E., & Kealey, S. B. (2011). Translating research evidence for WCET practice—Searching the sea of evidence: Part III. *WCET Journal, 31*(1), 30–35.

Levin, R. F., Kealey, S. B., & Burke, R. E. (2011). Translating research evidence for WCET practice—Searching the sea of evidence: Part III. *WCET Journal, 31*(2), 26–29.

10

Synthesizing Evidence and Separating Apples From Oranges

Rona F. Levin

The one real object of education is to have a [person] in the condition of continually asking questions.

—Bishop Mandell Creighton

Synthesizing evidence to answer a burning clinical question is a difficult task for many of us, particularly students. So one of the first assignments I give students in a graduate research course is to formulate a burning clinical question and then find a sample of evidence that bears on this question.

A major challenge we face as faculty is helping students to think critically. The task of deciding whether or not research studies belong in the same evidence base (i.e., are relevant to the clinical question being asked) is a daunting one for many students. They seem to have particular trouble identifying the specific protocol of an intervention (what we used to call the operational definition) and the outcome variables of interest. When I started teaching a graduate research course from an evidence-based practice (EBP) perspective, I thought this learning task would be one of the simpler ones. I was wrong.

I realized the error of my thinking when students began showing me articles to approve for an assignment on finding evidence that was relevant to their clinical question. More often than not, neither the independent (e.g., intervention, prognostic factor, risk factor) nor dependent (outcome) variables in several studies matched. Many students went through this process several times before they understood that if one is trying to find related articles on treatment effectiveness, at the very least the treatment needed to be the same in all of the studies.

After students learn how to identify clinical problems and focus clinical questions, they need to find the evidence that bears on that clinical question. The first step is for students to access the abstracts of the studies they find. Based on the abstract, they are to determine whether or not the dependent or outcome variables and independent or treatment variables in the studies are the same, similar, or not related at all. If they determine the latter to be the case, then they know the study is not relevant and there is no need to access the entire study.

I ask them to show me three abstracts they believe are relevant to their clinical question. If I approve the abstract, then they retrieve the full study. If I see that the abstract is not relevant to their question, I direct them to search further. This is an essential first step to point students in the right direction for finding the appropriate evidence for their clinical question. If students do not complete this portion of the assignment correctly, they cannot possibly write a coherent paper synthesizing the relevant evidence on a clinical problem and determining its readiness for application to practice.

LEARNING ACTIVITY 1: APPLES, OR APPLES AND ORANGES?

As part of a class prior to directing students to find evidence on a clinical problem, I use the following interactive exercise to help them determine whether or not studies belong in the same evidence base; that is, to differentiate apples from apples and oranges. Students read the abstracts of two studies in class. I choose to have them read the abstracts in class because when I previously assigned two entire studies for students to read prior to class, they rarely completed the assignment. By using the abstracts only, students are able to read the material in 5 to 10 minutes during break or class time. You may use either the abstracts of actual studies, write your own abstracts of actual studies, or create fictional abstracts. I have found that using the latter two approaches allows you to incorporate all the relevant details needed for students to judge the comparability of studies. Also, I choose two abstracts that do not belong to the same evidence base.

After reading the abstracts, I ask students to identify the following components for each study:

- Clinical problem as identified by the author(s)
- Dependent variable(s) or outcome variable(s)
- Independent variable(s) or interventions/prognostic factors/risk factors
- Population being studied

Next, I ask students to make judgments about similarities and differences for each of these components by asking the following questions:

- Are the dependent or outcome variable(s) in each study the same, similar, or different? If similar, describe the variations.

- Are the independent variable(s) in each study the same, similar, or different? If similar, describe the variations.
- Is the population the same in each study?
- Is the clinical problem in each study the same, similar, or different?

After answering the first three questions, students are prepared to answer the last question in a PICO (population, intervention, comparison, outcome) format, which I require them to do. Having the clinical question for each study in such a format makes the final question of the exercise much easier to answer: Do studies 1 and 2 belong in the same evidence base? Students should now be prepared to develop their own clinical questions and look for relevant, related evidence.

LEARNING ACTIVITY 2: ANSWERING A CLINICAL QUESTION

Before embarking on a full-blown synthesis of evidence, a product many faculty members require in a nursing research or other nursing course, students need to master the process. In order to do so, they need practice in synthesizing evidence on a small scale. Therefore, the first graded assignment in a nursing research course could consist of sampling three studies on a particular clinical question and learning how to critique an evidence base (i.e., critique the three studies as a whole rather than individually). Exhibit 10.1 provides readers with the actual assignment I have used to accomplish this learning goal. As stated in the beginning of this chapter, students do not proceed with the assignment until they have (a) developed and I have approved their clinical question and (b) accessed three studies that we have agreed are indeed all apples. Of course, they could all be oranges as well.

In addition to providing practice in learning the basic skills needed to develop a successful synthesis paper, I provide students with a sample paper demonstrating how to critique an evidence base. In the past I have used a paper I developed for this purpose. Currently, a colleague who teaches the graduate research course uses a synthesis paper written by Garrelts and Melnyk (2001), which is an excellent example of this type of paper (refer to Exhibit 10.2).

To summarize, the main purposes of this learning exercise are to help students develop skill in (1) finding the evidence to answer a burning clinical question; (2) critiquing an evidence base; and (3) determining whether or not the evidence justifies a change in practice. Providing students with learning exercises that give them practice in the above skills builds confidence in their ability and thus facilitates successful completion of a synthesis paper.

EXHIBIT 10.1 SYNTHESIZING EVIDENCE ON A CLINICAL PROBLEM

Student Assignment

1. Select a *clinical nursing problem.*
   Example. You are working on a surgical unit and observe that patients who undergo certain types of surgical procedures are not achieving effective pain relief with regularly prescribed pain medication. What nursing interventions, other than administering analgesics, can be used to achieve effective pain relief in postoperative patients?
2. Identify the *outcome variable* of interest (dependent variable).
   In the above clinical problem, the outcome variable is postoperative pain.
3. Conduct a *literature search* focusing on research that addresses the effects of nursing interventions on postoperative pain.
4. Choose *at least three studies* that have a *similar problem* or *purpose.* An example is, "What is the effect of music on postoperative pain in a population of women who have had abdominal surgery?"
5. *Critically read* these studies to determine their scientific merit.
   Use the critique guidelines contained in the course syllabus.
6. *Write a 5- to 8-page, typed, double-spaced paper* that includes the following:
   (a) A narrative statement of the clinical nursing problem
   (b) The burning clinical question in PICO format
   (c) Identification of studies reviewed
   (d) Summary of the evidence base (as per sample)
   (e) Strengths and limitations of the evidence base
   (f) How these limitations affect the readiness of the new intervention for use in clinical practice
   (g) A conclusion that addresses the state of the art on your topic

Teacher Evaluation Criteria

1. The clinical nursing problem is identified and stated according to PICO criteria. 10%
2. The summary is succinct, yet includes sufficient information about the studies for the reader to determine their overall validity. 30%
3. Strengths and limitations are accurately identified and related to application of findings in practice. (This section reflects the writer's knowledge of the research process and critiquing ability.) 30%

4. The paper concludes with the writer's opinion about whether or not the findings are ready to be implemented in practice. Sufficient rationale is clearly presented in relation to the overall strengths and limitations of the research base. 10%
5. The paper reflects clarity of thought, logical progression of ideas, and is grammatically correct. 10%
6. The paper adheres to APA guidelines. 10%

EXHIBIT 10.2 PACIFIER USAGE AND ACUTE OTITIS MEDIA IN INFANTS AND YOUNG CHILDREN

Laurie Garrelts and Bernadette Mazurek Melnyk

Acute otitis media (AOM) is a commonly encountered pediatric illness that affects approximately 70% of children by 3 years of age, with one-third experiencing more than three episodes (Pichichero & Cohen, 1997). AOM is the most frequent diagnosis for office visits in children under the age of 15 years and is the primary reason that children receive antibiotics (Andrews, 2001). The estimated cost of treatment for AOM in the United States is $8 billion annually (Fitzgerald, 1999). If not properly treated, AOM can lead to hearing loss, middle-ear disorders, and delayed speech development (Petersen-Smith, 2000). Simultaneously, overly aggressive treatment with antibiotics has led to increased antibiotic resistance in children (Fitzgerald, 1999).

Illness prevention through anticipatory guidance is an important element of pediatric primary health care. Therefore, clinicians should become familiar with the risk factors for AOM so that parents can be educated about prevention strategies. Studies have indicated that several variables increase the risk for AOM, including: (a) bottle-feeding infants, (b) feeding infants in the supine position, (c) passive smoke exposure, (d) attendance at group child daycare, and most recently, (e) pacifier usage (Fitzgerald, 1999).

Pacifier use is a common practice, as it is estimated that approximately 75% to 85% of all children in western countries use or have used a pacifier (Victora, Behague, Barros, Olinto, & Weiderpass, 1997). Use of a pacifier is typically thought of as a comforting and harmless habit, with only a temporary effect on dentition and occlusion. However, this habit may not be as risk free as once thought, as

(*continued*)

EXHIBIT 10.2 (*continued*)

some researchers contend there is a relationship between otitis media (OM) and pacifier use in children (Niemela, Pihakari, Pokka, Uhari, & Uhari, 2000).

Laurie Garrelts, BSN, RN, is a pediatric nurse practitioner/care of children and families graduate student, University of Rochester School of Nursing, Rochester, NY; and staff nurse, Neonatal Intensive Care Unit and Pediatric Emergency Department, Children's Hospital, University of Rochester Medical Center, Rochester, NY.

Bernadette Mazurek Melnyk, PhD, RN-CS, PNP, is associate dean for research and director, Center for Research & Evidence-Based Practice and Pediatric Nurse Practitioner Program, University of Rochester School of Nursing, Rochester, NY. (At the time of publication of this information the information was current.)

Source: Garrelts, L., & Melnyk, B. M. (2001). Pacifier usage and acute otitis media in infants and young children. *Pediatric Nursing, 27*, 516–519.

CLINICAL QUESTION

Is there a relationship between pacifier usage and AOM in infants and young children?

SEARCH FOR THE EVIDENCE

The search for evidence began by accessing the Medline database and entering the key words "otitis media" and "pacifier." These key words were combined using the term "and" and the search was limited to humans, the English language, and the years 1995 through 2001. Only four of the 10 articles located were studies that addressed pacifier usage and OM. Three articles were selected to be included as evidence in this report; the fourth article was excluded because it was an older publication that analyzed several risk factors for AOM.

THE EVIDENCE

Study #1

The purpose of the first study by Niemela and colleagues (2000) was to evaluate the association between pacifier use and the occurrence of AOM through an intervention that educated parents on restricting pacifier use in their infants and young children. This study was a randomized, controlled, prospective clinical trial that was conducted at 14 well-baby clinics in Oulu, Finland between December 1996 and February 1997. The clinics were paired according to their size and the area they served, after which one clinic from each pair was randomly assigned to either the experimental or control group.

A total of 484 healthy children less than 18 months old were included in this study. There were no statistically significant differences between the experimental and control group children at baseline on variables such as age, gender, day care, history of AOM, adenoidectomy, tympanostomy, pacifier use, parental smoking, atopic eczema, and breastfeeding.

The educational intervention used in the study by Niemela and colleagues (2000) was delivered by clinic nurses and consisted of providing parents with verbal and written information about the adverse effects of pacifiers, including an increased risk for AOM, oral candidiasis, dental caries, and malocclusion. Nurses in the experimental clinics informed the parents that the need for sucking during the first 6 months is often great and reflexive, therefore, pacifiers may be used as often as necessary during this time period. However, parents were advised to limit pacifier usage after 6 months and discontinue its use after 10 months of age (Niemela et al., 2000). The parents who attended the control clinics received standard care, which did not include counseling or educational materials about pacifier usage.

Parents at both clinics were instructed to document the occurrence of AOM on a daily symptom sheet that they mailed to the clinic on a monthly basis. During this time period, if a child was evaluated by a physician for an illness, the parents also were instructed to have their physician write the child's diagnosis and medication prescribed on the daily symptom sheet. In addition, parents recorded the dates that pacifier usage by the child changed (e.g., a change from using a pacifier continuously to use only while falling asleep). The effect of the intervention on pacifier use was evaluated by calculating the time for which children over 6 months old used a pacifier continuously, only when falling asleep, or not at all during the monitoring period (Niemela et al., 2000).

Follow-up data collection was successful in 91% of the children who were enrolled in the study. Reasons for attrition were that five families moved away geographically, and 45 families did not return the symptom sheets. The time frame in which monitoring of data occurred ranged from 1 to 6 months with a mean of 4.6 months.

Findings indicated that at the end of the study 68% of the children in the intervention group and 66.5% of the children in the control group were still using a pacifier. However, time spent using a pacifier continuously was significantly reduced for children in the intervention group. For intervention group children who were 6 to 10 months of age, they spent 35% of their monitoring time using pacifiers continuously compared to 48% in the control group (Niemela et al., 2000).

Study findings also indicated that the occurrence of AOM was 29% less in the group that received the intervention compared to the control group. In addition, the occurrence of AOM was 33% higher in the group of children who continuously used the pacifier when compared to those children that only used the pacifier when falling asleep or not at all. Based on their findings, Niemela and colleagues concluded that health care providers should encourage parents to terminate pacifier usage in infants after 10 months of age. The rationale provided was that an infant's physiological need to suck is greatest in the first 6 months of life, and the incidence of AOM prior to 10 months is low (Niemela et al., 2000).

Study #2

Niemela, Uhari, and Mottonen (1995) used a prospective, correlational, longitudinal design to investigate the relationship between the independent variable of pacifier use and the dependent variable of AOM over a 15-month period of time. The convenience sample consisted of 845 White children attending a daycare center full time in Oulu, Finland between March 1991 and June 1992. The ages of the children ranged from 0.25 to 7.24 years, with a mean age of 3.29 years and a mean monitoring time of 10 months, with a range of 1 to 15 months.

Parents of the children were asked to record daily signs and symptoms of infectious disease in their children on monthly symptom sheets. Visits to their primary care provider, along with the child's diagnosis, medications, and number of days absent from day care also were to be recorded on the symptom sheets. In the last month of the study, parents were asked to complete a questionnaire addressing their child's use of a pacifier at the start of the study, number of months in which the pacifier was used during the monitoring period, number of adenoidectomies and tympanostomies, duration of breastfeeding, parental smoking practices, and social class of the parents. The authors did not indicate how many hours per day a child needed to suck on a pacifier in order for them to consider the child a "pacifier user." The authors defined the dependent variable as more than three episodes of AOM during the monitoring period and controlled statistically for age and other possible confounding variables (i.e., parental smoking) in their analyses. Relative risk ratios and 95% confidence intervals were used to determine if children who used pacifiers had a statistically significant higher occurrence of AOM than nonpacifier users.

Findings indicated that more than three episodes of AOM occurred in 29.5% of children younger than 2 years of age using pacifiers compared to 20.6% of children who were not using pacifiers (relative risk of 1.6). In children 2 to 3 years of age, the incidence of AOM was 30.6% in pacifier users and 13.2% in nonpacifier users (relative risk of 2.9), which was statistically significant ($p = .01$). In addition, the use of a pacifier led to a statistically significant increase in the annual rate of AOM in children less than 2 years old and in children 2 to 3 years of age (Niemela et al., 1995).

Niemela and colleagues (1995) concluded that their study supports the theory that the use of a pacifier is a risk factor for AOM, especially for recurrent attacks. These authors also suggested that pacifier usage should be restricted to the first 10 months of life, when the need for sucking is the greatest and AOM is uncommon. The authors did address some study limitations, such as the lack of consistent diagnostic criteria between physicians and the fact that all children attended a daycare center, where infection rates are high due to the close contact among many children. They stated that pacifier use may not be such a potent risk for children that do not attend daycare centers (Niemela et al., 1995).

Study #3

Jackson and Mourino (1999) also sought to examine the relationship between pacifier use in 200 children, aged 12 months or younger, and the incidence of OM. Since the authors used the general term of OM, it is unknown whether OM was used to indicate only AOM or both AOM and OM with effusion. The study was conducted at a pediatric practice that was part of a university medical center in Virginia. The mean age of the children in the study who had been diagnosed with at least one episode of OM was 8.3 months. Seventy-five percent of the sample was African American, 22% White, 2% Hispanic, and 0.5% Asian. Seventy-six percent of the parents were reported as having a low education level.

The authors reviewed the children's past medical records and recorded the number of episodes of OM experienced by each child. The diagnosis of OM was made by practitioners that employed similar criteria via physical exam coordinated with reports of signs and symptoms. In addition, parents or guardians completed a questionnaire that elicited data regarding pacifier habits, length of time the pacifier was used per day, daycare utilization, breastfeeding practices, bottle feeding, parental smoking, thumb sucking, and parental educational level. The authors defined a "pacifier user" as a child who sucked on a pacifier for more than 5 hours a day. The parent questionnaire and definition of pacifier use was based upon information gleaned from previous pilot studies (Jackson & Mourino, 1999). Findings indicated that the prevalence of OM in pacifier users (36%) was larger than the prevalence of OM in nonpacifier users (23%; $p < .05$). This association remained significant after controlling for other confounding variables (e.g., parental smoking). Children who used a pacifier were twice as likely to develop OM. There were no associations between OM and gender, race, breastfeeding, parental smoking, and parent education level. Based on their study's findings, the authors concluded that there is an increased risk for OM in children who use pacifiers versus those who do not. As a result of their findings, Jackson and Mourino (1999) suggest that parents should be encouraged to discontinue the use of pacifiers with their infants before 10 months of age.

CRITIQUE OF THE EVIDENCE

A strength of all three of the studies reviewed was that they had large sample sizes, which provided sufficient power to detect statistically significant results (Brown, 1999). However, the samples used in the studies were not randomly selected. In addition, the first two studies were conducted with exclusively White children in Finland, and the third study's sample was predominately comprised of African American children whose parents had a low level of education. Therefore, external validity of these studies is weak, and caution must be used in generalizing the results of these studies to other populations, such as those comprised of varied ethnicity and social classes (Brown, 1999).

Each study provided a detailed methodology section with a concise description of their research design. Although there is a paucity of research pertaining to this topic, Jackson and Mourino (1999) provided background information and a thorough literature review.

The first study by Niemela and colleagues (2000) was a randomized, prospective, controlled clinical trial, the strongest design for testing cause and effect relationships (Polit & Hungler, 1999). Although the investigators were not able to use true random assignment, they used cluster randomization to allocate the well-baby clinics to study groups in order to decrease the probability of contamination between the intervention and standard care groups. Because the second and third studies used correlational designs, findings only support that there is a relationship between pacifier usage and OM, not that pacifier usage causes OM.

A strength of the first two studies also is that both employed prospective designs, which are generally stronger than a retrospective design, as used by Jackson and Mourino (1999) (Polit & Hungler, 1999). Since the third study used a retrospective chart review, the authors were unable to determine if the pacifier habit had occurred before, concurrently, or after the first episode of OM (Jackson & Mourino, 1999). All three studies relied upon parental completion of symptom sheets or questionnaires for their data collection. As a result, parent self-report may have resulted in "response bias," as subjects may have distorted their answers to provide more favorable responses, which may have led to inaccurate study results (Polit & Hungler, 1999). In addition, parent reporting of symptoms may not be a valid strategy for documenting the incidence of AOM, which is a major limitation of the first two studies. All three studies reviewed also relied heavily upon parental memory of infant pacifier-sucking patterns, which may not be accurate. However, only Jackson and Mourino (1999) recognized this issue as an inherent limitation of their study.

Jackson and Mourino (1999) were the only researchers who attempted to develop some form of interrater reliability in their study in that they developed a predefined set of criteria for OM on which physicians were to base their diagnosis. These researchers also used pilot studies to test their questionnaires. No information is provided regarding the validity or reliability of the data collection methods used in either the Niemela et al. (2000) or Niemela et al. (1995) studies. However, a strength of all three studies is that each used appropriate statistical measures to analyze their data.

Future studies should use random samples that are heterogeneous and representative of the population at large so that results may be generalized. In addition, more valid and reliable methods for documenting episodes of AOM should be used in future research on this topic.

IMPLICATIONS FOR PRACTICE

OM is a common pediatric illness that can have significant complications, such as hearing loss and speech delay. Therefore, it is critical for pediatric nurses and other pediatric health care providers to have knowledge regarding factors that may increase risk for AOM in children. Based on the studies reviewed, evidence is accumulating to indicate that there is a relationship between substantial pacifier usage (i.e., continuous usage or usage more than 5 hours a day) and AOM in infants and young children. Therefore, it is important to assess the extent to which parents use pacifiers with their infants at routine well-child care visits early in infancy and to educate parents regarding the potential for increased risk of AOM with substantial pacifier usage, especially after 6 to 10 months of age.

Simultaneously, parents need to be educated about the mechanism by which pacifier usage may contribute to AOM. Specifically, sucking on a pacifier lifts the soft palate in the mouth causing the contraction of the tensor veli palatine muscle. Contraction of this muscle results in the Eustachian tube becoming actively patent and provides an ideal medium for bacteria and viruses from the nasopharynx to be swept into the middle ear (Jackson & Mourino, 1999). In addition, sucking on a pacifier increases the amount of saliva in the mouth, which is an excellent medium for microorganisms. Thumbsucking, on the other hand, has not been shown to produce this same pathophysiological mechanism, and studies have not supported its relationship to AOM (Niemela et al., 1995).

If parents are using pacifiers with their young infants continuously or with their infants who are older than 10 months of age, they should not be made to feel guilty about this practice. Instead, sensitive interventions that support these parents in gradually weaning their children from the pacifier are needed. Nurse practitioners and nurses are in an ideal position to routinely incorporate assessment and appropriate anticipatory guidance related to pacifier usage with parents of young infants. Early intervention is important in that it could prevent costly physical, psychological, and financial negative outcomes associated with OM in children.

GLOSSARY OF TERMS

Confidence intervals: The range of values in which a population parameter lies.

Convenience sample: A sample that is obtained by convenience (i.e., the most readily available subjects to participate in the study).

Dependent variable: The outcome variable.

External validity: The extent to which the results of a study can be generalized from the sample to the population.

Independent variable: The variable that is thought to cause or influence a change in the dependent or outcome variable.

Interrater reliability: The extent to which two raters assign the same ratings for a variable that is being measured.

$p = .01$: The probability that the study results are due to chance is 1 in 100.

$p < .05$: The probability that the study results are due to chance is less than 5 in 100.

Randomized, controlled, prospective trial: A true experiment in which subjects are randomly assigned to either the experimental or control group and the outcomes are studied over time.

Relative risk ratio: The probability of contracting the illness.

REFERENCES

Andrews, J. S. (2001). Otitis media and otitis externa. In R. A. Hoekelman (Ed.), *Primary pediatric care* (pp. 1702–1706). St. Louis: Mosby.

Brown, S. J. (1999). *Knowledge for health care practice: A guide to using research evidence.* Toronto: W.B. Saunders.

Fitzgerald, M. A. (1999). Acute otitis media in an era of drug resistance: Implications for NP practice. *The Nurse Practitioner, 24*(10), 10–14.

Garrelts, L., & Melnyk, B. M. (2001). Pacifier usage and acute otitis media in infants and young children. *Pediatric Nursing, 27,* 516–519.

Jackson, J. M., & Mourino, A. P. (1999). Pacifier use and otitis media in infants twelve months of age or younger. *Pediatric Dentistry, 21,* 256–260.

Niemela, M., Pihakari, O., Pokka, T., Uhari, M., & Uhari, M. (2000). Pacifier as a risk factor for acute otitis media: A randomized, controlled trial of parental counseling. *Pediatrics, 106,* 483–488.

Niemela, M., Uhari, M., & Mottonen, M. (1995). A pacifier increases the risk of recurrent acute otitis media in children in daycare centers. *Pediatrics, 96,* 884–888.

Petersen-Smith, A. M. (2000). Ear disorders. In C. E. Burns, M. A. Brady, A. M. Dunn, & N. B. Starr (Eds.), *Pediatric primary care: A handbook for nurse practitioners* (2nd ed.) (pp. 783–806). Philadelphia: W. B. Saunders Co.

Pichichero, M., & Cohen, R. (1997). Shortened course of antibiotic therapy for acute otitis media, sinusitis and tonsillopharyngitis. *Pediatric Infectious Disease, 16,* 680–695.

Polit, D. F., & Hungler, B. P. (1999). *Nursing research: Principles and methods* (6th ed.). New York: Lippincott.

Victora, C. G., Behague, D. P., Barros, F. C., Olinto, M. T., & Weiderpass, E. (1997). Pacifier use and short breast-feeding duration: Cause, consequence, or coincidence? *Pediatrics, 99,* 445–453.

11

Evaluating Clinical Practice Guidelines

Rona F. Levin, Lorraine Ferrara, and Mary Jo Vetter

True genius resides in the capacity for evaluation of uncertain, hazardous, and conflicting information.

—Winston Churchill

This chapter reflects the evolution of a teaching strategy to evaluate clinical protocols. Two prior publications focused on this topic. First is a column by Levin and Vetter (2007) that took readers through the process of assessing a clinical practice guideline (CPG) for dementia using the original AGREE instrument. At the time we had to print the appraisal tool and calculate scores for each aspect of the tool by hand. Although this process required a lot of work on the part of evaluators and several hours for workshops on how to use this critical appraisal tool, all those who participated in workshops on how to assess CPG's with the AGREE instrument found this method of guideline assessment relevant and useful. A second column by Levin and Ferrara (2011) focused on the exceptional and useful refinements made to enhance the original instrument and the process for its use, which resulted in the AGREE II (see www.agreetrust.org). Not only has the *Rigour of Development* domain for guideline assessment been enhanced, but the entire process of guideline evaluation can now be conducted online. The current chapter combines parts of these two columns to best demonstrate how to evaluate CPGs using the AGREE II.

First it is important to define what we mean by CPGs. There are three relevant terms to consider: *guidelines, protocols,* and *recommendations,* which are often used interchangeably by health professionals. A recommendation is a suggestion for practice, not necessarily sanctioned by a formal, expert group. A CPG is an official recommendation or generally prescribed approach to diagnose and manage a broad health condition, such as heart failure, smoking cessation, pain management, or dementia. A protocol is a more detailed guide for approaching a clinical problem or patient health condition and is tailored to a specific practice situation. The validity of any of these practice guides can vary depending on the type of evidence upon which they are based, as well as other factors such as the composition of the group charged with their development (Rich & Newland, 2006). How does one begin to tackle this challenging task?

In 2001, the AGREE instrument for the appraisal of CPGs was released in its initial form. The process that led to its development began in 1992 with the creation of an appraisal instrument for the National Health Services supported by the United Kingdom National Health Services Management Executive. Funding for the AGREE instrument, an international effort, was later provided by the European Union (AGREE Collaboration, 2001). The instrument then contained 23 items categorized into six quality domains: scope and purpose, stakeholder involvement, rigor of development, clarity and presentation, application, and editorial independence. For example, when evaluating scope and purpose, evaluators responded to three items with a 4-point Likert scale. Today, the AGREE II has been enhanced in terms of editing items for clarity and has included a 7-point Likert scale for finer distinctions in evaluation (Figure 11.1). Important then, as well as with the new, revised AGREE II, is to increase the reliability of the evaluation. To do this, there must be more than one appraiser for each guideline. Initially, the tool used a 4-point Likert scale, from strongly disagree to strongly agree, to score for each item within a domain. Individual domain scores are the outcome, which, based on a review of domain scores, allow the appraiser to give a subjective assessment of the guideline. We can come to a subjective conclusion related to the overall assessment, but the instrument does not recommend averaging domain scores for a total quantitative rating.

Since its first iteration, the tool has been refined in a number of ways. First, the 4-point Likert scale on the original tool has been replaced with a

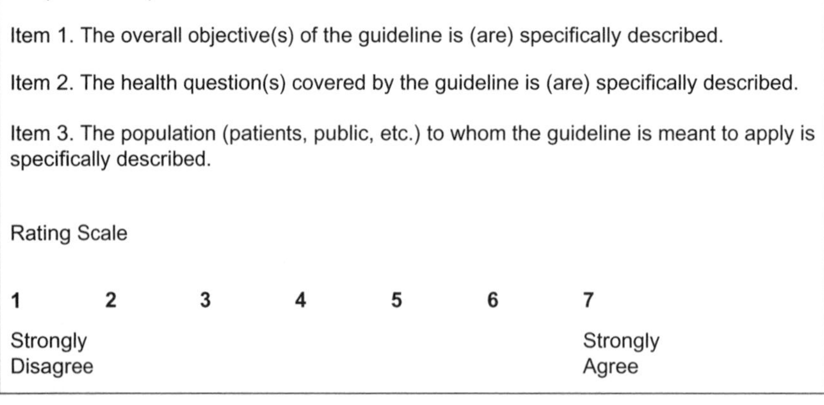
Scope and Purpose

Item 1. The overall objective(s) of the guideline is (are) specifically described.

Item 2. The health question(s) covered by the guideline is (are) specifically described.

Item 3. The population (patients, public, etc.) to whom the guideline is meant to apply is specifically described.

Rating Scale

1	2	3	4	5	6	7
Strongly Disagree						Strongly Agree

FIGURE 11.1 Sample domain and items from the AGREE II instrument for critical appraisal of clinical practice guidelines with rating scale.

7-point scale to allow for finer distinctions in evaluation. Next, modifications, additions, and deletions have been made to approximately half of the original core items. One major change is the addition of Item 9: "The strengths and limitations of the body of evidence are clearly described" (AGREE Next Steps Consortium, 2009, p. 2). The last change is that the new AGREE II tool includes a newly restructured user's manual. The manual is part of the complete agree tool document and includes information and guidance for completing each of the items. The remainder of this chapter focuses on practical hints for using this amazing new tool.

PRACTICAL HINTS

First, go to the AGREE Trust website, www.agreetrust.org. Next, create a User ID and your own confidential password by clicking on "Register here" (Figure 11.2). There is no charge for this (that in itself is amazing in this day and age!). Next, download the AGREE II PDF (Figure 11.3). Before reading the AGREE II Users' Manual, you may want to familiarize yourself with the tool by viewing the AGREE II Overview Tutorial, an avatar-guided tutorial that takes approximately 10 minutes to complete.

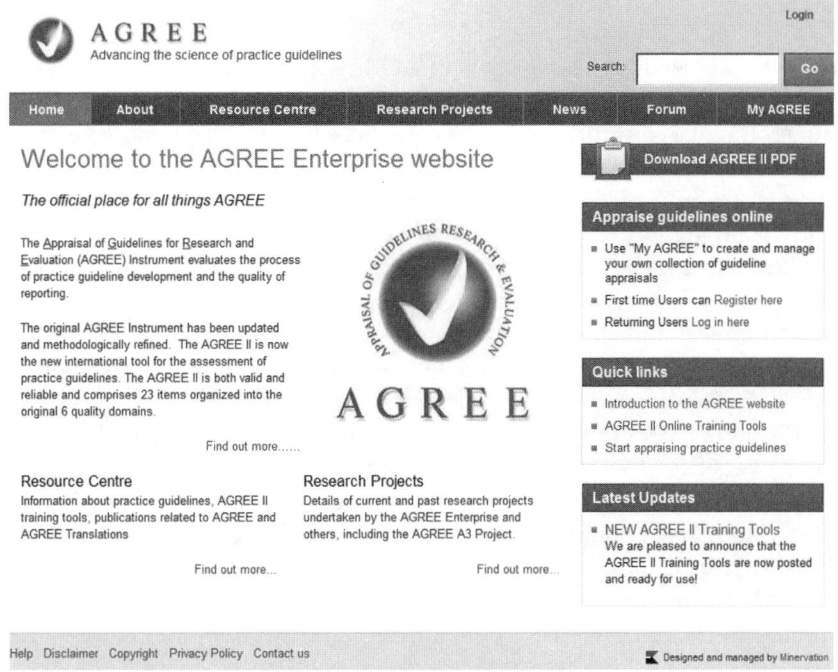

FIGURE 11.2 AGREE II home page.

AGREE
Advancing the science of practice guidelines
Search:
Go
Home
About
Resource Centre
Research Projects
News
Forum
My AGREE
AGREE Enterprise website > Resource Centre > Training > Introduction
AGREE II Training Tools
AGREE II Translations
AGREE-related publications
Practice Guidelines
AGREE II
The Original AGREE Instrument
AGREE II Training Tools
The AGREE A3 Research Team has developed two training tools to assist AGREE II users to effectively apply the tool. The tools are currently being evaluated in a randomized research study.
AGREE Publications
Browse our library of publications related to AGREE
Download AGREE II
Download the latest AGREE tool as a PDF
AGREE II Overview Tutorial
Launch the tutorial
This tool provides an Avatar-guided overview of the AGREE II tool. This tool takes approximately 10 minutes to complete.
It will open in a new browser tab when you click the link.
AGREE II Practice Exercise
Launch the exercise
Expanding upon the Avatar-guided tutorial, the "Practice Exercise" tool provides trainees with the opportunity to appraise a test practice guideline with the AGREE II; upon submitting their ratings, the training tool system provides immediate feedback to how the trainees responses compares with those of expert ratings.

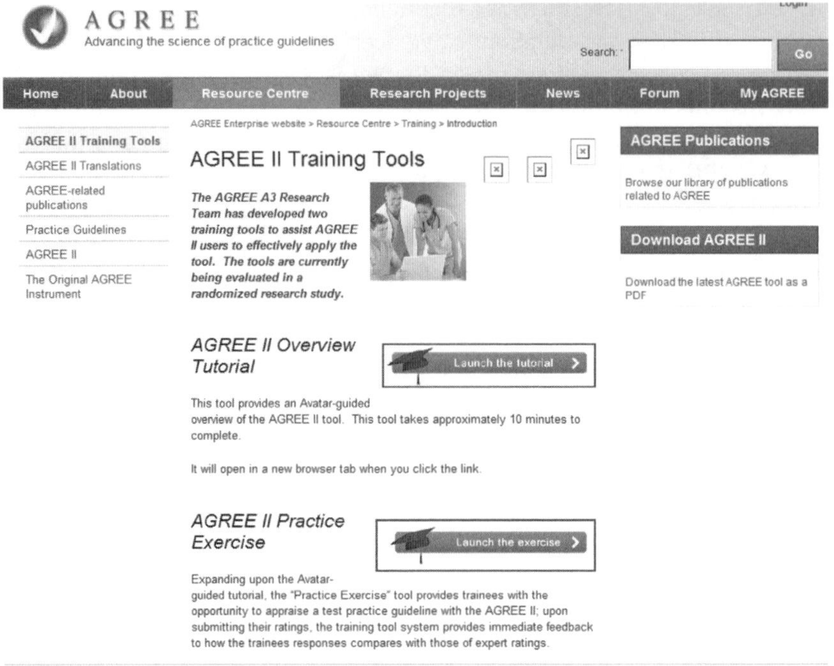

FIGURE 11.3 AGREE II training tools.

The tutorial provides an overview of AGREE II and how to use it. To view the tutorial, click on "AGREE II online Training Tools" (Figure 11.2) and launch the above tutorial. This tutorial is one of two training tools that help users apply the AGREE II to the evaluation of CPGs.

Once you have digested the process by viewing the tutorial and reading about the tool and how to use it, go to the second tool, the "AGREE II Practice Exercise" (Figure 11.2). This new development allows you to rate a sample practice guideline that experts have reviewed and appraised and then compare your score with theirs, a totally online experience. Two of the authors have used the evaluation of CPGs using the AGREE instruments for workshops at the Visiting Nurse Service of New York (VNSNY) and in classes with graduate students at several different universities. The most successful approach is for each participant to have a computer and rate the practice guideline during the workshop or class. (Students and clinical nurses alike were asked to read the guideline that was to be evaluated prior to the workshop or class.) After participants complete the exercise, we discuss only those items for which participants differed by more than 1 or 2 points from the experts' opinions. We have received very positive feedback on this process to evaluate CPGs from both students and clinical nurses.

Important to note is that not every guideline you may be interested in appraising has experts who have already weighed in on it. But, once you have practiced with the guideline that is on the website, you are ready to venture into your own appraisals with your students and colleagues. This website also allows for more than one person to appraise the same guidelines, save your ratings, and then display all appraisal scores. This will be very helpful to teaching a class of students or group of nurse colleagues, followed by a discussion of areas of agreement and discrepancy, and then "agree" (pun intended) on the recommendations that would be made for using any of the appraised guideline recommendations for clinical practice that you want.

REFERENCES

AGREE Collaboration. (2001). *Appraisal of guidelines for research & evaluation (AGREE) instrument*. Retrieved September, from http://www. agreecollaboration.org

AGREE Next Steps Consortium. (2009). *Appraisal of guidelines for research & evaluation II*. Ontario, CA: The AGREE Research Trust.

Levin, R. F., & Vetter, M. (2007). Evidence-based practice: A guide to negotiate the clinical practice guideline maze. *Research and Theory for Nursing Practice, 21*(1), 5–9.

Levin, R. F., & Ferrara, L. (2011). Using the appraisal of guidelines for research and evaluation II to assess clinical practice guidelines. *Research and Theory for Nursing Practice: An International Journal, 25*(3), 16–162.

Rich, E. R., & Newland, J. A. (2006). Creating clinical protocols with an APGAR of 10. In R. F. Levin & H. R. Feldman (Eds.), *Teaching evidence-based practice in nursing: A guide for academic and clinical settings* (pp. 121–132). New York: Springer Publishing.

12

Teaching Evidence-Based Practice Statistics

Priscilla Sandford Worral

Statistical thinking will one day be as necessary for efficient citizenship as the ability to read and write.

—H. G. Wells, 1866–1946, British novelist, teacher, historian, journalist

Few terms in academia or science within the health care environment evoke a stronger emotional response than does the term "statistics." How many students face their statistics courses with trepidation, focused not on mastering the content, but rather on simply surviving the course with a passing grade? How many clinicians who read their professional journals limit their attention to the abstract and conclusions, skipping over anything that relates to discussion of statistical procedures or results of data analysis? Today, most health profession students and clinicians are aware of the importance of basing practice decisions on current best research evidence. A clinician's ability to make the best evidence-based decisions relies in part upon that clinician's ability to identify and critically appraise relevant research. When relevant research includes quantitative studies, critical appraisal of that research requires the ability to understand and accurately interpret results of statistical analysis.

A BRIEF BACKGROUND: LITERATURE ON TEACHING STATISTICS

Epstein, Santa Mina, Gaudet, Singh, and Gula (2011) recently published an integrative review of international nursing literature from 1980 to 2010 to identify best practices for teaching statistics to undergraduate nursing students. Among the 12 studies that met their inclusion criteria for review, only two were reports of research. Both were described by reviewers (Epstein et al., 2011) as informative, but of low quality. The remaining

10 articles were anecdotal reports in which instructors shared their experiences in the classroom. The reviewers conclude that research on the pedagogy of teaching statistics to nurses is needed and suggest that nurse educators look to nonnursing statistics literature to guide research efforts as well as to inform their teaching.

In light of the importance of nurses understanding how to interpret statistics for evidence-based practice (EBP), it is worth noting that studies reviewed by Epstein and colleagues (2011) addressed two aspects of teaching statistics that might be considered to be indirectly related to EBP: the importance of sequencing the statistics (students further along in their program achieved better course grades), and the benefit of teaching statistics and research concurrently together rather than separately (students achieved better grades). While no claim of cause-and-effect can be made from any of the articles and studies reviewed, it is interesting to note that students who were more successful in their statistics courses were those who also were more likely to have had extensive time in the clinical setting and who learned statistics within the context of other aspects of the research process.

As is the case in nursing, much of the literature specifically focused on teaching statistics to undergraduate medical students also can be described as informative, but nonexperimental (Bland, 2004; Freeman, Collier, Staniforth, & Smith, 2008; Jacobson, 2007; Miles, Price, Swift, Shepstone, & Leinster, 2010; Morris, 2002). Consistent across these articles was the focus on the need to teach statistics in a way that would help students to relate what they were learning to their clinical practice. Miles and colleagues surveyed physicians who had graduated from the same medical school and were now practicing in the United Kingdom to learn how these physicians viewed their statistics training and whether they thought what they had learned was useful in daily practice. The 130 (29% response rate) who provided feedback noted that they had not recognized the value of statistics during training, but had since found statistical knowledge relevant in their work. A frequent suggestion from respondents was to focus training on integrating statistics with clinical practice.

Rao and Kanter (2010) conducted a review of literature published from 1999 to 2009 that described how evidence-based medicine is taught to medical students. They, too, concluded that statistics need to be taught so that physicians can accurately interpret research results. Based on his own experiences with medical students at the Mayo Clinic, Jacobson (2007) suggests that students be taught how to read studies, extract relevant empirical findings such as means and standard deviations, actually calculate effect sizes and other statistics used in treating patients, and then apply these statistics in the clinical setting. Similarly, Welk (2007) suggests teaching statistics to nursing students by using scenarios that enable the student to personally calculate relevant statistics—an example would be an effect size—and to do so in a small group setting so students could learn from one another.

This brief background from the literature is not intended to be comprehensive, but to give you some idea of the context within which the remainder of this chapter is written. No meta-analyses of randomized control trials or clinical practice guidelines based even on quasi-experimental studies could be found upon which to base strategies for teaching statistics. What the literature does provide is a wealth of experiential data blended with results from surveys and a few interventional comparative and before-and-after studies. In a similar fashion, findings and suggestions from relevant articles will be included in the five strategies to be presented here; however, most of what will be described in suggesting these strategies will be based upon my own experience as both a hospital-based nurse–scientist and adjunct faculty member at a number of institutions throughout my career. I have had the pleasure of teaching statistics to undergraduate, master's, and doctoral nursing students—and a few medical and graduate studies students—for more than 20 years. I do not know who first coined the phrase "the best way to learn something is to teach it," but I certainly have found that to be true.

The intent of this chapter is to encourage those of you who teach statistics in health care to feel more comfortable and confident in the experience, whether you are facing a class of students before you, your peers, and colleagues around you, or yourself in the mirror. The following strategies are focused on teaching students and colleagues who need to know how to interpret statistics in their critical appraisal of research as a basis for making EBP decisions. As you will notice, these strategies are neither mutually exclusive nor exhaustive, but are intended to complement one another.

STRATEGY #1: BE POSITIVE

However you landed in the position of teacher, instructor, or coach, here you are. Your positive attitude—both toward the usefulness of statistics and toward the ability of your students or colleagues to learn statistics—is perhaps the single most important ingredient in successfully imparting sustainable knowledge of statistics to the learner. The first time you mention statistics to students or colleagues, make your introduction positive and involve the learner. For example, you might begin by asking for a show of hands in response to the question, "How many of you skip over the statistics—especially the tables—when you read a study?" You are likely to see raised hands from the majority of learners. Regardless of whether 5% or 95% of those present raise their hands, assure them that they all have the ability to learn how to use statistics correctly to improve patient care.

One very simple, time-efficient method for demonstrating your positive attitude to students is to use a combined form of scripting and use of analogies. Start with your favorite phrase to encourage your family, friends, or yourself, such as "You/I can do this!," and develop the habit of using that phrase in every class or session. Over time, learners will connect that phrase with course content. If you are not teaching an entire statistics course, but rather one in-service or continuing education session, use your favorite encouragement phrase with an analogy added to give more emphasis as a substitute for repetition. For example, if you are presenting a session on how to read a Forest plot to a group of ICU nurses, you might use the analogy of the number of mini-bags hanging from IV poles and attached the pump. If those nurses can handle what looks like an over-decorated Christmas tree of IV medications one of which is a vasopressor, they certainly can handle the point estimates, confidence intervals, and line of no effect shown in a Forest plot! Among the hundreds of students, clinical staff, and other colleagues with whom I have worked over the past two decades, almost all have improved their ability to understand and use statistics, not because of their instructor, but because they met their own positive expectations.

STRATEGY #2: BE LEARNER-FOCUSED

Teach From the Familiar to the Foreign

If a positive attitude of the teacher is the most important ingredient in successfully teaching statistics, maintaining a learner-focus is a close second. The example given above of the analogy of hanging mini-bags with point-estimates and confidence intervals is one example of being learner-focused. If you were introducing Forest plots to a group of nursing unit managers, you might use the analogy of a master staffing schedule. Just as the ICU nurse is titrating and flushing multiple medications, the unit manager is weaving multiple individual schedules, each with time requests, into an overall plan that one hopes will cover every shift for every day for the period of that schedule. If all shifts are covered, each individual schedule is a positive addition to that coverage. Each example connects statistical terms and concepts with terms and concepts already understood by the learner. These examples also demonstrate how the strategies addressed in this chapter complement one another. Teaching from a learner-focused perspective includes using examples that are relevant to the learner as well as teaching from the familiar (e.g., multiple mini-bags of IV medication) to the foreign (e.g., point estimates and confidence intervals). Teaching statistics within a context that is relevant to the learner is a strategy to be discussed later in this chapter.

Use Multiple Strategies to Address Multiple Learning Styles

Teaching with a focus on the learner means using a variety of teaching strategies and types of media to meet the needs of learning styles of students and colleagues. Sredl (2006) conducted a one-group pretest/posttest study testing an intervention that incorporated visual, auditory, and kinesthetic learning styles into a technique for teaching medication calculations to pediatric nurses. Results demonstrated that use of multiple strategies incorporating all three learning styles improved students' accuracy of mathematical problem solving. Markowitz and DuPré (2007) found that graduate biomedical science students positively evaluated coursework that incorporated the importance of learning styles in developing methods they might use themselves in teaching others.

Most adult learners are able to use more than one learning style with relative ease, however, understanding and retention of new information is likely to be most successful if learning activities include a preferred style. In the simplest sense, this means that you do include some lecture to introduce new information to auditory learners, do include PowerPoint slides for visual learners, and do use worksheets that can be completed manually by kinesthetic learners. For online learning, do use voice-over discussion of slides and provide the opportunity for open-text responses to questions that are integrated into completion of course content. One online resource for learning statistics that is especially geared for kinesthetic as well as for visual learners is Seeing Statistics (McClelland, 1999) at http://www.seeingstatistics.com). This program uses graphs and animation to visually display how variation in numbers entered into a statistical procedure by the learner affect such calculated statistics as Pearson's *r* correlations.

Use of more than one textbook is another strategy to meet learners' diverse styles and needs. Most statistics courses have a required textbook. By all means, use the required text as a method for supporting consistent content throughout the course; just do not limit yourself to only the definitions and descriptions used in that one textbook. If you are teaching a graduate course that has completion of an undergraduate course in statistics as a pre-requisite, invite students to use their undergraduate text to review basic content if that text was helpful to them. Journal articles on statistics are another additional source of content. Even the most experienced and expert statistics instructor, no matter how talented, is unlikely to teach statistics in a way that fits the preferred learning style of every student. A few examples of articles that might be helpful are included in a Resources section at the end of this chapter.

Related to the subject of textbooks is the subject of how many pages students are assigned and how many they are likely to read. What I have suggested to students in past graduate research and EBP courses is that they focus on what they need to learn rather than on how many pages they are reading. Their weekly assignments include topics with suggested texts, journal articles, occasional worksheets, and/or Internet sites to review to help them to learn.

One strategy I consistently have found to be successful in motivating students to review undergraduate statistics in preparation for critical appraisal of research at the graduate level is to offer an online multiple choice, matching, and short-answer test that they can practice as many times as they wish for 3 to 4 weeks prior to taking essentially the same test as an in-class closed-book exam. Students have the option to submit their test answers for feedback each week during the pre-exam period. I do not directly provide the correct answer, but offer suggestions for consideration and reading. The in-class exam does have the items and optional responses reordered from the pre-test, some variation in wording, and additional short answer bonus questions to enable the student to earn additional points beyond 100. Students may use those points to improve any other graded assignment in the course. The exam itself is worth 10% of the course grade. An example of variation in wording would be to ask on the pre-test which of four responses describes nominal level of measurement, and to ask on the in-class exam which of four responses describes interval level of measurement.

Just as individuals vary in their preferred style or combination of styles for learning, learners vary in the method of evaluation most likely to demonstrate their acquisition of knowledge. While my experience has been to work with graduate students and clinicians who prefer papers to tests, some students are more comfortable with and successful on tests. For those students, the pre-test followed by the in-class exam is an opportunity to demonstrate knowledge acquisition using a preferred method of evaluation.

Offer Mathematical Detail for Those Who Prefer It

Some learners will continue to ask questions of their instructor until they are able to understand new information at the "cellular level." A clinical example of this is the nurse who wants to know how the active ingredient in a medication is transported across the cell membrane. A statistical example is the nurse who wants to know exactly how a beta weight is calculated so one can better understand how to interpret that statistic in terms of relative influence of one factor versus another on an outcome. The point here is that not all learners will be overwhelmed by inclusion of mathematical principles and statistical formulae. Creating supplemental handouts and suggestions of additional resources should be a routine plan when you are preparing to teach statistics.

If you as the teacher are hesitant to provide additional detail about the mathematics underlying statistics, by all means find a consulting statistician or colleague who enjoys statistics rather than decide that learners do not need that level or type of detail.

STRATEGY #3: BE RELEVANT

Integrating Statistics, Research, and Practice

Even the most cursory review of the literature will reveal articles speaking to the importance of integrating statistics and research with practice. While integration can be operationalized as including a statistician and researcher as co-course instructors, the focus in this chapter is on integrating course content.

A well-worded research hypothesis and knowledge of how each variable is operationalized essentially dictates the appropriate statistical procedure(s) for testing the related null hypothesis. During preparation for teaching course content, find current studies that can serve as accurate examples of use of each statistic you plan to cover. After your introductory description of the statistical procedure, invite students to find that procedure in the article and describe in their own words how the statistic is used. If students are completing an EBP paper or project as part of their coursework, ask them to share studies they are including in their project that also include use of the statistical procedure under discussion. If the students' articles exemplify an incorrect use of the statistic, ask the students whether they can identify any differences in how the statistical procedure is used in their article versus use of the statistic in the article you have assigned. One common misuse of statistics can be found when investigators choose to conduct multiple *t*-tests rather than analysis of variance to test the effect of an intervention on three or more comparison groups.

If you are teaching statistics to practicing clinicians, by all means use studies on topics of interest to them as examples of statistical procedures you want them to learn. If you are teaching statistics to students with little or no practice experience, use studies on topics that are being covered in their other courses. Promise yourself enough time to update the articles you use every time you teach a course, continuing education program, or class on statistics. Remaining current will keep your course current, keep both you and the students engaged, plus will keep you on top of the statistics currently found in the literature. Statistics is a young science, with advances in computer technology geometrically increasing the potential for conduct of statistical procedures that can account for multiple differences in characteristics of study subjects as well as accounting for multiple outcomes of interest.

Statistical Significance Versus Clinical Relevance

Statistical significance and clinical relevance are not synonymous with one another. Clinical relevance of an intervention to affect a desired outcome may be important in practice even if it does not reach statistical significance from a research perspective. This is an especially important distinction when one or more studies testing the effectiveness of an intervention report(s) nonsignificant results. Clinicians still have to provide care and patients cannot wait for an adequate number of studies to be conducted before they receive that care. An important point to be made when results are determined to be clinically relevant, but not statistically significant is that any practice decisions must be made with caution. The fewer the studies supporting a practice decision and/or the less statistically significant the results are, the more carefully patients must be monitored in case outcomes are different from those expected.

The warning "don't throw the baby out with the bath water" can be applied to teaching statistics. In other words, do not discount statistical significance in your effort to promote the importance of research findings as possibly clinically relevant, even if statistically significant differences or relationships are not demonstrated. Instead, have students discuss why results of a study were not statistically significant. Using small groups for this discussion is one excellent method for giving learners the opportunity to integrate their understanding of statistics with what they have learned about other steps in the research process.

Most textbooks include PowerPoint presentations and other teaching aids to support content presented in a lecture format. If you teach statistics in an academic setting, use your own examples to supplement teaching aids provided. As noted earlier, if you teach in a clinical setting, use examples that are relevant to your colleagues. Statistics are likely to be most easily understood if they are discussed within the context of a currently meaningful clinical situation.

If you are in the position of teaching content with which you have had no hands-on or clinical experience, invite your students to provide examples of situations in which statistics are used. Giving students the opportunity to provide examples that you then use to teach content is likely to require you to think on your feet. The advantages are that the students will be more involved in their learning and are more likely to engage in discussion with one another as well as with you as the instructor. Remember, however, to be prepared with an article that correctly uses the statistical procedure(s) under discussion in the event that your students have an article that incorrectly or incompletely discusses data analysis. If ever you are in doubt about whether an article is accurate or inaccurate, never doubt the benefit of having colleagues. One comment I invariably make, especially to my graduate students, is that they do not have to be statisticians, but they should make every effort to know one.

STRATEGY #4: STRESS ACCURACY IN MEASUREMENT AND STATISTICS

Statistics is the grammar of science.

—Karl Pearson, 1857–1936, father of mathematical statistics

Being "user-friendly" does not mean "dummy-down." The literature is consistent in describing knowledge of statistics as important for health care professionals to accurately understand and interpret research results in making EBP decisions (Jacobson, 2007; Morris, 2002; Pursell & While, 2010; Rao & Kanter, 2010). Just how an accurate understanding of statistics is to be accomplished, however, is approached in the literature from a variety of perspectives, some of them in direct opposition to one another. Rao and Kanter argue that statistics should be taught independently from discussion of critical appraisal to ensure accurate and comprehensive understanding among undergraduate medical students. In contrast, Morris argues that integrating statistics into teaching critical appraisal is "the best opportunity yet for teaching medical statistics" (2002, p. 969). From yet another perspective, Pursell and While argue that undergraduate health care students should not be taught probability statistics at all because they are too likely to misunderstand and misinterpret the results of analysis.

The language of statistics is a precise language, but precision does not mean indecipherable. Perhaps the greatest challenge in teaching the language of statistics correctly is when you as the instructor are confronted with a publication in which terms are used incorrectly.

Define what statistics are, what they are not, and why they are important. Simply defined, a statistic is "a numerical value obtained from a sample" (Burns & Grove, 2011, p. 447). Polit and Beck (2012) define a statistic as "an estimate of a parameter, calculated from sample data" (p. 743). While not identical, these definitions are consistent with one another. Both definitions are beneficial because they each provide an introduction to one of the two major uses of statistics: description and inference. Limiting students to only one definition raises the risk of confusion once students move from defining the term to actually using statistics in the clinical setting. That said, if you are teaching statistics to clinicians in a nonacademic setting, do not assume that first defining the term is unnecessary. Learning what statistics are provides a logical segue to what statistics—especially inferential statistics—are not. An inferential statistic that by definition is an estimate means that an inferential statistic is not "truth."

Descriptive statistics such as percentage, median, and mean are important because they organize numbers (data) from a sample into information that can be used to describe that sample. Descriptive statistics use data from a sample to which the data collector has direct access. If you are teaching statistics to students or colleagues who have not already completed a statistics course, start with descriptive statistics so students can identify a sample of interest to them, collect data from that sample, and use data they actually have collected to calculate percentages, medians, means, and so forth. Those who learn best by having concrete examples will be especially grateful, but even those students who are comfortable in an abstract world may find inferential statistics easier to understand if they begin by learning descriptive statistics. Why? The answer lies in the definition of statistics as an "estimate of a parameter" (Polit & Beck, 2012, p. 743).

Inferential statistics such as confidence interval or alpha as a level of significance are important because, if appropriately used, they provide an estimate of results for a population in which you are interested based upon results from a sample to which you or another data collector has access. Inferential statistics are estimates of how effective an intervention might be for people not actually included in a study but who are similar to those who were. Teaching inferential statistics begins with teaching students that these are estimates of what outcomes of an intervention might be and reminding them that "might be" and "will be" are not necessarily synonymous terms.

Because clinically relevant results should not be discounted, this does not mean that statistical significance is consequently not important. Knowing how patients might respond to an intervention is certainly important. Rarely if ever does a researcher have the resources necessary to test the effectiveness of an intervention on every person in every location now and in the future who might benefit from that intervention. The importance of statistical significance—the likelihood that study results will be replicated in a similar situation—cannot and should not be discounted. Nonsignificant study findings can be the result of many weaknesses in study design, sample selection, study conduct, and/or instrumentation. When study findings are statistically significant, rather than discounting the findings as more mathematical than clinical, give examples of how these results still have value.

Teach semantics and principles from a consumer perspective. A majority of clinicians are consumers of statistics who need to know what a Pearson correlation coefficient or a beta weight tells them, but do not need to know how to calculate one.

STRATEGY #5: BE PERSISTENT AND PATIENT

As noted at the beginning of this chapter, your positive attitude toward statistics and toward the learners' ability to better understand and correctly use statistics is of critical importance. Equally important are your persistence and patience in maintaining the expectation that the learner can and will master the essentials of course or class content. Peter Safar, acknowledged as the "father of CPR," coined one of my favorite phrases: "Patience is a virtue, but persistence to the point of success is a blessing." This phrase is useful both for you and for your students during and even after they have completed their statistics course or program. Many students may tell you at the end of a course that they still are not certain that they understand statistics, that they need more class time learning them. Assure students that if they are willing to be patient and persistent they will discover that statistics are no longer a foreign language. If students actually read the data analysis section of articles now that no course grade is attached to how correctly they interpret what they are reading, they might be surprised at how much they have learned. Perhaps most reassuring is the fact that a health professional does not need to become a statistician or commit to memory the many statistical procedures one will encounter in the literature. Several excellent resources exist online for clinicians to use when they critically appraise research (see Box 12.1).

BOX 12.1 ONLINE STATISTICS RESOURCES

Cochrane open learning material, includes descriptions of statistics relevant to systematic reviews: http://www.cochrane-net.org/openlearning/index.htm

Statistics software program analogous to SPSS or SAS, but open access: http://www.gnu.org/software/pspp/get.html

Studying a Study online, includes tutorials for all aspects of appraisal including statistics: http://www.studyingastudy.com/ss_main.html

Thanks to Jeanne Grace, PhD, RN, C, University of Rochester, for creating these fables as a way to teach students about research and

(*continued*)

BOX 12.1 (*continued*)

statistics: http://www.son.rochester.edu/student-esources/research-fables/index.html

Seeing Statistics is an excellent web-based learning site for students to learn about statistics by interacting with the content: http://www.seeingstatistics.com

Similar to other basic statistics software programs, StatTools is an open access tutorial with useful statistics tools: http://www.stattools.net

SUMMARY

Despite the emotional aversion to statistics experienced by many, today's health care professionals must be able to critically appraise and appropriately use statistics if they are to make practice decisions based upon current best evidence. Whether you are a health care professional who is teaching statistics to others or teaching them to yourself, this chapter provides both evidence-based and experientially based strategies for helping you to make learning statistics successful and positive—perhaps even enjoyable!

Remember to be *positive,* because you *can* master this content! Be *learner-focused,* by using familiar concepts and learner-preferred styles to exemplify and teach statistical procedures. Be *relevant* by using articles that address current clinical situations important to learners and reminding students, colleagues, and yourself that both statistical significance and clinical relevance are important in providing quality care to patients. Stress *accuracy* in use of statistics by defining terms, using concrete examples of use of statistics, and reminding fellow learners that patients are depending on your ability to interpret results of research to provide the care they need. Finally, be *persistent and patient.* To paraphrase a quote attributed to Margaret Meade: never doubt that those determined to learn statistics can succeed; indeed, they are the only ones who ever have!

REFERENCES

Bland, J. M. (2004). Teaching statistics to medical students using problem-based learning: The australian experience. *BMC Medical Education,* 4(31), DOI: 10.1186/1472-6920-4-31.

Burns, N., & Grove, S. K. (2011). *The practice of nursing research: Conduct, critique, and utilization* (6th ed.). St. Louis, MO: Elsevier Saunders.

Epstein, I., Santa Mina, E. E., Gaudet, J., Singh, M. D., & Gula, T. (2011). Teaching statistics to undergraduate nursing students: An integrative review to inform our pedagogy. *International Journal of Nursing Scholarship, 8*(1), DOI: 10.2202/1548-923X.2234.

Freeman, J. V., Collier, S., Staniforth, D., & Smith, K. J. (2008). Innovations in curriculum design: A multi-disciplinary approach to teaching statistics to undergraduate medical students. *BMC Medical Education, 8*(28), DOI: 10.1186/1472-6920-8-28.

Jacobson, R. M. (2007). Teach medical students evidence-based practice statistics—to calculate them and immediately apply ro their patients. *Minnesota Medicine, 90*(11), 37–38, 46.

Markowitz, D. G., & DuPré, M. J. (2007). Graduate experience in science education: The development of science education course for biomedical science graduate students. *CBE—Life Sciences Education, 6*, 233–242.

McClelland, G. (1999). *Seeing statistics*. Retrieved from Duxbury Press website: http://www.seeingstatistics.com

Miles, S., Price, G. M., Swift, L., Shepstone, L., & Leinster, S. J. (2010). Statistics teaching in medical school: Opinions of practising doctors. *BMC Medical Education, 10*(75), DOI: 1472-6920/10/75.

Morris, R. W. (2002). Does EBM offer the best opportunity yet for teaching medical statistics? *Statistics In Medicine, 21*, 969–977.

Polit, D. F., & Beck, C. T. (2012). *Nursing research: Generating and Assessing Evidence For Nursing Practice* (9th ed.). Philadelphia: Wolters Kluwer.

Purssell, E., & While, A. (2010). P = nothing, or why we should not teach healthcare students about statistics. *Nurse Education Today*, DOI: 10.1016/j.nedt.2010.11.017

Rao, G., & Kanter, S. L. (2010). Physician numeracy as the basis for an evidence-based medicine curriculum. *Academic Medicine, 85*(11), 1794–1799.

Sredl, D. (2006). The triangle technique: A new evidence-based educational tool for pediatric medication calculations. *Nursing Education Perspectives* March/April 21(2), 84–88.

Welk, D. S. (2007). How to read, interpret, and understand evidence-based literature statistics. *Nurse Educator, 32*(1), 16–20.

RESOURCES

Frick, K. D., Milligan, R. A., & Pugh, L. C. (2011). Calculating and interpreting the odds ratio. *American Nurse Today, 6*(3), 24–25.

Hedges, C., & Bliss-Holtz, J. (2006). Not too big, not too small, but just right: The dilemma of sample size estimation. *AACN Advanced Critical Care, 17*(3), 341–344.

McHugh, M. L. (2007). Clinical statistics for primary care practitioners: Part I—incidence, prevalence, and the odds ratio. *Journal for Specialists in Pediatric Nursing, 12*(1), 56–60.

McHugh, M. L. (2008). Clinical statistics for primary care practitioners: Part II—absolute risk reduction, relative risk, relative risk reduction, and number needed to treat. *Journal for Specialists in Pediatric Nursing, 13*(2), 135–138.

13

Teaching Treatment Effectiveness Formulas

Rona F. Levin

To understand God's thoughts, we must study statistics, for these are the measure of His purpose.

—Florence Nightingale

This chapter is largely a reproduction of articles published in the *World Council of Enterostomal Therapists Journal*. The intent of the original articles was to provide a "user-friendly" description of statistical approaches that are applied in clinical research to determine the effectiveness of interventions. I realize that many of the readers may not be familiar with some of the concepts and statistical approaches to the data analysis techniques that authors use to present their results. In meta-analyses of clinical studies that look at treatment effectiveness, you will see summary statistics, such as weighted mean, odds ratios, relative risk (RR), relative risk reduction (RRR), absolute risk (AR), and number needed to treat (NNT). To be an intelligent consumer of evidence presented in meta-analyses, you need to be able to have a good understanding of these concepts and formulas. The first part of the chapter defines types of outcome variables and presents definitions and formulas for RR and RRR.

WHAT DO CLINICAL EFFECTIVENESS FORMULAS MEAN? PART I

Dichotomous and Continuous Variables

It is important to initially distinguish between dichotomous and continuous outcome variables. This is important because the type of variable under analysis determines the appropriate statistical approach. A dichotomous variable can be divided into two aspects, for example, a good outcome or bad outcome. In other words, the choice of either one or the other outcome is possible; there is no middle ground. Since a dichotomous variable either is or is not that situation, use of a statistical average is meaningless. In clinical wound studies you might consider healing within 3 months a "good" outcome and not healing within 3 months as a "bad" outcome. You are not measuring the time to healing as 3 months, so you cannot average 3 months; instead you are measuring good healing as occurring by 3 months and bad healing as not occurring by 3 months. Therefore, in this study there is no other outcome option that you are measuring, as there is no average between good or bad. These are two distinct outcomes.

Unlike a dichotomous variable, a continuous variable is not an either or situation, or as we say in research language, "discrete." There are lots of points between the variable that can be measured, hence the name continuous. A continuous outcome variable is one for which you can derive an average or mean. For example, the measurement of a wound area in centimeters is a continuous variable. For this type of variable you do not compare a "good" versus "bad" outcome, but the exact difference in the change in the size of wounds receiving an experimental treatment to those treated with standard care.

Appropriate Statistical Tests

Once you can identify the type of outcome variable being studied, you can then determine if the appropriate statistical tests are being used. For continuous variables, a weighted mean is often the summary statistic of choice. Relative and absolute risk or odds ratios are the most common summary statistics used in meta-analyses when dichotomous outcome variables are being evaluated. Number needed to treat, used not as frequently, is also an important concept for making clinical practice decisions.

Relative and Absolute Risk

In order to calculate and interpret relative and absolute risk, we need to begin with two other fundamental concepts, experimental event rate (EER) and control event rate (CER). EER is the percent of patients in the experimental group who have an outcome occur. Remember the dichotomous variable example of wound healing above; using EER we could determine the rate of wound healing in 3 months. The CER is the percentage of patients who were in the placebo or control group (not healing within 3 months) and had that same outcome. Both of these numbers need to be calculated before we can determine risk (Exhibit 13.1).

Once we have these numbers we can determine risk ratios. RR is the relative chance of experiencing a bad outcome due to the experimental treatment. RRR is the proportional reduction in rates of bad outcomes between experimental and control groups (Exhibit 13.2).

EXHIBIT 13.1 CALCULATION OF EER AND CER WITH A HYPOTHETICAL EXAMPLE

Hypothetical Calculation of EER and CTR

Let us say in a research study there were a total of 1,383 persons who were treated with a new dressing. You wanted to see how many people who used this dressing had their wound heal in 3 months. At the end of your study, 172 persons had their wounds heal in 3 months.

- EER = number of persons in treatment group who had a wound healing with a particular dressing within 3 months = 172/ 1383 = .125 (12.5′X)*
- CER = number of persons in control group (standard care) with a wound healing with a particular dressing within 3 months = 176/ 1383 = .127 (12.7%)**

The EER* and CER** as calculated here will be used to calculate relative risk (RR)*** and relative risk reduction (RRR) as illustrated in Exhibit 13.2.

EXHIBIT 13.2 CALCULATION OF RR AND RRR WITH A HYPOTHETICAL EXAMPLE

- Relative risk (RR)
  The formula for calculating relative risk (RR) is to divide experimental event rate (EER) by control event rate (CER).

  Formula: RR = EER/CER.98*** = 12.5%*/12.7%**

  * Remember this number was calculated in Exhibit 13.1.
  **Remember this number was calculated in Exhibit 13.1.
  Now we can use the relative risk (RR)*** as calculated above to calculate the relative risk reduction (RRR) as seen below:
- Relative risk reduction

The formula for calculating relative risk reduction (RRR) is the number one minus the relative risk (RR)***.

Formula:	RRR = 1	1
	Relative risk	−.98***
	RRR = .02	.02

***Remember this number for relative risk was calculated above by dividing experimental event rate (EER) by CER percent of people in control group.

Now what do the numbers tell us? In statistical language, they tell us that the reduction in risk of having a wound heal within 3 months is .02%. Of course we need to look at the fact that a reduction in risk in the case of a desired positive outcome simply means the difference in effect between the experimental and control group. We are not looking at a bad versus a good outcome, but simply wishing to determine if there is a difference in wound healing between the two groups. Looking also at the EEE (12.5%) and the CER (12.7%), you can see that there is barely a difference between these groups.

Thus the appropriate conclusion in our hypothetical example is that the experimental intervention, a particular new dressing, did not have a clinically significant effect on wound healing.

PART II

The second part of this discussion focuses on the definitions and formulas for absolute risk (AR), absolute risk reduction (ARR), and number needed to treat (NNT). I include hypothetical scenarios to exemplify the use of these approaches to data analysis and build upon the previous discussion.

You may remember that relative risk (RR) gives us an indication of the relative chance of experiencing a bad outcome in one group versus another group (e.g., experimental versus control group) and that relative risk reduction (RRR) provides information about the proportional decrease in rates of bad outcomes between groups. Exhibit 13.3 provides a review of those formulas. Refer to Part I above if you need to review how they are calculated.

You may also remember that I used an example of wound healing to show how these formulas are applied to clinical practice. In the above example, then, we learn that the RRR is 2% (see Exhibit 13.2) I, meaning that the chance of having a wound heal within 3 months with the new

EXHIBIT 13.3 CALCULATION OF RR AND RRR WITH HYPOTHETICAL DATA

- RR

  Formula: RR = EER/CER = .98 = 12.5%/12.7%

- RRR

  Formula: RRR = 1 − RR = .02 = 1 − .98

treatment is hardly worth considering given such a minimal clinical effect. RRR, however, does not tell the whole story.

Since we are now armed with the above information, why use AR and ARR to further analyze our data? The answer is that RRR fails to discriminate huge absolute treatment effects from those that are trivial. In addition, RRR ignores how rarely or commonly an outcome in question, for example, wound healing or not healing, occurs anyway in patients who may be part of any trial to test a new treatment.

Let us assume, hypothetically, that another new treatment for wound healing has an RRR of 70%. In other words, the new treatment reduced the risk of not healing within 3 months by 70%. Further, let us say that the actual study percentages were 77% in the control group (standard treatment) who did not have a wound heal within 3 months, whereas 23% in the experimental (new treatment group) has this negative outcome. Also, let us say that this difference was statistically significant and that the conclusion reached was that the new treatment was more effective for wound healing. This result could be misleading. Let us see how.

Suppose that the event rates were 10 times less than in the actual study. That is, the 77% is really 7.7% and 23% is really 2.3%. The RRR would still be 77%, despite the difference in numbers, because this formula deals with relative proportions. Thus, this conclusion can be misleading and give an overestimate of treatment effectiveness. Using ARR, which is the absolute difference in experimental versus control rates, you would look at the actual rather than relative rates in the experimental and control groups (Exhibit 13.4). Thus, in this hypothetical trial, the ARR is the risk in the experimental group minus the risk in the control group. If, however, the percentages were 10 times less, 7.7% to 2.3%, then the ARR would be only 5.4%, a vast difference in treatment effectiveness.

Another treatment effectiveness formula in common use is NNT. The NNT is the number of patients we need to treat with the experimental treatment for the duration of the trial to prevent one additional bad outcome (e.g., wound not healing within the specified time frame). The formula

EXHIBIT 13.4 CALCULATION OF ARR IN TWO HYPOTHETICAL EXAMPLES

- ARR 1

  Formula: ARR = CER − EER = 77% − 23% = 54%

- ARR 2

  Formula: ARR = 7.7% − 2.3% = 5.4%

for NNT is 1/ARR. Using the above example, the NNT with the experimental treatment to heal one wound would be 1/ARR = 1/.54 = 1.85. Of course, we cannot speak about 1.85 persons; thus the result is rounded to the nearest whole number. Doing that we see that for every two wounds treated with the experimental intervention, one case of a bad wound outcome would be averted. In other words, we need to treat two people with the experimental intervention for every individual positive outcome achieved. This information is important to consider in deciding whether or not to institute a new treatment. We can also then calculate the cost benefit of adopting the new treatment.

PART III

The first two parts were devoted to the meaning and use of clinical effectiveness formulas (Levin, 2009a, 2009b). Part III covers the meaning and interpretation of odds ratios (OR). As in the previous two parts, I include hypothetical scenarios to exemplify the use of this treatment effectiveness statistic.

You may recall from Part I that variables may be categorized as dichotomous or continuous (Levin, 2009a). When considering treatment outcomes with dichotomous variables, we think of a good versus bad outcome. This is in contrast to using means (averages) to compare two groups on a continuous outcome variable, such as the size of a wound measured in centimeters. With a continuous variable, then, we would measure the amount of reduction in wound size, for example in centimeters. On the other hand, a dichotomous variable in relation to the outcome of an experimental treatment would measure whether or not a wound healed in 3 months (i.e., the good versus the bad outcome).

An OR is a common statistic that is used often in health care studies, particularly in case–control studies or as an effect size in meta-analyses and therefore important for us to understand. The OR is a statistic used to compare the efficacy of a treatment for an exposed group (e.g., experimental treatment) versus an unexposed group (control). For example, an OR of 2:1 might indicate that twice as many wounds were healed in the experimental group versus the control group.

Exhibit 13.5 provides a numerical example of how ORs are calculated. Let us use the hypothetical example of a new innovative treatment for wound healing (maybe ultraviolet light). One outcome measure is wound completely healed in 3 months versus not completely healed in 3 months. We have 100 patients in each of the treatment and control (standard treatment) groups. Of the 100 patients in the treatment group, 25 demonstrate complete wound healing within the 3-month time frame. Of

EXHIBIT 13.5 CALCULATION OF OR IN A HYPOTHETICAL EXAMPLE

Treatment	Control
$N = 100$	$N = 100$
$N_{\text{Successes}} = 25$	$N_{\text{Successes}} = 20$
Probability (success)	Probability (success)
25/100 = .25	20/100 = .20
OR calculation	
1 success **to 3 failures**	**1** success **to 4 failures**
OR = .33	**OR** = .25
Overall OR = .33/.25 = 1.32	

the 100 patients in the control group, 20 demonstrate complete wound healing in the same time frame. This means that we had one success for every three failures in the treatment group and one success for every four failures in the control group. Given the odds of having successful outcomes in the treatment (.33) versus control (.25) groups, we can now calculate the overall OR, which turns out to be 1.32. This means that the treatment is 1.32 times more likely to achieve wound healing than the standard treatment (Barnes & Levin, 2006).

So what does this all mean? Consider that if the OR was 1, or nearly 1 (e.g., .98), that would mean that there is really no difference between the odds of achieving success with the new treatment over the standard treatment. That tells us a great deal. For example, if a new treatment had a wonderful marketing campaign and espoused more successful results than a current or comparative treatment and it was more expensive, yet the research indicates that the chances of successful outcomes are equivalent between the two treatments, why would anyone opt for the new treatment? What do you think?

PART IV

This fourth part discusses means and Cohen's *D* as a measure of treatment effect (Levin, 2009d). The past three parts were about those statistics that are used to determine effect sizes for dichotomous variables (Levin, 2009a, 2009b, 2009c). You may remember from the first column in this series that dichotomous variables are those that can be divided into two aspects or categories; for example, a good or a bad outcome of a treatment. On the other hand, continuous variables are those that can be measured with a tool that has many points on a scale and has equal intervals between those points; for example, temperature measured with a thermometer, or a wound measured in centimeters (Levin, 2009c).

Means

The most common metric used for determining the value of continuous variables is the average or mean score on a measurement tool; that is, average temperature, average blood pressure, or average wound size. A mean may be *standardized* or *unstandardized*. A *standardized* mean is used when the same variable is measured in different ways; for example, in a study where more than one tool is used to measure depression or quality of life. On the other hand, when the same tool or measurement scale is used to measure the effect of a treatment, an *unstandardized mean* is used (Levin, 2009a).

Let us say we want to determine the effect of a new treatment for wounds. The outcome variable in which we are interested is wound healing. One measure of that outcome is wound size determined in centimeters with the same ruler. We decide to measure the wounds of two groups, receiving different treatments, before treatment and after 1 month, to determine if treatment A was more effective than treatment B in healing the wounds. In this example, we would use the same tool or scale to determine in centimeters either the diameter or circumference of the wound. In this case we would use standardized mean of centimeters to measure differences between groups and differences in each group before and after treatment. If we subtract the standardized mean of the control group from the standardized mean of the treatment group, we get the mean difference between groups and for each group from baseline to post-treatment. If this difference results in a number greater than zero, we could say that treatment A was better than treatment B in achieving the desired outcome. If, on the other hand, the difference between the two group means is less than zero, the reverse would be true; that is to say, treatment B is better than treatment A. Of course when there is no difference between the two treatment groups, no difference about the effect of the treatment on the outcome can be inferred (Barnes & Levin, 2006).

Cohen's *D*

Once we determine whether or not there is a difference between groups and that the treatment in which we are interested or the experimental treatment appears better than the control or comparative treatment, we next need to find out the magnitude or strength of that effect. In order to find this, researchers often use Cohen's *D*. The following criteria are often used to guide a discussion of the strength of an effect:

If *d* is less than .50, the strength of the effect is considered weak.

If *d* is .50 but less than .50, the strength of the effect is considered moderate.

If *d* is greater than .50, the strength of the effect is considered strong.

Weighted Mean

One last point is that in a meta-analysis you will often read that a *weighted mean* was used to determine effect size when continuous variables are being studied. A *weighted mean* gives more consideration to the means found in certain studies compared to others in the analysis. The most common reason for weighting is sample size; that is, the results of a study with a larger sample is usually more externally valid or more generalizable beyond the specific sample in the study. Another reason for weighting might be the quality rating that reviewers conducting a meta-analysis give to individual studies (Levin, 2009a). Under any circumstance, the researchers need to indicate why they are using a weighted mean if they do so.

REFERENCES

Barnes, M. J., & Levin, R. F. (2006). Teaching meta-analysis: Summarizing quantitative research. In: R. F. Levin, & H. R. Feldman (Eds.), *Teaching evidence-based practice in nursing: A guide for academic and clinical settings* (Chapter 7, pp. 105–110). Springer.

Levin, R. F. (2009a). Clinical effectiveness formulas: Part I. *World Council of Enterostomal Therapists Journal*, 2010, *29*(3), 25.

Levin, R. F. (2009b). Clinical effectiveness formulas: Part II. *World Council of Enterostomal Therapists Journal*, *29*(4), 38–39.

Levin, R. F. (2009c). Clinical effectiveness formulas: Part lII. *World Council of Enterostomal Therapists Journal*, *30*(1), 34–35.

Levin, R. F. (2009d). Translating research evidence into WCET practice—Appraising a systematic review. *World Council of Enterostomal Therapists Journal*, *30*(2), 39–40.

14

Determining Sensitivity and Specificity of Assessment Tools for Formulating "At Risk" Nursing Diagnoses

Rona F. Levin

All assessment is a perpetual work in progress.

—Linda Suske

Over the years much has been presented and published about ways to study diagnostic validity of the NANDA I nursing diagnoses. A good deal of the validation research has used Fehring's models (1987), which use "expert nurse opinion" to ascertain content and clinical validity of nursing diagnoses. The most recent diagnostic validation studies published in the *International Journal of Nursing Terminologies and Classifications* continue to use Fehring's model as a gold standard for methodology (e.g., Carmona & Baena de Moraes Lopes, 2006; Guirao-Goris & Duarte-Climents, 2007). Yet in many instances we still lack the desired precision (sensitivity and specificity) of assessment tools for gathering the needed information upon which to make accurate nursing diagnoses.

In relation to nursing diagnoses, sensitivity may be defined as the number of clients who are determined, using certain assessment measures, to have a particular diagnosis and who really have that diagnosis. Specificity has to do with those who do not really have the diagnosis and whose assessment parameters indicated that they in fact do not. The evidence-based practice (EBP) medical literature has a good deal to offer us about how to measure these two validity parameters of "diagnostic tests" (assessment tools) in order to increase the validity of the nursing diagnoses we formulate in clinical practice.

The concepts of sensitivity and specificity come from evidence-based epidemiologic frameworks and are the more practical ways to assess the reliability and validity of diagnostic and screening tests than those applied to measuring outcome variables in research. The purpose of this chapter is to demonstrate how to apply the concepts of sensitivity and specificity to the evaluation of assessment tools to formulate nursing diagnoses, specifically "at risk" nursing diagnoses, and how to teach those tools to students and/or health care professionals in practice (see Chapter 16).

BACKGROUND

Traditional assessment methods in nursing have focused on nurses' clinical judgments about the presence or absence of defining characteristics of a nursing diagnosis. Often, no standardized validated assessment tool is used to determine defining characteristics and then formulate an "at risk" diagnosis, for example, "at risk for falls."

As mentioned above, diagnostic validity studies in nursing have used a preponderance of "expert opinion" to determine diagnoses upon which nurses act to reach patient care goals. Varying definitions of experts exist in the nursing diagnosis literature (Levin, 2001). As we all know, "expert opinion" is among the lowest level of evidence for practice. Fehring's models of establishing diagnostic validity were developed in the 1980s and refined in the 1990s (Fehring, 1986, 1987, 1994) prior to the movement toward EBP. Recent studies (Carmona & Baena de Moreas Lopez, 2006; Guirao-Goris & Duarte-Climents, 2007) also use Fehring's work as the gold standard for studies seeking to validate diagnostic criteria.

More recently, an evidence-based approach to determining the sensitivity and specificity of diagnostic tools has been proposed and explained, from a medical diagnosis perspective by Straus and colleagues (2005), and by Gordis (2009), from an epidemiological perspective. These approaches seem much more in keeping with an evidence-based approach to diagnostic assessment for both medical and nursing practice.

CHOOSING THE BEST ASSESSMENT TOOL

In choosing the best assessment tool to inform practice we need to consider several factors: validity—including sensitivity, specificity, positive predictive value, and negative predictive value—reliability, applicability, and practicality.

Validity

Validity is defined as a tool's ability to actually measure what it is we want to measure. When assessing an "at risk" diagnosis, we want to measure which patients are at risk for particular adverse health outcomes or incidents. A valid measure of such a state must be able to provide an accurate estimate of those patients who have the characteristics that would put them at risk for a particular diagnosis or incident (sensitivity) as well as those patients who are not at risk (specificity).

Positive predictive value or PPV refers to the proportion of patients who are identified as having a particular nursing diagnosis and who actually have that health condition or are "at risk" for developing it. Negative predictive value or NPV refers to the proportion of patients who are identified as not having a particular health condition or being at risk for an incident or health problem and do not have the health condition or will not encounter the high-risk incident.

Reliability

Another very important aspect of tool evaluation is its reliability. When we speak of reliability, we mean the ability of an instrument or test to give similar readings again and again. That statement, of course, assumes that all factors in the individual patient remain similar at each reading. An important component of an observational assessment tool is its interrater reliability, which refers to the consistency of different raters assessing or evaluating the same diagnosis or potential for risk of developing the health condition or incident.

Applicability and Practicality

Applicability (feasibility) and practicality (clinical utility) are also important but often neglected aspects of tool assessment. Applicability refers to the ability to transfer or extrapolate the findings from a study to a specific clinical setting, patient group, or caregiver (Gamel & van der Bijl, 2007). Practicality refers to "the clinical utility of the instrument." Although valid, reliable, and applicable, an instrument may not be practical for use in all clinical settings (Gamel & van der Bijl, 2007). For example, when conducting a study on the effect of relaxation exercises on postoperative pain and anxiety, Levin, Malloy, and Hyman (1987) found a well-supported tool for measuring anxiety (Spielberger State-Trait Anxiety Scale). This instrument, however, had 40 items that needed a response, each on a Likert-type scale. This type of instrument, although it had excellent psychometric properties and was well developed, was not applicable to or practical for use with a fresh postoperative patient. The instrument is not applicable because a postoperative patient population in the first 24 to 48 hours is usually in acute pain, receiving sensory altering analgesics, and is thus unable to focus on answering a 40-item self-administered questionnaire. Therefore, although the instrument is valid and reliable with the populations with whom and in the clinical settings where it was initially tested, the instrument does not have clinical utility on a postoperative inpatient unit in a hospital or in an ambulatory surgery setting during the recovery phase.

A CLINICAL EXEMPLAR: AT RISK FOR FALLS

A suburban community hospital noted from their quality report that the rate of patient falls exceeded the benchmark set for falls at the agency. Most patients were being assessed with a particular assessment tool used to identify at risk for falls. Upon review it was determined that the tool lacked needed sensitivity and specificity. Why is this important in clinical nursing practice? Using the example of *risk for falls,* if the assessment tool is not sensitive enough to correctly identify those patients who are truly at risk, the chance of patients falling becomes greater. On the other hand, if the tool is not specific enough, then too many patients are identified as being at risk. The resources available to implement preventive measures may compound the problem. For example, if all patients on an inpatient unit are considered fall risks and resources are limited in terms of personnel to implement preventive measures, the evidence-based protocol for this type of care may not be carried out because there just are not enough people and not enough time to institute these measures with every patient. Alternatively, by overestimating the extent of the problem, unnecessary additional and costly resources may be deployed. If we use a tool that is sensitive and reliable, however, the potential of patients for risk can be more appropriately assessed and only those patients who achieve a certain risk score are provided with the preventive measures—an evidence-based and more efficient way of instituting preventive care.

During an actual practice improvement project at the institution, nurses reviewed the evidence systematically and found an assessment tool that they believed was not only sensitive and specific but was also applicable and practical for their institution. This tool, the STRATIFY, was developed, by Oliver, Britton, Seed, Martin, and Hopper in 1997 is compared to other *risk for falls* assessment tools in a later systematic review (Oliver, Daly, Martin, & McMurdo, 2004). Table 14.1 presents the items of the STRATIFY.

Sensitivity and Specificity of the STRATIFY

To assess the sensitivity and specificity of the STRATIFY, Oliver and colleagues (1997) conducted a study to not only determine the risk factors for falls but also to derive an assessment tool and evaluate its predictive power. In Phase I of the study, they conducted a prospective case–control

TABLE 14.1 The STRATIFY

1. Did the patient present to hospital with a fall or has she or he fallen on the ward since admission? (Yes = 1, No = 2)

Do you think the patient is (questions 2–5)

2. Agitated? (Yes = 1, No = 2)
3. Visually impaired to the extent that everyday function is affected? (Yes = 1, No = 2)
4. In need of especially frequent toileting? (Yes = 1, No = 2)
5. Transfer and mobility score of 3 or more (Yes = 1, No = 2)

Total Score

Source: Oliver et al. (1997).

study to determine the risk factors for falling. In Phase II, the researchers conducted a prospective evaluation of the tool. The setting for this study was elderly care units in two United Kingdom hospitals. The sample of patients was 65 years of age and older and consisted of hospital inpatients.

Based upon data collected from "ward incident books" in Phase I, items were developed that were hypothesized to indicate a risk for falling. During Phase II, the items generated in Phase I were validated. Table 14.2 presents the risk assessment scores for "fallers versus non-fallers" in Phase II of the local validation study conducted by Oliver et al. (1997). This is the first step in determining the sensitivity and specificity of a tool. Table 14.3 presents the differential sensitivity and specificity for determining "risk for falling" at different cutoff scores.

The teaching strategy for reading the mathematical information regarding the concepts of sensitivity and specificity is crucial to facilitating students' understanding of these concepts. Over the many years I have taught research and EBP I have found that walking students through the formulas and mathematics with actual examples is key to understanding their meaning. Figure 14.1 and Tables 14.4 and 14.5 take the students through the way in which Oliver et al. (1997) arrived at the final numbers of sensitivity and specificity for the STRATIFY. Subsequent to

TABLE 14.2 Development of the STRATIFY: Risk Assessment Scores of Fallers Versus Non-Fallers

Risk Assess Score	Non-Fall ($N = 324$)	Falls ($N = 71$)
0	181	71
1	103	4
2	28	17
3	10	34
4	2	13
5	0	2

TABLE 14.3 Development and Evaluation of the STRATIFY: Sensitivity and Specicity

	Score ≥ 2	Score ≥ 3
Sensitivity		
(84.3 – 97.7)	93.0	
(56.9 – 79.5)	69.0	
Specificity		
(83.6 – 91)	87.7	
(93.6 – 98.1)	96.3	
PPV		
(52.3 – 71.5)	62.3	
(68.2 – 89.4)	80.3	
NPV		
(96.0 – 99.4)	98.3	
(90.2 – 95.8)	93.4	

presenting a "how to" lecture, I have either individual students or students working in small groups apply the formulas for calculating these indicators of validity for diagnostic tests/assessment tools to a problem and then discuss their results. In this way I can easily assess their understanding of the concepts and how to apply them, and evaluate what further support they may need to grasp these concepts.

CLINICAL APPLICATION

So what do reliability, validity, sensitivity, specificity, applicability, and practicality mean to students? Unless we bring this content full circle to an

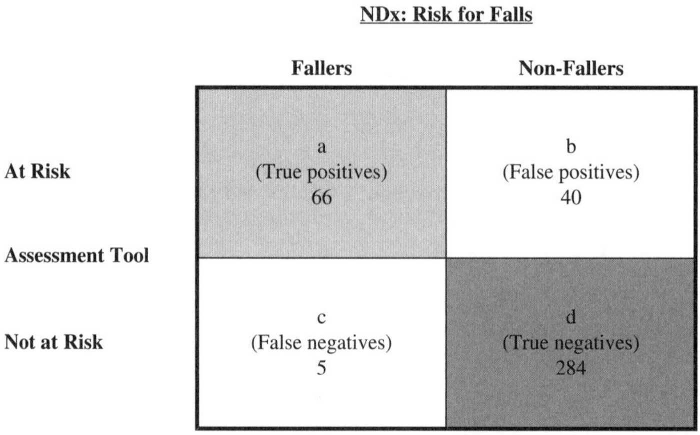

NDx: Risk for Falls

Assessment Tool	**Fallers**	**Non-Fallers**
At Risk	a (True positives) 66	b (False positives) 40
Not at Risk	c (False negatives) 5	d (True negatives) 284

Visual concept adapted from Gordis (2009).

FIGURE 14.1 Visual depiction of sensitivity and specificity.

TABLE 14.4 Calculating Sensitivity and Specicity

Sensitivity

- True Positives (TP) ÷ TP + False Negatives
- 66 ÷ (66 + 5) = .93

Specificity

- True Negatives (TN) ÷ TN + False Positives (FP)
- 284 ÷ (284 + 40) = .877

actual clinical scenario, students may simply consider this content an academic exercise and not actually a part of the professional clinical practice for which they are being groomed. Thus an actual clinical example follows.

> A group of nurses identified the clinical problem of not being able to reach their benchmark for patient falls. As an outgrowth of the agency's shared governance approach, a Falls Committee was established to investigate and take action on the issues. At an initial meeting with an EBP mentor, the committee shared the following information:
>
> - The current assessment of patients for fall risk was not systematic.
> - The current policy for how to assess risk for falls was not implemented consistently.

Important to note is that at this juncture it was determined that the inclusion of the quality management department was crucial to an understanding of the problem. Thus, going forward, the director of quality management attended all committee meetings. The group decided to develop a proposal for an EBP project in an effort to reduce the fall rate at the hospital. The overall project goals were to:

- Find the most sensitive, specific, applicable, and practical tool to measure risk for falls
- Develop an evidence-based protocol for fall prevention
- Reduce the fall rate at the hospital

TABLE 14.5 Calculating Positive and Negative Predictive Value

- PPV
  - # of falls with score of $\geq n(2)$ ÷ the # of all scores ≥ 2
  - 66 ÷ (66 + 40) = .623
- NPV
  - # of falls with a score $< n(2)$ ÷ the # of all scores $< n(2)$
  - 284 ÷ 289 = .983

The next step was for the committee to conduct a systematic review of the literature on several fronts—factors that predict falls, preventative interventions, and tools to assess risk for falling. How would we find the best fall risk assessment tool for the agency's purposes? After identifying from the literature the top five predictors of patient falls in a hospital setting, the committee searched for tools that included these predictors, and were sensitive, specific, applicable (relevant to the agency's setting and population), and practical (easy to administer). Interestingly, the agency was currently using an older, lengthier tool that did not include one of the five top predictors for falls, that is, toileting needs. This tool was eliminated as evidence supported the need for a new, more inclusive approach to assessment. The literature review and critical appraisal of the evidence led to the selection of the STRATIFY.

Following tool selection, we needed to determine interrater reliability of the nurses who were responsible for conducting falls risk assessments. After a small test of change in which nurses used the tool to assess patients, they found that they were able to obtain the same results with different nurses using the tool with the same patient. They also found that the tool was sensitive, accurately assessed fall risk, accurately identified patients who were not a fall risk (specificity), and was applicable and practical (the STRATIFY was much shorter than the assessment tool being used, making it more efficient). In fact, nurses could complete the assessment in 1 minute, a very practical finding. Based on these factors, a decision was made to implement the STRATIFY on a larger scale and then review the quality data about falls after 3 months.

In conclusion, when teaching content on sensitivity and specificity, important considerations are: (1) making the application of all these foreign statistical concepts real, and (2) providing exemplars that demonstrate the concepts of validity, reliability, sensitivity, specificity, applicability, and practicality are used to make decisions about the choice of an assessment tool to evaluate any nursing diagnosis, whether actual, potential, or "at risk."

REFERENCES

Carmona, E. V., & Baena de Moraes Lopes, M. H. (2006). Content validation of parental role conflict in the neonatal intensive care unit. *International Journal of Nursing Terminologies and Classifications*, *17*(1), 3–9.

Fehring, R. (1994). The Fehring model. In R. M. Carroll-Johnson, & M. Pacquett (Eds.), *Classification of nursing diagnosis: Proceedings of the tenth conference* (pp. 55–57). Philadelphia: J.B. Lippincott.

Fehring, R. (1987). Methods to validate nursing diagnoses. *Heart & Lung*, *16*, 627–629.

Fehring, R. (1986). Validating diagnostic labels: Standardized methodology. In M. E. Hurley (Ed.), *Classification of nursing diagnosis: Proceedings of the sixth conference* (pp. 183–190). St. Louis, MO: Mosby.

Gamel, C., & van der Bijl, J. (2007). *Establishing the practicality of an instrument*. Paper presented at Pace University. New York, NY.

Gordis, L. (2009). *Epidemiology*. Philadelphia: Saunders.

Guirao-Goris, J. A., & Duarte-Climents, G. (2007). The expert nurse profile and diagnostic content validity of sedentary lifestyle: The Spanish validation. *International Journal of Nursing Terminologies and Classifications*, 84–92.

Levin, R. F. (2001). Who are the experts? A commentary on nursing diagnosis content validation studies. *Nursing Diagnosis: The Journal of Nursing Language and Classification, 12*(1), 29–32.

Levin, R., Malloy, G., & Hyman, R. (1987). Postoperative pain management: The use of relaxation techniques with female cholecystectomy patients. *Journal of Advanced Nursing, 12*, 463–472.

Oliver, D., Britton, M., Seed, P., Martin, F. C., & Hopper, A. H. (1997, October 25). Development and evaluation of evidence-based risk assessment tool (*STRATIFY*) to predict which elderly inpatients will fall: Case–control and cohort studies. *British Medical Journal, 315*, 1049–1053.

Oliver, D., Daly, F., Martin, F. C., & McMurdo, M. E. (2004). Risk factors and risk assessment tools for falls in hospital inpatients: A systematic review. *Age Ageing, 33*(2), 122–130.

Straus, S. E., Richardson, W. S., Glasziou, P., & Haynes, R. B. (2005). *Evidence-based medicine: How to practice and teach EBM* (3rd ed.). London, UK: Elsevier.

15

Sensitivity and Specificity of Diagnostic Tests

Jason T. Slyer

Better to understand a little than to misunderstand a lot.

—Unknown

When teaching clinicians how to think about which diagnostic tests they will order for a patient, it is important to ask questions about what the test results actually mean, what they are going to do with the test results, and how the results will impact the care of the patient. The clinician should understand that the diagnostic decision-making process will not determine with complete certainty what condition a patient has but will help to determine the probability of a patient in a specific clinical scenario having a given diagnosis. Barriers to using current evidence related to a diagnostics test's accuracy may stem from the learner's difficulty in understanding concepts of sensitivity, specificity, and likelihood ratios. As teachers, it is important to keep in mind that, while the terms *sensitivity* and *specificity* may be familiar to the learner, their actual meaning and use may be more abstract. Mathematical formulas for calculating these statistics may be intimidating, further compounding the learner's ability to understand these concepts.

In teaching concepts related to sensitivity, specificity, and likelihood ratios of diagnostic tests, it is helpful to tailor the discussion to clinical experiences familiar to the learner. Using concrete examples and plotting values on a 2 × 2 table can assist the learner in understanding these concepts. The purpose of this chapter is to demonstrate how to teach clinicians to evaluate and apply the concepts of sensitivity, specificity, and likelihood ratios when ordering and interpreting diagnostic tests in clinical practice.

SELECTING A DIAGNOSTIC TEST

Diagnostic testing may be done to establish a diagnosis for a patient, screen for the presence of disease, provide prognostic information in patients with a particular condition, or monitor the effects of a particular therapy (Mulley, 2009). When clinicians are presented with a particular clinical scenario, they are often tasked with deciding which of a multitude of diagnostics tests should be ordered to answer questions and aid in the diagnosis and treatment of their patient. Diagnostic tests are performed to lessen the uncertainty a clinician has at labeling a patient with a particular condition (Straus, Glasziou, Richardson, & Haynes, 2011).

A reference or gold standard diagnostic test is the most accurate diagnostic test possible. Reference tests may be considered, although these tests are usually more costly, less widely available, and incur a greater risk to the patient. Surrogates for the reference test, therefore, are often performed. Clinicians must be able to interpret the results of these surrogate tests in a way that increases their ability to diagnose a particular disease or condition. A diagnosis is a hypothesis, and diagnostic tests help to increase the probability that the hypothesis is true (Scherokman, 1997).

No diagnostic test is 100% accurate. Accuracy is defined as how correct a diagnostic test result is compared to a reference standard (Mulley, 2009). Clinicians must evaluate the reliability and validity of a diagnostic test chosen. A thorough understanding of the concepts of sensitivity, specificity, positive predictive value (PPV), and negative predictive value (NPV) are essential for formulating accurate diagnoses (both medical and nursing). (Also see Chapter 14, "Determining Sensitivity and Specificity of Assessment Tools for Formulating 'At Risk' Nursing Diagnoses," as a companion to this chapter.)

When a diagnostic test has high sensitivity, clinicians can be fairly certain that a negative test will rule out the disease. When a diagnostic test has high specificity, clinicians can be fairly certain that a positive test will rule in the disease. When choosing diagnostic tests, clinicians want a test that minimizes the chance of false-positive and false-negative results. If a diagnostic test has a high PPV, there will be few false-positive results, reducing the chance that a patient without a disease would undergo more invasive testing or receive unnecessary treatment. If a diagnostic test has a high NPV, there would be few false-negative results, reducing the number of patients with a disease that would not receive necessary therapy.

When evaluating the validity of a diagnostic test in a particular clinical scenario, clinicians should be taught to first determine the pre-test probability or prevalence of the disease in a specific population. Pre-test probability is usually derived from prior knowledge of the prevalence of a disease in a patient population and from clinical expertise based on information obtained from the patient's history and physical examination.

CLINICAL EXAMPLE: DIAGNOSING HEART FAILURE IN THE EMERGENCY ROOM

A 55-year-old obese, African American female patient with a history of uncontrolled hypertension, asthma, and a 20-pack per year smoking history presents to the emergency room (ER) with a complaint of dyspnea on exertion worsening over the prior 3 weeks. The physical exam is significant for bilateral rales and wheezing, lower extremity edema, and a third heart sound. A chest x-ray is unremarkable and an electrocardiogram has nonspecific T wave abnormalities.

The clinician expects the patient has congestive heart failure (CHF); however, there is some level of uncertainty. Her symptoms could also be pulmonary in nature given her history of asthma and smoking. The clinician decides to order a B-type natriuretic peptide (BNP) blood test to aid in the diagnosis. The clinician probably knows that BNP is secreted from the heart in response to volume overload (McCullough et al., 2002). While the clinician has used the BNP test in the past to aid in diagnosing patients, his understanding of the properties of the BNP test has been based on common practice in the ER rather than on data from scientific testing.

Clinicians should be taught to derive clinical questions from common scenarios and to search the literature for evidence to support their decision. In this case the clinician asks: In patients presenting to the ER with a complaint of dyspnea, can the BNP test aid in supporting a diagnosis of CHF? A Medline search of the literature using terms "heart failure" and "BNP" and "sensitivity" and "specificity" results in an article by McCullough et al. (2002) titled "B-Type Natriuretic Peptide and Clinical Judgment in Emergency Diagnosis of Heart Failure."

When critiquing an article on the sensitivity and specificity of diagnostic tests, clinicians should be taught to ask:

1. Are the results of the diagnostic test valid?
2. Are the results of the diagnostic test important?
3. Can the valid, important evidence about the diagnostic test be applied to the clinical question at hand (Straus et al., 2011)?

When assessing for validity, the clinician should look to see if the comparison between the diagnostic test and an appropriate reference standard of diagnosis was blinded to the reviewers. The reference standard should be applied to all patients in the study, regardless of the diagnostic test result, in order to obtain a true level of disease prevalence in the population. The clinician should also assess whether the test was evaluated on an appropriate population of patients that would be seen in clinical practice, including those with mild, moderate, and severe forms of the disease, those with treated and untreated conditions, and those with alternative diagnoses for presenting symptoms.

In the study by McCullough and others (2002), the reference standard was defined as a diagnosis of CHF made by two independent cardiologists after a review of the clinical history, electrocardiogram, chest x-ray, echocardiogram, and other clinical tests or consultations performed, in addition to calculations of Framingham scores for CHF and National Health and Nutrition Examination Surveys for CHF. Agreement between the two cardiologists was needed to provide a diagnosis of CHF or no CHF. The cardiologists were blinded to the results of the BNP test. The population included a broad spectrum of patients presenting to the ER with dyspnea with a low, moderate, or high probability of CHF, reflective of a population that would present to any ER.

The importance of the diagnostic test results is determined by examining sensitivity, specificity, predictive values, and likelihood ratios. It is important for clinicians to learn how to fill in a 2 × 2 truth table to aid in the assessment of a diagnostic test's validity. One side of the 2 × 2 table represents the diagnostic test results and the other represents the results of the reference standard. The clinician wants to determine that, in performing a diagnostic test, the results of the test will significantly change what he thinks the diagnosis is before the test (pre-test probability or prevalence) compared with what he thinks the diagnosis is after the test (post-test probability or PPV).

These concepts and calculations can often become confusing and working from a 2 × 2 table can help reduce this confusion. A 2 × 2 table with the calculation for common statistical parameters is shown in Table 15.1. Many authors typically label these boxes *a, b, c,* and *d*. These

TABLE 15.1 2 × 2 Truth Table

	Disease as determined by gold standard		
	Disease	No disease	Row totals
Positive test result	True Positive (TP)	False Positive (FP)	Total positive test results (TP + FP)
Negative test result	False Negative (FN)	True Negative (TN)	Total negative test results (FN + TN)
Column total	Total patients with disease (TP + FN)	Total patients without disease (FP + TN)	Total number of patients in study (TP + TN + FP + FN)

Sensitivity = TP/(TP/FN)
Specificity = TN/(TN + FP)
Accuracy = (TP + TN)/(TP + TN + FP + FN)
Positive likelihood ratio = sensitivity/(1 − specificity)
Negative likelihood ratio = (1 − sensitivity)/specificity

Prevalence = (TP + FN)/(TP + TN + FP + FN)
Positive Predictive Value = TP/(TP + FP)
Negative Predictive Value = TN/(TN + FN)

TABLE 15.2 Calculating Positive and Negative Values

Sensitivity = TP/(TP + FN) 0.90 = TP/722 TP = 650	Specicity = TN/(TN + FP) 0.73 = TN/816 TN = 596
Positive Predictive Value = TP/(TP + FP) PPV = 650/870 = 0.75	Negative Predictive Value = TN/(TN + FN) NPV = 596/668 = 0.90
Accuracy = (TP + TN)/(TP + TN + FP + FN) Accuracy = (650 + 596)/1538 = 0.81	Prevalence = (TP + FN)/(TP + TN + FP + FN) Prevalence = 722/1538 = 0.47
Positive likelihood ratio = sensitivity/(1 − specificity) Positive likelihood ratio = 0.90/(1 − 0.73) = 3.33	
Negative likelihood ratio = (1 − sensitivity)/specificity Negative likelihood ratio = (1 − 0.9)/0.73 = 0.14	

Source: Data derived from McCullough et al. (2002).

labels may add to the confusion in performing the calculation. Referring to the boxes a *true positive (TP), true negative (TN), false positive (FP),* and *false negative (FN)* may alleviate some confusion in performing the calculations.

From McCullough et al. (2002) we are told that the BNP test has a sensitivity of 90% and a specificity of 73%. Out of 1,538 patients, there were 722 patients with a diagnosis of CHF and 816 without a diagnosis of CHF. Start by filling in what is known on the 2 × 2 table, and then work backward using the values of sensitivity and specificity the remainder of the 2 × 2 table can be filled in (see Table 15.2 and Figure 15.1).

The sensitivity gives us information about the ability of the diagnostic test to rule out a disease while the specificity gives us information about the ability of the diagnostic test to rule in the disease. In most clinical scenarios as well, it is important to note that the usefulness of the sensitivity and

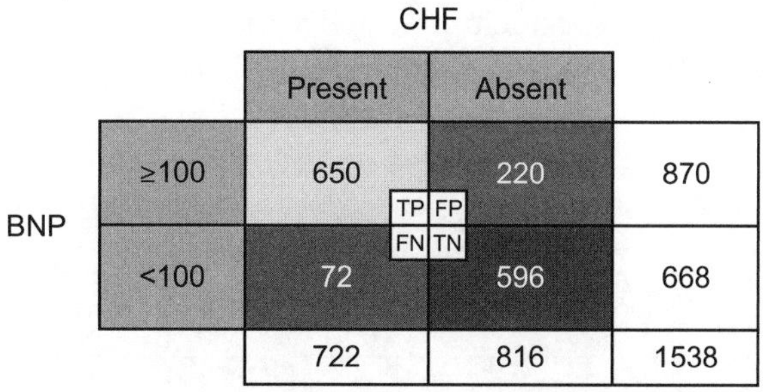

		CHF Present	CHF Absent	
BNP	≥100	650 (TP)	220 (FP)	870
BNP	<100	72 (FN)	596 (TN)	668
		722	816	1538

Source: Data derived from McCullough et al. (2002)

FIGURE 15.1 2 × 2 Table comparing BNP test results to the presence or absence of CHF.

		CHF		
		Present	Absent	
BNP	≥100	277	332	609
		TP	FP	
		FN	TN	
	<100	31	898	929
		308	1230	1538

FIGURE 15.2 Prevalence = 20%.

specificity is limited because we do not know the results of the reference standard test. The PPV can provide more useful information about whether a patient has the disease and the NPV provides information about whether a patient does not have the disease. The predictive values, however, can vary depending on the prevalence of the disease (Scherokman, 1997). Sensitivity and specificity are properties specific to a test and should remain constant across various populations regardless of disease prevalence.

As the prevalence of disease decreases, the PPV will decrease and the NPV will increase. Figure 15.2 shows what happens when the prevalence of CHF in the population decreases to 20% but the sensitivity and specificity of the BNP test remain unchanged. The PPV falls to 46% and the NPV increases to 97%. Figure 15.3 shows what happens when the prevalence of CHF in the population increases to 80% but the sensitivity and specificity of the BNP test remains unchanged. The PPV increases to 93% and the NPV decreases to 65%.

Let us say the patient from our scenario was found to have a BNP of 400. The clinician wants to know how likely it is for his patient with a BNP of 400 to have CHF. We know from the study that 90% of patients with a BNP ≥ 100 will have CHF; this is the sensitivity of the BNP test. We also know that 73% of patients with a BNP less than 100 will not have CHF; this is the specificity of the BNP test. Conversely 27% with a BNP less than 100 will actually have CHF; this is the false-negative rate.

		CHF		
		Present	Absent	
BNP	≥100	1107	83	1190
		TP	FP	
		FN	TN	
	<100	123	225	348
		1230	308	1538

FIGURE 15.3 Prevalence = 80%.

The prevalence, or pre-test probability, of CHF in patients presenting to the ER with dyspnea is 47%. If the BNP $\geq$ 100, the post-test probability of having CHF (PPV) is 75%. If the BNP is less than 100, the post-test probability of not having CHF (NPV) is 90%. We can see that in performing a BNP test, a BNP $\geq$ 100 increases the probability of a diagnosis of CHF from 47% to 75% and a BNP less than 100 increases the probability of not having CHF from 53% to 90%.

The clinician wants to know how likely it is for his patient with a BNP of 400 to have CHF. The positive likelihood ratio tells us how much a diagnostic test result will raise or lower the pre-test probability of having the disease. The positive likelihood ratio (+ LR) is:

$$+LR = \text{sensitivity}/(1 - \text{specificity})$$
$$+LR = 0.90/0.27 = 3.33$$

The negative likelihood ratio (−LR) is:

$$-LR = (1 - \text{sensitivity})/\text{specificity}$$
$$-LR = 0.10/0.73 = 0.14$$

A likelihood ratio of 1 indicates that the diagnostic test provides no additional information to the clinical scenario. The + LR should be greater than 1 and the −LR should be between 0 and 1. The greater the + LR the more certain a clinician can be that a positive test result will rule in the disease. The lower the −LR the more certain a clinician can be that a negative result will rule out the disease (Halkin, Reichman, Schwaber, Paltiel, & Brezis, 1998). This patient's BNP of 400 is 3.33 times more likely to occur in a patient with CHF than in someone without CHF. A BNP of less than 100 would only be 0.14 times more likely to occur in a patient with CHF than in someone without CHF.

The likelihood ratio can then be used to calculate the post-test probability of having CHF. We must first calculate the post-test odds using Bayes' theorem (Akobeng, 2006), which relates the probability of a particular condition in a group of people with specific characteristics (pre-test odds) to the likelihood of that condition occurring.

$$\text{Post-test odds} = \text{Pre-test odds} \times \text{Positive Likeliness ratio}$$

where, Pre-test odds = Prevalence/(1 − prevalence)

If the patient from our clinical scenario has a pre-test probability similar to that of patients from the study then,

$$\text{Pre-test odds} = 0.47/(1 - 0.47) = 0.89$$
$$\text{Post-test odds} = 0.89 \times 3.33 = 2.96$$

Post-test odds can then be converted into a post-test probability,

Post-test probability = post-test odds/(1 + post-test odds)
Post-test probability = 2.96/3.96 = 0.75

Note that this is identical to the PPV from the study. We can then conclude that this patient with a BNP of 400 has a 75% probability of having CHF. Performing the diagnostic test increases the patient's probability of having CHF from 47% to 75%.

Post-test probability can also be easily determined using the likelihood ratio nomogram developed by Fagan (1975, see Figure 15.4). The left column is the pre-test probability, the middle column is the likelihood ratio, and the right column is the post-test probability. Draw a line connecting the pre-test probability and the likelihood ratio for the study and extend this line to the post-test probability column to determine the results. The top line represents a patient from the McCullough et al. (2002) study

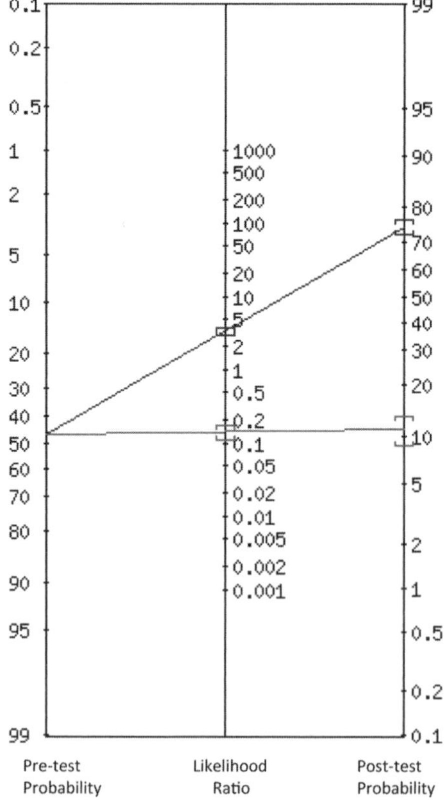

FIGURE 15.4 Likelihood ratio nomogram showing results from McCullough et al. (2002) with a pre-test probability of 47%.

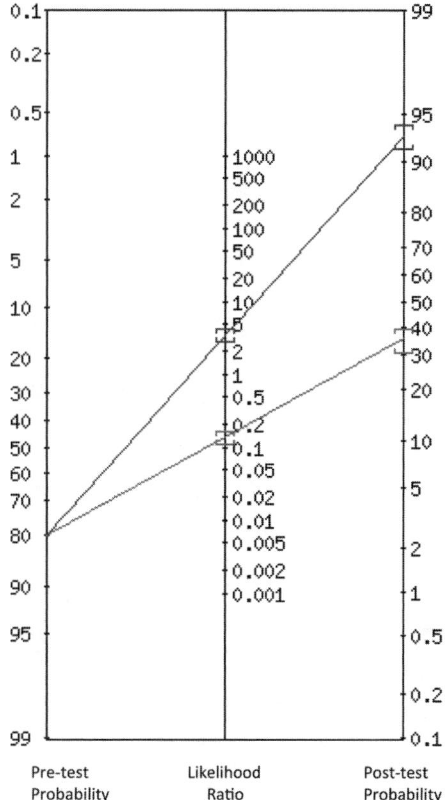

FIGURE 15.5 Likelihood ratio nomogram showing a pre-test probability of 80%.

with a pre-test probability of 47% and a +LR of 3.33. The post-test probability is found to be 75%. The bottom line represents −LR of 0.14 and corresponds to a post-test probability of 11%.

Figure 15.5 shows what happens when the pre-test probability of CHF increases to 80%. The post-test probability of CHF with a BNP ≥ 100 increases to 93% (top line) and the post-test probably of CHF with a BNP less than 100 increases to 36% (bottom line).

Figure 15.6 shows what happens when the pre-test probability of CHF decreases to 20%. The post-test probability of CHF with a BNP ≥ 100 decreases to 45% (top line) and the post-test probably of CHF with a BNP less than 100 decreases to 3% (bottom line).

CAUSES OF UNCERTAINTY

Once the importance of the diagnostic test results has been explored, the applicability of the diagnostic test in clinical practice should be assessed.

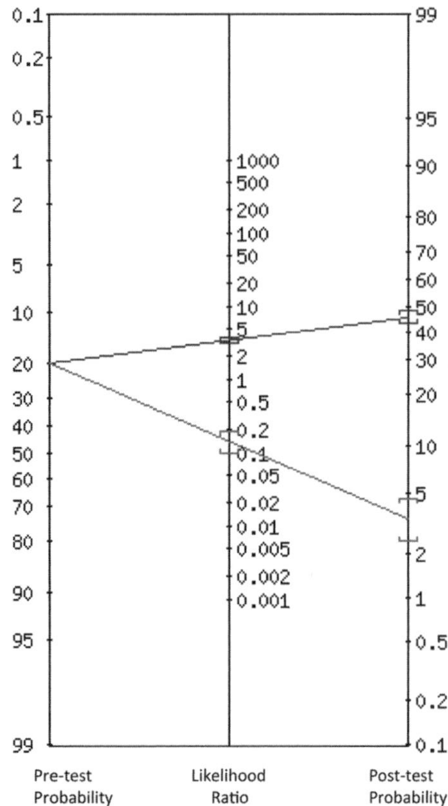

FIGURE 15.6 Likelihood ratio nomogram showing a pre-test probability of 20%.

Is the test applicable and practical for use in the clinical setting? Will the diagnostic test result affect patient management? Even if a test was found to be 100% sensitive, specific, and accurate, the results need to be relevant to diagnosing the clinical scenario at hand. For example, pulmonary angiograms are highly sensitive, specific, and accurate in the diagnosis of pulmonary embolisms; however, if the clinical suspicion for a pulmonary embolism is low, negative results of this invasive test will have little impact on determining an accurate diagnosis.

Clinicians need to consider the following points when evaluating the validity of diagnostic tests:

1. How will the results from the study be affected when the diagnostic test is applied to the general population? Variability may limit the applicability of the study results to the general population.
2. How is the diagnostic test conducted? Differences in the execution of the diagnostic test or the technology used to conduct the diagnostic test may influence the sensitivity and specificity of the results.

3. Will inter-observer variability result in differences in diagnostic test results based on who is interpreting the results?
4. Will clinical knowledge have an impact on the interpretation of the test results? Experienced clinicians may be able to successfully predict the presence of a disease from a patient's history and physical examination, increasing the pre-test probability of the patient actually having the disease. If an experienced clinician is able to say he is 90% certain a patient has CHF based on history and physical exam findings, ordering a BNP will not provide any further prognostic benefit as a positive BNP only tells us the patient has a 75% chance of having CHF.
5. Are there differences between the population used to study the sensitivity and specificity of a diagnostic test and the general population the test will actually be performed on? Studies evaluating the reliability of diagnostic tests need to be conducted on similar populations that the test is designed to be performed on. If a diagnostic test is studied on a sample of patients with more severe forms of a disease, the sensitivity will be falsely elevated, as will the positive predictive value of the test. The presence of comorbidities in patients without a disease may produce false-positive test results. If a diagnostic test is studied on a sample of healthy patients without typical comorbidities seen in the general population, the diagnostic test will be used, the specificity will be falsely elevated, and the positive predictive value will be increased.

In conclusion, when teaching clinicians how to interpret sensitivity and specificity of diagnostic tests it is important for the clinician to conceptualize and understand that diagnostic tests do not give absolute answers to clinical questions. Diagnostic tests help the clinician to understand the probability of a disease in a specific clinical scenario. An evidence-based practice perspective will allow clinicians to approach decision making from a more scientific methodology. Using clinical scenarios to teach the concepts of sensitivity, specificity, predictive values, and likelihood ratios, while plotting values on a 2 × 2 table, can help clinicians understand the applicability of diagnostic tests, the circumstances under which a diagnostic test should be used, and whether the results of the diagnostic test will actually help guide diagnostic decisions and improve patient outcomes.

REFERENCES

Akobeng, A. K. (2006). Understanding diagnostic tests 2: Likelihood ratios, pre- and post-test probability and their use in clinical practice. *Acta Pædiatric, 96*(4), 487–491.

Fagan, T. J. (1975). Letter: Nomogram for Bayes theorem. *New England Journal of Medicine, 293*(5), 257.

Halkin, A., Reichman, J., Schwaber, M., Paltiel, O., & Brezis, M. (1998). Likelihood ratios: Getting diagnostic testing into perspective. *QJM: An International Journal of Medicine, 91*(4), 247–258.

McCullough, P. A., Nowak, R. M., McCord, J., Hollander, J. E., Herrmann, H. C., Steg, P. G. et al. (2002). B-type natriuretic peptide and clinical judgment in emergency diagnosis of heart failure: Analysis from breathing not properly (BNP) multinational study. *Circulation, 106*, 416–422.

Mulley, A. G. (2009). Selection and interpretation of diagnostic tests. In A. H. Garoll, & A. G. Mulley (Eds.), *Primary care medicine: Office evaluation and management of the adult patient*. Philadelphia: Lippincott Williams & Wilkins. Retrieved from http://www.dermaamin.com/site/images/stories/fruit/Primarycaremedicine/Copyright.html

Scherokman, B. (1997). Selecting and interpreting diagnostic tests. *The Permanente Journal, 1*(2), 4–7.

Straus, S. E., Glasziou, P., Richardson, W. S., & Haynes, R. B. (2011). *Evidence-based medicine: How to practice and teach it*. Edinburgh: Elsevier.

16

Conducting a Gap Analysis

Bonnie Lauder

If you can not describe what you are doing as a process, you don't know what you are doing.

—W. Edwards Demming (1900–1992)

Organizational effectiveness is determined by many factors, the most important of which is the quality of available pertinent knowledge (evidence) and the ability to implement that knowledge into practice (performance improvement). The present health care system places great emphasis on explicit or scientific knowledge presented in the literature. There are approximately 400,000 articles added to the biomedical literature each year (Davenport & Glaser, 2002). Although evidence-based practice (EBP) is identified as the most effective management approach for many health conditions, much of the available evidence is not acted on in everyday practice. The reason for this is that most strategies to bridge the gap between research and practice have focused almost exclusively on the production, presentation, and distribution of codified knowledge when knowledge utilization research has demonstrated that getting evidence into practice takes both explicit and implicit knowledge. Implicit knowledge is referred to as the "know how," where explicit knowledge is the "know what" (facts). The Evidence-Based Practice Improvement Model (EBPI) developed by Levin et al. (2010) has overcome this challenge by focusing on the continuous identification and elimination of gaps in knowledge and processes, resulting in improvements in clinical practice. The model uses action learning cycles of plan, do, study, and act (PDSA) or small tests of change (Langley, Nolan, Nolan, Norman, & Provost, 1996). Action is focused and measured around specific strategic goals. The goal or goals is (are) what the team is working toward to improve and is frequently identified through external regulatory agencies and benchmarking trends. Goals are translated to outcome and process measures; practice protocols are developed from evidence-based guidelines and tested; data are collected and shared during the action periods to determine if the goals are being met. During these action periods both explicit and implicit knowledge are shared and tested.

WHAT IS A GAP ANALYSIS?

Within this framework, a gap analysis is a method of understanding the current and desired state (best practice) of a process, and bridging the differences between the two. Perfecting the process of implementing an improvement is key to being able to attribute outcomes to the new practice. The goal of the new practice protocol is to increase quality at no additional cost by making processes more efficient and effective, removing redundant rework and standardizing workflow; integrating the best available evidence into current practice; and creating innovation by re-designing processes or implementing new practice protocols. The EBP protocol and flowchart are tested and evaluated through the action periods of the plan, do, study, and act cycles. It is through the small test of changes that the new practice protocol becomes standardized and sustainable within the existing system. Until processes are perfected, we cannot expect to achieve desired outcomes.

WHY CONDUCT A GAP ANALYSIS?

An organization's capacity to change is directly related to its knowledge of current processes and ability to standardize operations. Organizations looking to improve performance frequently implement specific interventions without fully understanding the problem they are trying to solve. The high failure rate in implementing new practices is mainly attributable to not understanding the current system in which the new practice/ process is being integrated. In traditional organizations, like health care agencies, there is a large gap between what a task looks like in a procedure manual and what it looks like in reality. Actual work practices are full of tacit improvisations that employees would have trouble articulating (Brown & Duguid, 2000). During a gap analysis, these gaps and improvisations, which are not standardized and result in varying levels of quality, are captured and are negotiated as to whether they should be considered part of the current practice. This chapter provides readers with strategies and tools needed to teach learners how to conduct a gap analysis.

HOW DO YOU CONDUCT A GAP ANALYSIS?

Prior to conducting a gap analysis, the strategic objective to focus the improvement work has been identified, usually through industry benchmarking, regulatory quality indicators, organizational scorecards, and staff and customer (client) feedback. Project aims are then stated in measurable terms. What is usually not well-defined is the scope of the process to be improved. Preliminary literature reviews and formation of the clinical question start defining the scope of the practice to be evaluated. A practice is made up of a number of specific processes. It is early on in the gap analysis that it is very important to drive toward narrowing the scope of the processes to match the practice to be improved. If you do not narrow the scope, you will end up trying to improve everything and end up not improving anything. The steps in a gap analysis are as follows:

- Understanding current state through workflow analysis and flowchart development
- Comparing current state to target state (best practices) and identifying opportunities for improvement
- Integrating the improvement opportunities into the current state flowchart, to create an EBP protocol and flowchart of desired processes

In addition, it is important to understand the organization's culture when managing performance. How an organization views its poor performance will determine its willingness and ability to change. Traditional organizations who blame poor performance on people and finger point when things go wrong have difficulty with understanding processes, standardizing workflows, and experience increased challenges when implementing change. Process-oriented organizations identify methods and structure as the cause for poor performance, and, therefore, work at improving processes. Thus these organizations are more effective in implementing change than traditional organizations. What is interesting is that the majority of organizational problems are related to methods (processes) and structure, and only 15% are people related (Madison, 2005). It will take more time to understand current state in traditional organizations. Additional time is needed to build trust in sharing information without staff feeling there will be negative repercussions and to facilitate conversations focused on work improvement processes instead of what people are doing wrong. Creating a process-oriented organization with a culture of improvement is a slow process, which starts with staff understanding how they work together.

When staff is brought together to develop a current state flowchart, ground rules and a process for consensus are established. All staff is given the opportunity to participate in improvement efforts, regardless of position. During this time staff is given the freedom to express both agreement and disagreement, improvement efforts become more feasible. During the development of the flowchart, consensus must be reached on the scope, steps, and sequences of steps that make up the process. It is not until staff tests the flowchart in practice that the accuracy of the flowchart can be determined. After initial testing of the flowchart, the process of flowchart development may need review and refinement, gaining consensus on the steps, and the sequence of steps again.

One of the most challenging aspects of a gap analysis, which will have a negative impact on the effectiveness or even prevent the use of the new practice, is not adequately identifying the needed inputs. Input into a process consists of informational handovers, environment factors, culture, performance capacity (skill and available), and knowledge gaps. An example of each type of input gap is as follows:

- Informational handovers: Is the patient's ejection fracture known to the home care clinician in order to begin the heart failure protocol at admission?
- Environmental factors: Do the physicians who order home care services for their patients understand that the home care agency will not get paid if the physician does not sign its orders timely?
- Culture: Does the staff feel they are able to share their opinion and errors openly without repercussion from leadership?
- Performance capacity: Is the staff willing and able to learn a new skill (e.g., assessing the appropriateness and adequacy of a medication regimen)?
- Knowledge gaps: Does the staff know how to administer the new evidence-based innovation?

HOW DO YOU CONSTRUCT AND INTERPRET FLOWCHARTS?

To help learners understand how to conduct a gap analysis you must first teach learners how to construct and interpret a flowchart. A flowchart is a visual diagram of a process or algorithm, representing the sequence steps and decisions to be made. As an organization becomes more and more comfortable with using flowcharting as a tool, it will move from being traditional to more process-oriented, increasing its ability to change and implement best practices. Whether the goal is to improve quality and/or decrease cost with increased efficiency of processes, flowcharting is a powerful process improvement tool for meeting that type of goal. Flowcharting is best accomplished by bringing together representatives from all levels and roles/functions in the organization who are directly involved in the process to be documented. This is very important for building understanding and gaining consensus of the current processes on which the EBP will be compared and integrated. Too often, understanding of the current process does not occur, creating difficulty or preventing spread of the EBP improvement across what turns out to be a nonstandardized system where results will vary.

Flowcharts serve many purposes. They help teams see how a process works including the flow of steps/events, people, and materials and their relationships to each other. In addition, these charts show unexpected complexity, bottlenecks, delays, redundancies, and places where simplification and standardization may be possible. They are used to compare the actual versus the ideal flow of a process to identify improvement opportunities. They define scope by determining the start and end point of the improvement work.

Flowchart Symbols and Conventions

To facilitate the use of flowcharts there are standard symbols and conventions, which learners must be able to refer when developing one. Just as one may keep an APA manual at hand when writing a manuscript, having a glossary of flowchart symbols in your pocket or on your computer is an essential tool for learning flowchart development. Exhibit 16.1 shows standard symbols and what they represent.

Using standard conventions make a flowchart easier to read. The following is a list of common conventions:

- Process name and date of creation
- Arrows on all lines to show direction
- Verbs to label tasks and activities
- Questions to label decision diamonds
- Clear starting and ending point
- Clear direction of flow from top to bottom, left to right
- Consistent level of detail
- Numbered steps

The two conventions that are more than labeling standards but take skill and practice are "clear direction of flow from top to bottom, left to right" and "consistent level of detail."

Different Types of Flowcharting and Their Use

The most common types of flowcharts used in improvement work are macro, top-down, deployment, and workflow. Macro, top-down, and deployment flowcharts are commonly used while conducting the gap analysis. Remember, the goal of the gap analysis is to develop the new

EXHIBIT 16.1 FLOWCHART SYMBOLS AND DEFINITIONS

Symbol	Definition	Detail/Example
	Start/End Input/Output	Request for proposal, Request for new hire, Create medication list
	Task, Action, Execution point, Process	Hold a meeting, Make a phone call, Open a box, Assess functional status
	Decision Points	Yes/No Accept/Reject Criteria Met/Not Met
	Document	Job request, Meeting minutes
	Arrow	Shows direction
A	Continuation	Go to another page or to another part of the chart
	Delay	Waiting for service, Report sitting on desk
	Shadow signifies additional flowchart for this task	A major task has subtasks not needed for this study

practice protocol to be tested and evaluated within the PDSA cycles. During the PDSA cycles the process becomes more refined and the details of a workflow flowchart should emerge. Each flowchart type services a specific function.

1. Macro flowcharts show only sufficient information to understand the general overall process steps. It is with the identification of the overall process steps that the Macro flowchart (see Exhibit 16.2) ultimately determines the *scope* of the process the improvement project is focused on.
2. Top-down flowcharts picture major steps in a work process. It minimizes the detail to focus only on the essential steps. In evidence-based performance improvement, brainstorming how the new EBP can be incorporated into current practice can be facilitated by the use of a top-down flowchart. The top-down flowchart helps teams visualize the practice change by systematically rearranging and labeling current steps at a higher enough level where the inserted new or changed steps will not get lost in the

EXHIBIT 16.2 MACRO FLOWCHART EXAMPLE

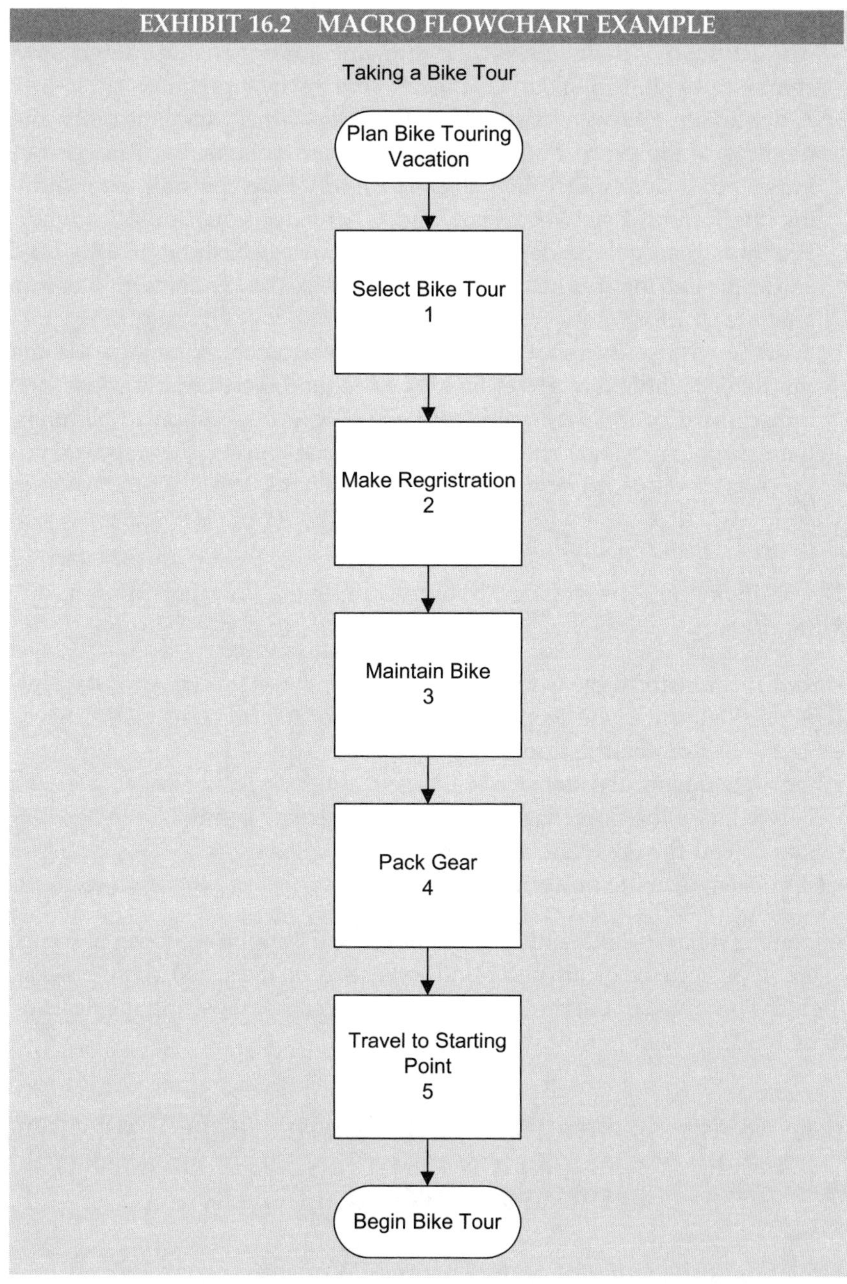

details of more complex workflow diagrams. Top-down flowcharts are effective visuals in communicating desired practice changes to leadership who only need to approve the practice from a framework of current practice, focusing them on the important decisions to be made and not distract them with details of their implementation. The top-down flowchart (see Exhibit 16.3) depicts the *vision* of the new practice.

3. A deployment flowchart shows staff or department responsibility and the flow of the process steps or tasks they are assigned with decisions indicated. It clearly identifies the *relationships* between staff, by indicating the handoffs between staff and where decisions must be made. For these reasons, the deployment flowchart (see Exhibit 16.4) is used as the visual for the EBP protocol, which is the outcome of the gap analysis process.
4. Workflow flowcharts show the flow of people, materials, paperwork, and machinery within a work setting. When redundancies, duplications, and unnecessary complexity are identified, people take action to eliminate these problems. They are generally not used during the gap analysis process; therefore, we will not get into detail here.

How to Diagram a Flowchart

The following are the steps on how to complete a flowchart (Brassard & Ritter, 1994):

- Step 1: Brainstorm the activities
- Step 2: Determine the scope or boundaries of the process
- Step 3: Determine the steps
- Step 4: Sequence the steps
- Step 5: Draw the flowchart using the appropriate symbols
- Step 6: Test the flowchart for completeness
- Step 7: Finalize the flowchart

As the flowchart (see Exhibit 16.5) indicates, it is important to review each of the steps with the group and build consensus on the scope of the process, the steps involved in the process, the sequence of the steps, and the decision to be made in each part of the process.

GAP ANALYSIS PROCESS EXAMPLE: THE DEVELOPMENT OF A PATIENT MEDICATION LIST USING THE PROCESS OF MEDICATION RECONCILIATION

Understanding Current State Through Workflow Analysis and Flowchart Development

To illustrate the gap analysis process we will use the development of a patient medication list using the process of medication reconciliation as an example. The process of developing a patient medication list took

EXHIBIT 16.3 TOP-DOWN FLOWCHART EXAMPLE

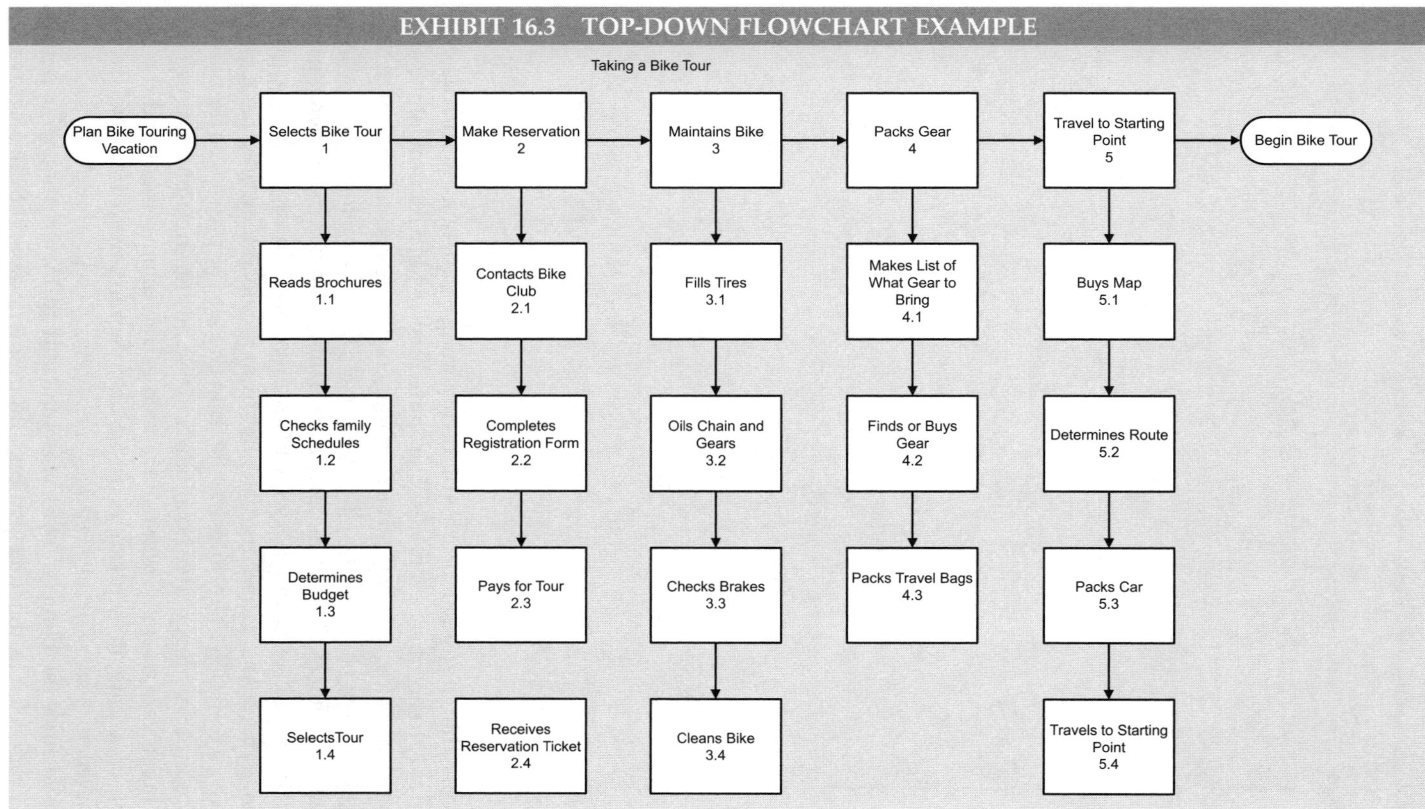

EXHIBIT 16.4 EXAMPLE OF A DEPLOYMENT FLOWCHART

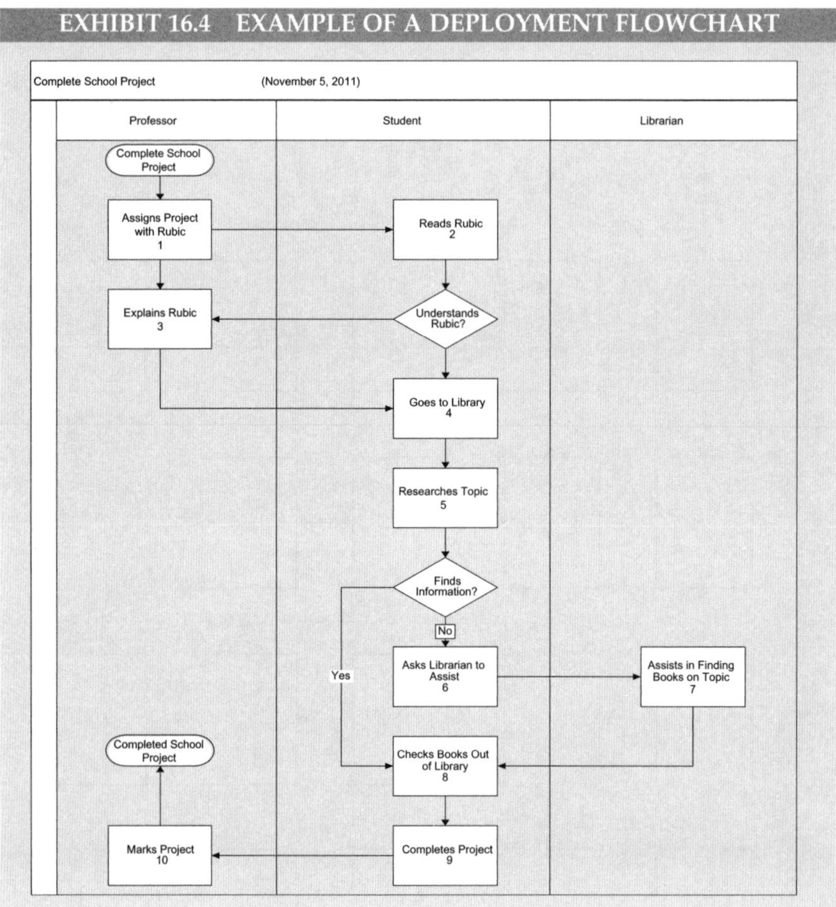

place within the overall process of transitioning a patient from an acute hospital stay to home care services. The team consisted of a referral intake staff, clinical director, patient service managers in charge of clinical teams, quality management staff, clinical specialist, and clinicians from a large home care agency. The home care referral intake staff worked from the hospital from where the patients were to be transferred. Ideally, having a physician, patient, and a discharge planner from the hospital would have made the team complete. The outcome the team chose to improve was decreasing the number of preventable hospitalizations. The literature cited a key driver for home care hospitalizations was medication management and the creation of a patient medication list as an intervention to improve patient adherence.

At first, the clinician staff was reluctant to the creation of a patient medication list as the intervention, citing how long and difficult it was to

EXHIBIT 16.5 FLOWCHARTING AT A GLANCE (BRASSARD, 1995)

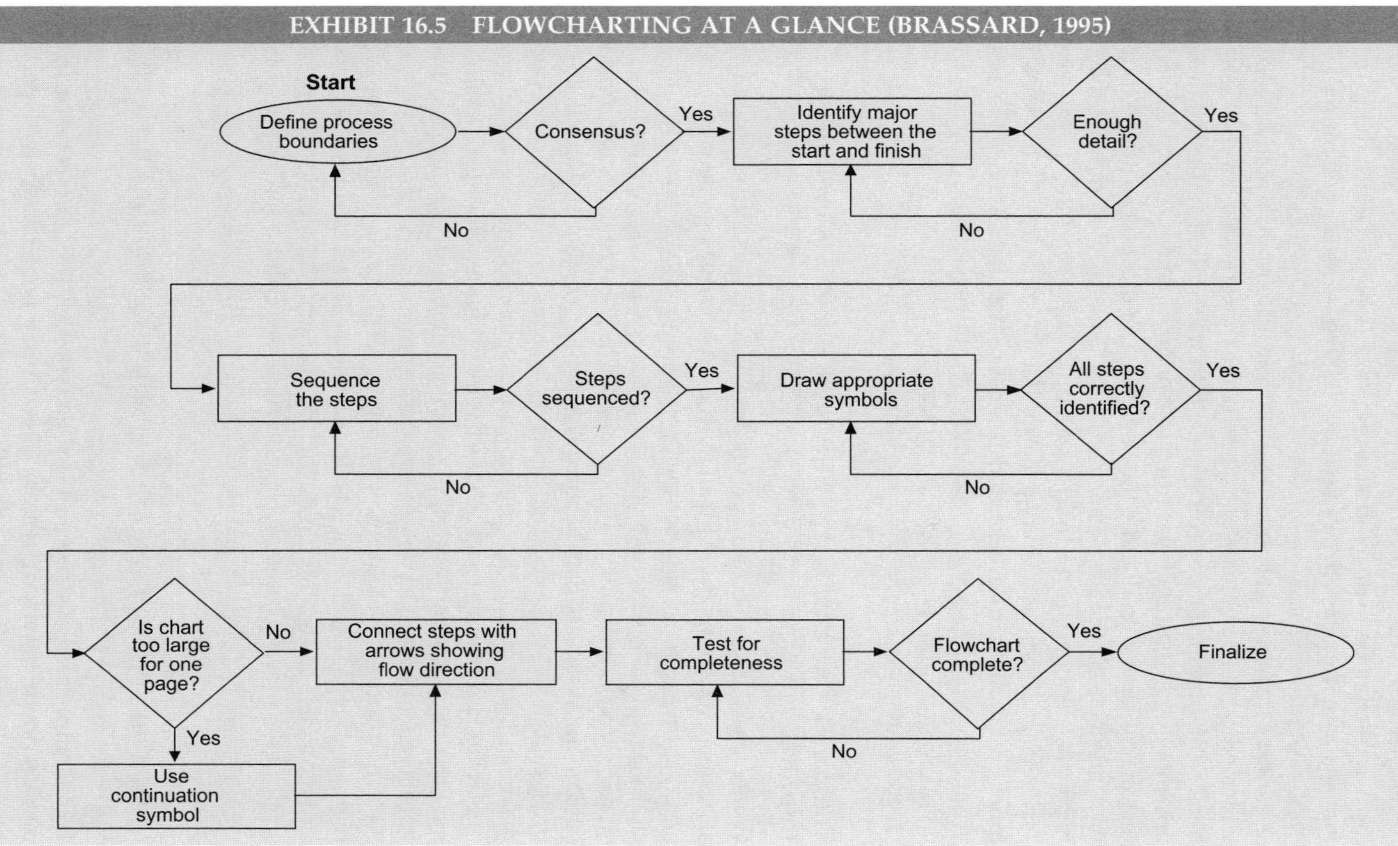

develop an accurate list. To further understand the challenges and barriers, it was agreed upon to develop a current state flowchart (see Exhibit 16.6) of the medication process from the time a patient is discharged from the hospital through the first 2 weeks of the home care services.

As the flowchart in Exhibit 16.6 illustrates, there were many challenges with medication management process at the transitional period of care. The intake staff obtained the medication list from the inpatient hospital record, not knowing if they changed prior to discharge. The agency policy stated that the clinician would verify the home care medications with the community physician on the first home care visit. Especially, from large teaching hospitals, the home care clinicians had difficulty reaching a physician to verify the medications, resulting in multiple attempts to call a doctor, sometimes over more than 2 weeks, and at times re-hospitalization of the patient. What also became apparent was that present practice and the documentation system did not support a clear definition of what medication reconciliation was.

Comparing Current State to EBP Identifying Opportunities for Improvement

What turned this project around for the clinicians was the recognition from all team members of how difficult the medication management process was and that the responsibility for the process cannot solely live with the field clinicians. It was agreed upon that the process was going to have to be redesigned incorporating an evidence-based definition of medication reconciliation; an accurate patient medication list as the end result of the process; and that there needed to be shared responsibility across departments and staff roles. This change in perception from "the clinicians are not trying hard enough to reach the doctor" (finger pointing) to evaluating the process opportunities for improvement moves an organization from a traditional culture to a process-oriented culture.

The process of medication reconciliation is broken down into three high-level steps. The three steps clarifies medications, verifies medications, and reconciles medications, along with documents medications focused the scope of the redesign project. The flowchart (see Exhibit 16.7) represents the macro-level flowchart that was developed by the team.

Integrating the Improvement Opportunities Into the Current State Flowchart, to Create EBP Protocol Flowchart

To visualize the recommended practice changes the team constructed on the top-down flowchart below. The current more detailed steps were organized under the more general steps of the medication reconciliation

EXHIBIT 16.6 CURRENT STATE: MEDICATION RECONCILIATION DEPLOYMENT FLOWCHART

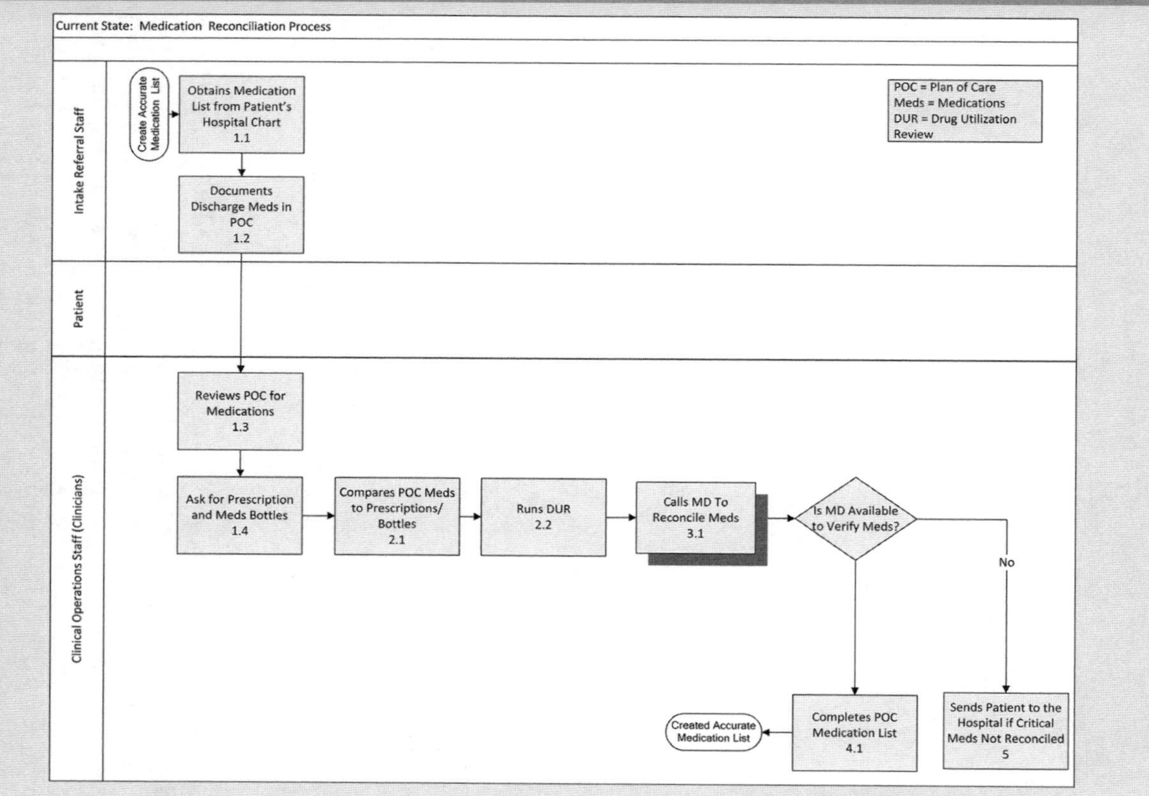

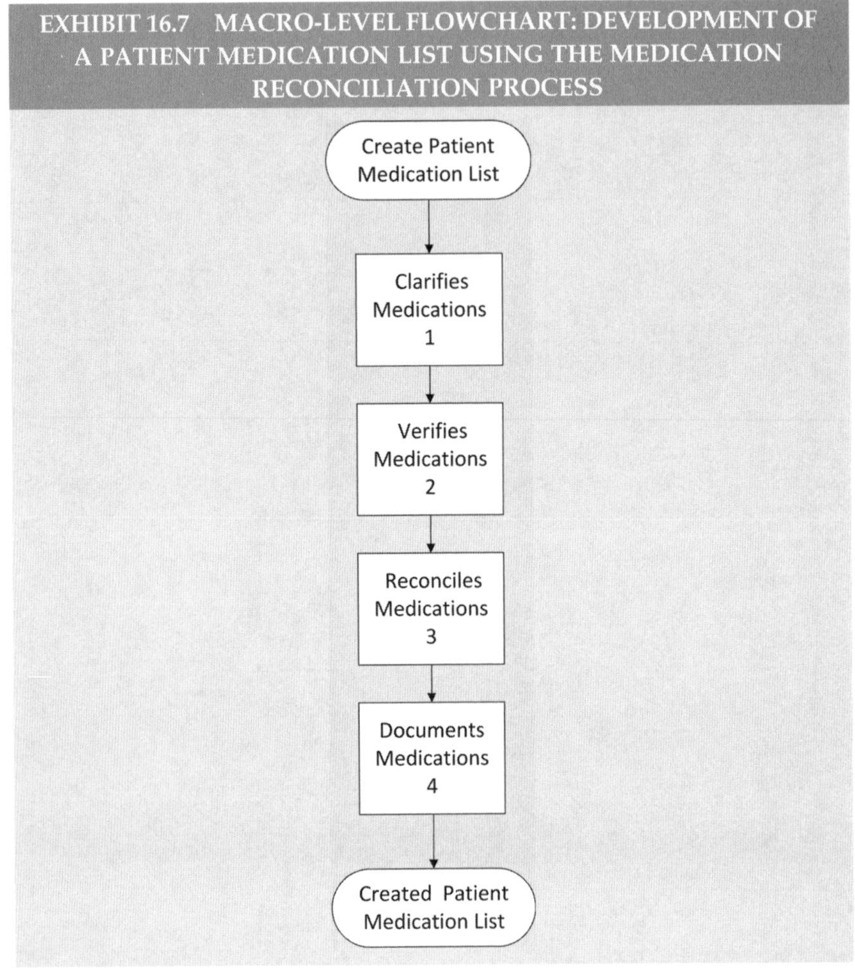

process, which gave the process an evidenced-based structure. The need to move the clarification of the medications further up-stream to prevent the need to clarify, verify, and reconcile the medications, all at once, at the point of calling the physician, became apparent. The use of the hospital discharge forms in clarifying medication is well documented in the literature and was incorporated into the practice change. In the flowchart (see Exhibit 16.8), "Ask for Signed Discharge Meds List" represents this added step.

When testing a new process the deployment flowchart is the best to use. As stated above, it clearly identifies roles, responsibilities, handoffs between staff and decision points. The flowchart, along with a data collection sheet, for measuring the success of each part of the new process, is used

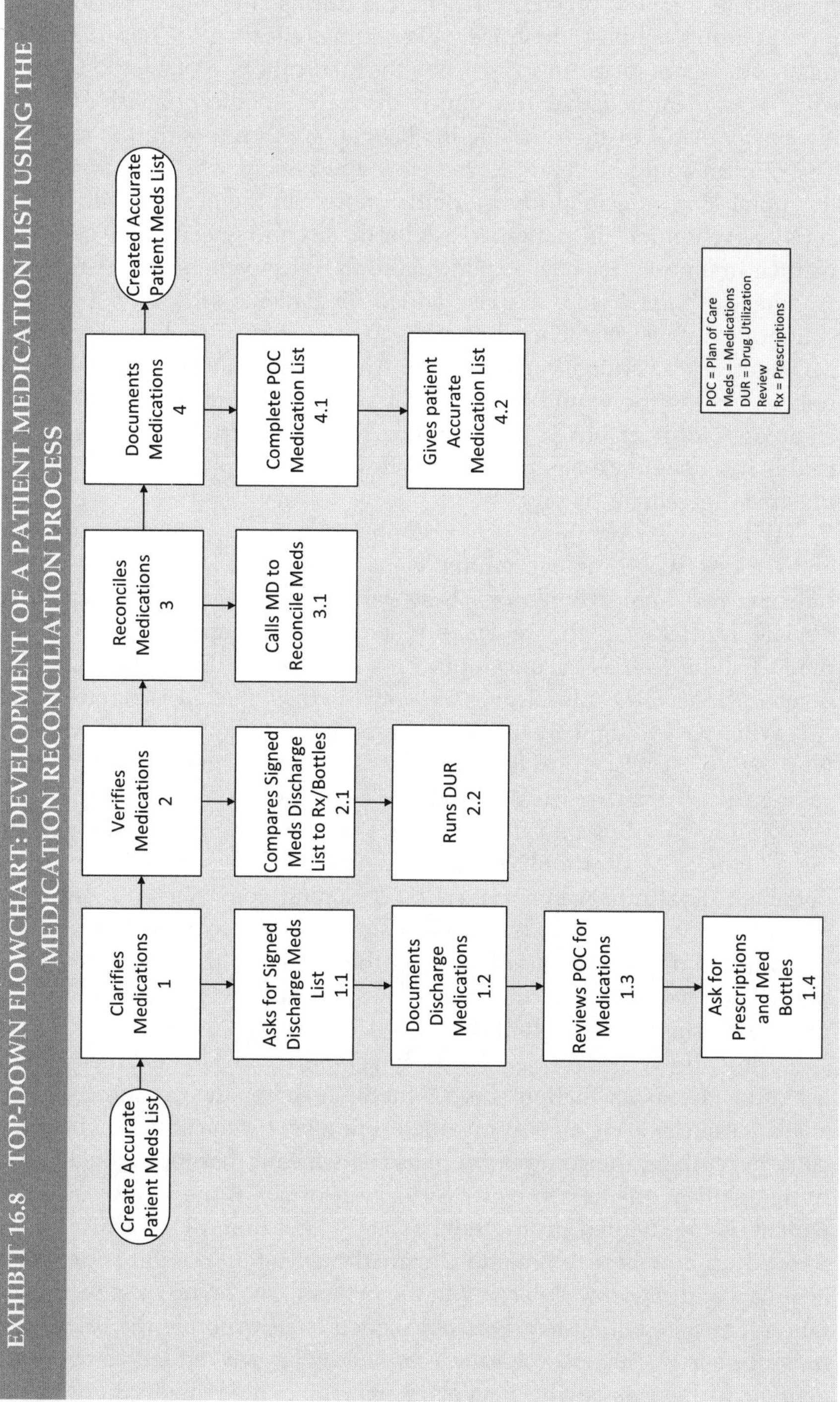

EXHIBIT 16.8 TOP-DOWN FLOWCHART: DEVELOPMENT OF A PATIENT MEDICATION LIST USING THE MEDICATION RECONCILIATION PROCESS

to evaluate the new practice change. It is during this testing period that gaps in inputs are best identified. When initially testing the new development of a patient medication list using the medication reconciliation protocol it was identified that the signed discharge medication list was not always available at the time the intake staff was processing the referral. The referral could be made days before the patient was discharged. At this point it was decided to include the patient in the process. The intake staff was to remind the patient to ask for the list and give it to the clinician on their first visit. This new step increased the effectiveness of the protocol. Another additional step was also added for patients who do not have a community physician. For these patients, the step of making a visiting MD referral was added to the process. An example of a patient who does not have a doctor would be a patient who has a scheduled follow-up clinic appointment but is homebound. The flowchart (see Exhibit 16.9) is the new evidence-based protocol flowchart developed through the illustrated gap analysis process.

When reviewing a process it is important to identify the path of steps and actions where, if everything went right, you would achieve the outcome you were striving for. These steps are "value added." Steps that deviate from this path are areas where further improvement can be made. Exhibit 16.10 is the development of a patient medication list deployment with the value-added steps indicated in the boxes shaded dark gray.

When reviewing the value-added process you may be asking yourself why the step "Calls MD to Reconcile Meds" is not included, knowing that calling the physician is very important at the start of home care services. Well, calling the physician at admission is very important but not for creating a "Patient Medication List" if the signed discharge medication list is obtained. The improvement idea of obtaining the "Signed Discharge Meds List" prevents the waits, delays, and rework of trying to reach the physician in the community. Involving the patient in their own care definitely adds value, but in this process we probably would not be able to control the standardization of this step.

The improvement project for the development of a patient medication list using the reconciliation process highlighted for the organization the challenges in creating an accurate medication list for the patient. The difficulty in reaching the community physicians meant that the reconciliation of the medications had to occur further upstream at the point when the patient is discharged from the hospital. The first two PDSA cycles focused on how best to obtain the signed medication discharge list from hospitals and *engaging the patient* in the process. The home care documentation management system was redesigned to incorporate the *medication reconciliation process* and the *patient medication list* was added as an intervention to help assist the patient in managing their medications. Both

EXHIBIT 16.9 DEPLOYMENT FLOWCHART: DEVELOPMENT OF A PATIENT MEDICATION LIST USING THE MEDICATION RECONCILIATION PROCESS

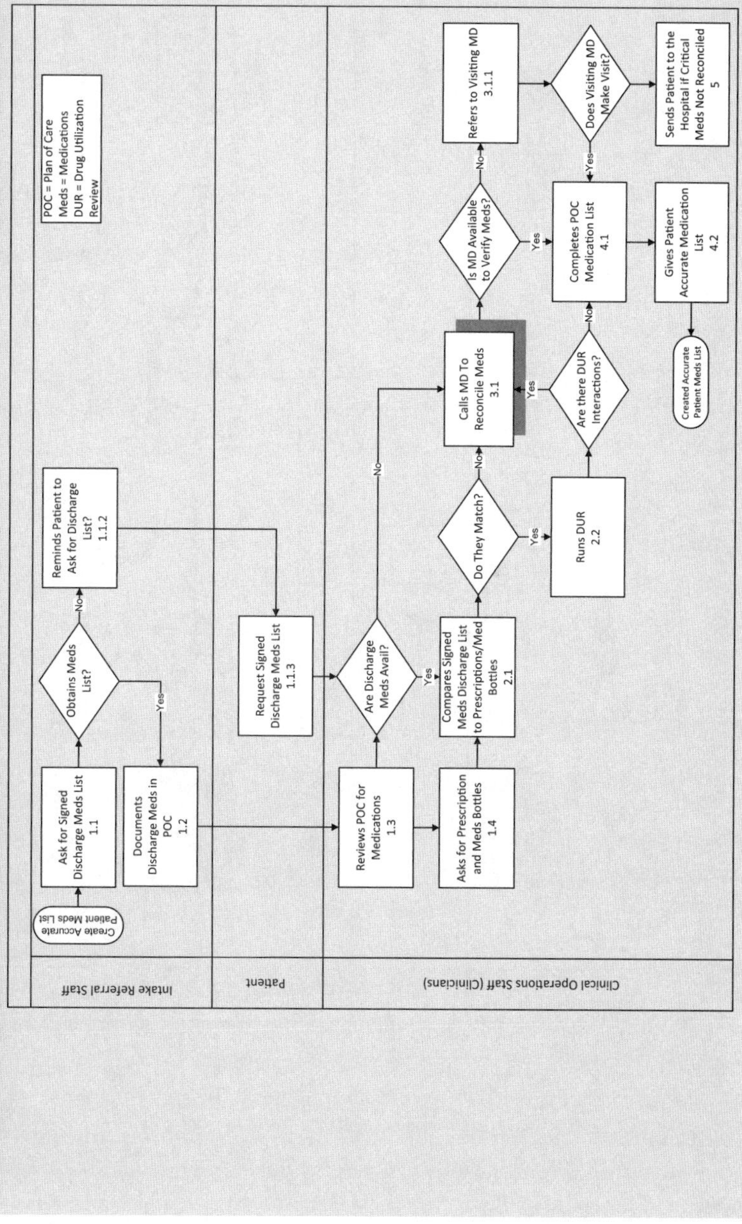

Intake Referral Staff

Create Accurate Patient Meds List

Ask for Signed Discharge Meds List 1.1

Obtains Meds List?

No

Reminds Patient to Ask for Discharge List? 1.1.2

Yes

Documents Discharge Meds in POC 1.2

POC = Plan of Care
Meds = Medications
DUR = Drug Utilization Review

Patient

Request Signed Discharge Meds List 1.1.3

Clinical Operations Staff (Clinicians)

Reviews POC for Medications 1.3

Are Discharge Meds Avail?

No

Yes

Asks for Prescription and Meds Bottles 1.4

Compares Signed Meds Discharge List to Prescriptions/Med Bottles 2.1

Do They Match?

No

Yes

Calls MD To Reconcile Meds 3.1

Runs DUR 2.2

Are there DUR Interactions?

Yes

No

Is MD Available to Verify Meds?

No

Yes

Refers to Visiting MD 3.1.1

Completes POC Medication List 4.1

Does Visiting MD Make Visit?

Yes

Gives Patient Accurate Medication List 4.2

Sends Patient to the Hospital if Critical Meds Not Reconciled 5

Created Accurate Patient Meds List

EXHIBIT 16.10 DEPLOYMENT OF VALUE-ADDED FLOWCHART: DEVELOPMENT OF A PATIENT MEDICATION LIST USING THE MEDICATION RECONCILIATION PROCESS

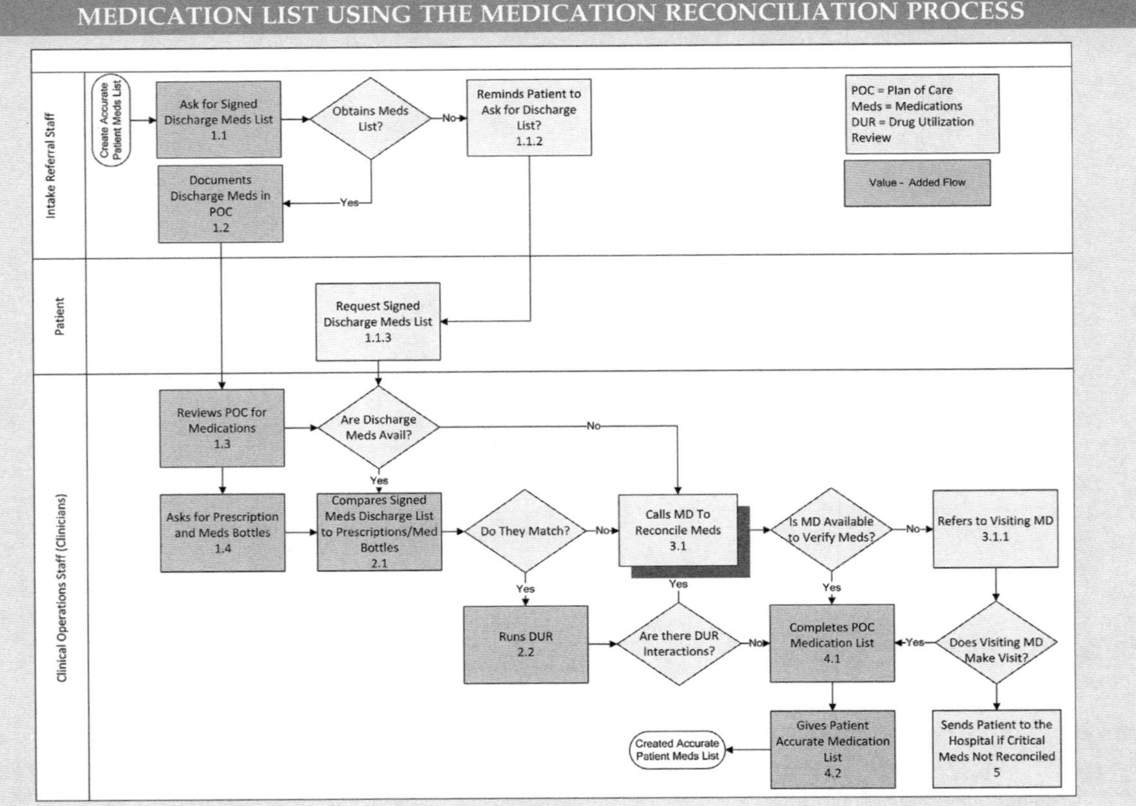

the awareness of the problem and the four improvement interventions have improved the overall outcome for medication management. Designing and standardizing a Visiting MD process is next in the improvement cycle.

SUMMARY

It is through the gap analysis process that an organization can effectively integrate EBP into their current operations. Too often organizations do not take the time to develop the skill in how to standardize their current processes, resulting in failed attempts in bringing change to their organizations. The gap analysis process as presented here is a systematic approach, using workflow analysis to understand current practice, bridge the gap between current and EBPs and develop a practice guideline that integrates EBP into current practice. It is in the innovation of integrating the EBP that an organization creates the necessary knowledge necessary to improve outcomes and remain competitive.

REFERENCES

Brassard, M., & Ritter, D. (1994). *The Memory Jogger II: A pocket guide of tools for continuous improvement & effective planning*. Salem: Goal/QPC.

Brown, J., & Duguid, P. (2000, May/June). Balancing act: How to capture knowledge without killing it. *Harvard Business Review*, 73–80.

Davenport, T., & Glaser, J. (2002, July). Just-in-time delivery comes to knowledge management. *Harvard Business Review*, 107–111.

Langley, G. J., Nolan, K., Norman, C. L., & Provost, L. P. (1996). *The improvement guide: A practical approach to enhancing organizational performance*. San Francisco: Jossey-Bass Publishers.

Levin, R. F., Keefer, J. M., Marren, J., Vetter, M., Lauder, B., & Sobolewski, S. (2010). Evidence-based practice: Merging two paradigms. *Journal of Nursing Care Quality*, *25*(2), 117–126.

Madison, D. J. (2005). *Process mapping, process improvement and process management: A practical guide for enhancing work and information flow*. Chico, CA: Paton Press LLC.

17

Outcome Evaluation for Programs Teaching EBP

Ellen Fineout-Overholt

One of the great mistakes is to judge policies and programs by their intentions rather than their results.

—Milton Friedman

As the seventh critical step of the evidence-based practice (EBP) process (Melnyk & Fineout-Overholt, 2011), evaluation of outcomes is integral to best practice and best education. Therefore, this imperative applies to learners (i.e., clinicians or students), educators, and programs. For clinician educators identifying criteria for evaluating a new orientee's performance, and academic instructors attempting to develop a "good" test item, evaluation of EBP principles is essential. In addition, evaluation of EBP education must span entire curricula. To relegate one class in orientation or one course in an academic program to EBP does the learner a disservice. Indeed, EBP must be integrated throughout clinical and didactic courses to maximize student assimilation of these principles (Coomarasamy & Khan, 2004; Fineout-Overholt & Johnston, 2005). All health care educational courses and programs need to integrate EBP into every offering/course. Subsequently, throughout the curriculum, courses must evaluate how well the learner learns, the educator educates, and the program conveys EBP principles. Most traditional evaluation techniques focus on evaluation of knowledge retention. While this type of evaluation is important, it is insufficient to provide educators with the full scope of how learners are integrating the knowledge desired for them to apply to their practices.

The mandate by the Institute of Medicine that 90% of health care decisions must be evidence based within the next few years (IOM, 2007) challenges educators in traditional health care education, academic, and clinical arenas to carefully evaluate whether or not clinicians are prepared to practice based on the best available evidence. Outcome evaluation of EBP learning must be one focus of health care education, and this evaluation must be consistent with methods that are used to teach EBP. Traditional methods of evaluation focus primarily on assessing knowledge retention and, therefore, do not provide enough scope to evaluate integration and application of EBP principles into students' and clinicians' practices. Both educator and learner need to fully understand the scope of EBP and then appropriate evaluation methods can be utilized.

The EBP paradigm should provide a framework that serves as the foundation for health care education. For this paradigm to be operational, clinical decision making must be based on a melding of (a) the best scientific evidence that is available; (b) the clinicians' expertise, which involves an understanding of how science (external evidence), the clinical environment, patient populations, practice-generated data (internal evidence), health care resource utilization, and life experiences influence clinician decision making; and (c) patients' choices, desires, and values for the current health care encounter. This paradigm allows for a dynamic clinician–patient relationship and focuses on unique outcomes for that patient. This dynamic aspect of the EBP paradigm allows for the myriad of patients who encounter and providers who work in, the health care system to receive and give individualized and best care (see Figure 17.1).

Every student must understand this paradigm and apply evidence-based decision making throughout their educational journey. It requires rethinking the usual evaluation methods used in nursing education as well. Educators must consider the most effective methods for evaluating

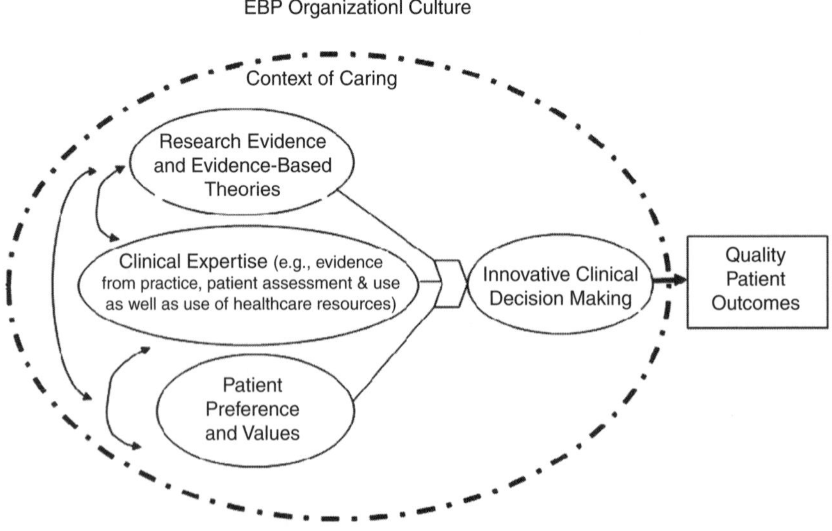

Source: © Melnyk & Fineout-Overholt, 2003.

FIGURE 17.1 EBP paradigm for evaluating learners.

how clinical decisions are made, with a particular emphasis on clinicians' integration of evidence, both internal and external, *in combination with* the impact of their expertise and the family/patient's values and preferences. Often, students and clinicians will be faced with how well they inform patients' preferences, so that their values are honored and best outcomes are achieved. Current health care educators must evaluate whether or not they are embracing these foundational principles in their educational philosophies and translating them to their curricula. These aspects of evidence-based decision making are important to teach and to evaluate; however, their evaluation is not likely to be encompassed in traditional educational outcome evaluation methods. Therefore, in this chapter, we are discussing a conceptual model to frame EBP evaluation, explore the infrastructure necessary to evaluate EBP principles, and offer practical methods for evaluating knowledge, skills, and application of EBP knowledge to practice.

A CONCEPTUAL MODEL FOR EVALUATION OF EVIDENCE-BASED PRACTICE

There are many ways to conceptualize evaluation in education. First, let us consider Kirkpatrick's (1994) foundational work that provided four levels of evaluation: reaction, learning, transfer, and results. Each of Kirkpatrick's levels of evaluation builds upon the next. Often in continuing education, *reaction* is the only level of evaluation (e.g., were the participants satisfied, did they feel whether the program met their objectives). The *learning* level encompasses the evaluation of knowledge and skills, and is often assessed via a written test or observation of activity (e.g., learners may be asked to demonstrate a skill). Evaluation of the extent to which a learner integrates EBP principles is called *transfer*. Transfer of knowledge and/or skill is not readily evaluated when teaching EBP. Researchers, however, have repeatedly demonstrated that individuals whose knowledge and beliefs in EBP increased after specific types of learning activities were more likely to transfer their knowledge to others (Melnyk, Fineout-Overholt, Giggleman, & Cruz, 2010; Melnyk et al., 2004; Wallen et al., 2010). Despite this positive learning opportunity, in a Cochrane systematic review, Parkes and colleagues (2004) found a dearth of evidence aimed at evaluating the effectiveness of teaching EBP, that is, how learners integrated EBP principles. In their review of 47 studies on teaching EBP, they found one randomized controlled trial (RCT) that met their criteria for evaluating the effectiveness of teaching critical appraisal of outcomes. Furthermore, Horsley and colleagues (2011), in their Cochrane review, found that the body of research that spoke to the impact on patient outcomes of teaching critical appraisal to health professionals was methodologically inadequate to draw a firm conclusion. Opportunity abounds for improving how educators evaluate learners' integration of EBP into their decision making.

For transfer of knowledge and skills, the EBP paradigm and principles must be diffusely integrated across the curriculum, both in clinical or academic settings; otherwise, a "disconnect" may be perceived by learners between the EBP paradigm and process and their practice, increasing the challenge of accurate evaluation. For learners to grasp the need for integrating EBP principles and to effectively evaluate this transfer of information, the culture must be imbued with EBP. Evaluation of Kirkpatrick's *results* demonstrates that principles of EBP are not only integrated but applied. For learners of EBP, this level of evaluation would indicate that they have fully internalized the paradigm shift and now operate in a culture and mindset underpinned by EBP principles. The challenges increase for educators as they strive to adequately evaluate at the *transfer* and *results* levels of evaluation.

Kirkpatrick's (1994) levels of evaluation focus primarily on the learner. For comprehensive information on how well EBP is being taught, the educator and the program need to be evaluated as well. Program and educator evaluations may influence each other. For example, the program may be well designed; however, the educator may have difficulty in communicating principles to learners and evaluation of the program may not reflect the excellence in design. For successful, accurate evaluation of programs, educators need to be skilled in EBP and other content areas that they are responsible to teach to learners. A faculty member indicated the following wisdom in an EBP workshop for educators, "we cannot teach what we do not know" (D. Hrabe, 2005, personal communication). Educators need to be mentored to set their own evaluation goals and be encouraged to take time to self-reflect to determine if they are meeting them. As an initial step, it is helpful to ask self-evaluation questions to assist in determining factors that may influence educators' effectiveness (see Exhibit 17.1). In addition, learner and program evaluation data can assist educators to know how well they are meeting their goals. These important steps to evaluation of how well a program is comprehensively meeting its completion goals are graphically represented as a suggested conceptual framework in Figure 17.2. This EBP model for educators is built upon the highly successful ARCC clinical practice model (see Chapter 1) and is titled, Advancing Research and Clinical Practice through Close Collaboration and Education (ARCC-E).

To determine the effectiveness of educational programs, goals first must be determined. Program goals would reflect the evaluation results expected of the learner, which should be based on the curricular philosophy and paradigm. In addition, these goals would determine the

EXHIBIT 17.1 INITIAL QUESTIONS FOR EVALUATION OF EDUCATOR EFFECTIVENESS

1. To what extent is the care that I deliver to my patients evidence-based?
2. How much do I believe that basing my care on the best evidence will lead to the highest quality outcomes for my clients and their families?
3. How much knowledge of the EBP process do I possess?
4. Do I have strong knowledge and skills related to EBP?
5. What is my personal commitment to EBP?
6. Do I model EBP in clinical settings?
7. Do I have adequate computer skills?
8. Do I have a relationship with librarians who have knowledge of EBP who can assist with EBP?

outcomes to be evaluated. For example, if the program goal was to produce nurses who practiced based on evidence in conjunction with their clinical expertise and with data about patient values and preferences (see Figure 17.1), then the outcomes to be measured could be the: (a) extent to

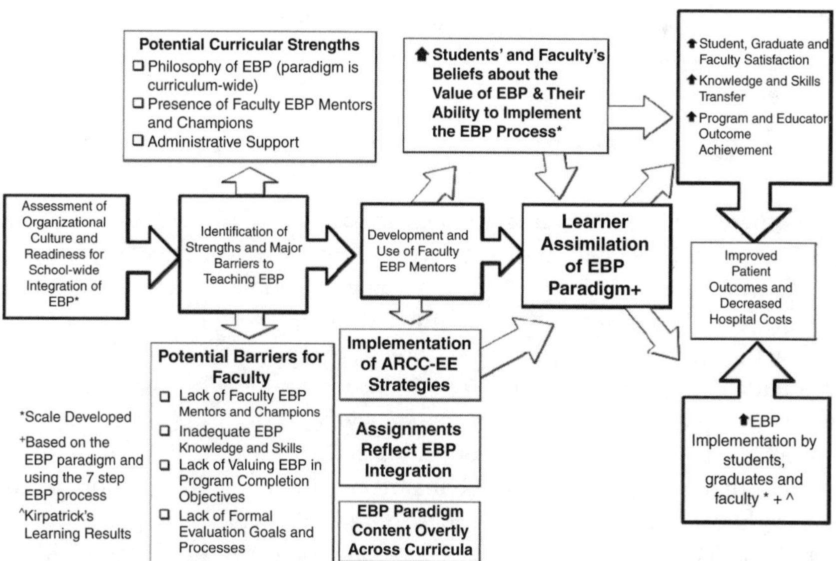

Source: © Fineout-Overholt & Melnyk 2011.

FIGURE 17.2 ARCC-E (Advancing Research and Clinical Practice through close Collaboration and Education) conceptual model for teaching EBP.

which clinicians' practices are based on the best available external and internal evidence; (b) extent to which clinicians seek assistance in using the evidence as needed; and (c) extent to which clinicians gather and use information about patient preferences and values.

Key stakeholders are essential to evaluating the process by which EBP is taught, and each stakeholder must have the opportunity to provide input into what the process should be, including consideration of how this process impacts the product of the program, how the EBP paradigm underpins the program, and how the process influences the overall difference the program makes in the professional community. For example, if the EBP teaching program is in the clinical setting, the educator may gather perspectives from those in administration, care providers, receivers of care, and other educators about what the outcomes of the program need to be to meet these key stakeholders' expectations. Their expectations may assist in determining the content and methods chosen for the program. In addition, the perspectives of those who will receive the program, its participants, will provide the educator with a preliminary estimate of the proposed impact of the program. This impact will then need to be evaluated to determine if it was realized. Other outcomes will become evident through discussions with key stakeholders about what impact they view the EBP teaching program will have on the community or agency. Measurement of these outcomes will indicate the program's success to the educator, the key stakeholders, and others. It is important to remember that measures of outcome, process, and impact must consider cultural, language, and gender differences (Bakken, 2002).

INFRASTRUCTURE TO SUPPORT EVALUATION

Congruence between the mission and philosophy of the organization and an EBP program's goals and objectives is imperative for effectively evaluating these principles in teaching. Having a designated cadre of educators whose focus is primarily on evaluation strategies for learners, educators, and entire programs facilitates a consistent approach toward program evaluation and enhancement. Yet, in order to function at the desired level, designated resources are necessary for educators to be able to collect data on their teaching effectiveness and learners' integration of content that is taught. Clear mechanisms need to be delineated for educators to know the procedure to collect data in the least biased manner. In addition, feedback loops must be evident for how those data will be returned to educators, who subsequently will use them to improve their courses/classes. Cultivating enthusiastic educators is essential for effective role models in EBP who set the stage for effective evaluation of EBP principles. Some of the resources necessary to evaluate teaching programs are computers and database software to house and analyze data about individualized programs, educator goals, and learner goals. In addition, ongoing educator development programs are necessary to provide the latest and best evidence in strategies for teaching EBP (Kiessling, Lewitt, & Henriksson, 2011; Krugman, 2003).

How faculty development is approached generally can make a difference in outcomes (Gruppen, Frohna, Anderson, & Lowe, 2003). For example, educators responded positively to a collaborative, cutting-edge program that fostered faculty development through mentorship (Fineout-Overholt, Stillwell, Cox, Robbins, & Williamson, 2010; Murad et al., 2009; Pololi, Knight, Dennis, & Frankel, 2002). Part of mentorship consists of assisting educators to shift their paradigm toward EBP, including turning data produced during normal educational activities into program improvements. Specified mechanisms for data to be consistently returned to the educator contribute to a positive culture of using data for program improvement.

STRATEGIES FOR LEARNER EVALUATION

Methods of learner evaluation are the backbone of knowing how well a curriculum reflects EBP and how well educators teach this paradigm and its principles. Review of a few of the available methods to evaluate learners' EBP knowledge and skills as well as their application and integration, particularly those related to planning and reflection, is timely.

Planning

One of the first steps to successful curricula is to plan for evaluation from the beginning. For example, before educators offer a program and then apply for continuing education credit, they must identify their objectives, methods to meet them, and measures that will evaluate whether or not they are met. The measures of evaluation and accompanying successful criteria must be clearly identified. Educators must consider what assignments they will use to evaluate learners' knowledge, skill, and application of EBP information presented in health care professions' programs. These assignments need to be clearly articulated for the learner. Learners do not need to be using their energy trying to decipher what are the successful criteria for evaluating their learning. Rather, they need to be fully engaged in the EBP paradigm and process and demonstrate their integration and proficiency in them both.

In planning for evaluation, budget considerations are important. It is also essential that all key stakeholders have "buy-in" on how evaluation methods will be used as well as the feedback of data for the purpose of improving EBP education. An attitude of continuous improvement in educational courses/classes provides a context for data collection and interpretation (Beecroft, Kunsman, Taylor, Gevenis, & Guzek, 2004).

Reflection

Another method to evaluate the learning of EBP that I want to touch on in this chapter is reflection. Reflection, according to Sparks and colleagues (1991), is being aware of one's thoughts, feelings, beliefs, and behaviors and how these influence one's interpretation of health care situations. Cole and colleagues (2004) discussed the need for education to have an experiential aspect that includes reflection. Using reflection to assist learners in their integration of EBP stretches them to dig deeper into ownership of their learning and to determine, by their own yardstick, their growth and progress. This intrinsic evaluation is key to sustainable paradigm shift and integration of EBP principles into learners' daily decision making; however, it is often perceived as requiring too much time for the return on investment. For educators to use reflection appropriately, this evaluation method must be both formative (i.e., used along the way) and summative (re-reflection of the formative reflection). Reflection aids learners to better engage the process of becoming professionals (Branch, 2011; Kelly, 2011). As learners use reflection to evaluate their own progress, they will better understand what they have learned and how far they have come.

Learners' capacity for understanding each step of the EBP process needs to be evaluated, for example, how a learner formulates the clinical question; if the question drives the search strategy; whether or not the search strategy is streamlined and focused. Also important for educators is the evaluation of how the learner gathers evidence other than research. For example, evidence from the history and physical exam enters into the decision-making process and the accuracy and efficiency of gathering this evidence need to be evaluated (Munro, 2004). How well learners assess patients' preferences and what they value in life is important to determine. In addition, integration of evidence-based theories to inform practice is essential to learners' evidence-based decision making. While in recent years, there have been several scales developed to measure EBP outcomes, for individual clinicians and for organizations, there is a paucity of information about how to evaluate these aspects of EBP. Since the primary focus of clinical education and academic EBP courses is on interpretation of research, the evaluation strategies tend to focus on this aspect as well. The evaluation methods of a well-rounded EBP program will reflect all aspects of evidence-based clinical decision making.

To assist educators and learners with evaluation, in 2009 Tilson and colleagues (2011) conducted a consensus building project at the International Conference of Evidence-based Healthcare Teachers and Developers to establish a rubric for evaluating different measures of EBP. "CREATE" (Classification Rubric of EBP Assessment Tools in Education) was thus born. From this work, the team suggested that areas of evaluation include benefits to patients, behaviors, skills, knowledge, self-efficacy, attitudes, and reaction to educational experiences. Furthermore, this team provided an overview of seven different EBP measures and how they met the established rubric: Berlin Scale (Fritsche, Greenhalgh, Falck-Ytter, Neumayer, & Kunz, 2002); EBP Attitudes Scale (Aaron, 2010); EBP Beliefs Scale and EBP Implementation Scale (Melnyk, Fineout-Overholt, & Mays, 2008); Evidence-based Practice Confidence (Salbach & Jaglal, 2010); Knowledge, Attitudes, Access, and Confidence Evaluation (Hendricson et al., 2011) and the Fresno Scale (Ramos, Schafer, & Tracz, 2003).

While these more standardized, established measures can be used across settings, other evaluation strategies may differ depending on the setting of the learner. For example, in the clinical setting, an evidence-based performance improvement project can provide evaluation of transfer of knowledge and skills to a clinical situation. Levin et al. (2010) offer a blended EBP and performance improvement paradigm as a framework for this daily focus on quality outcomes. Performance or quality improvement projects offer an opportunity to evaluate learners' ability to apply the evidence-based knowledge to a clinical issue clearly substantiated by internal evidence. These issues tend to be smaller in scope and focused on a single issue or problem. A successful outcomes management program can be used to determine if the learner has reached the results level of integration of knowledge and skill. This type of program focuses on continuous improvement of practice by monitoring specified outcome data and using those results for practice improvement.

In an academic setting an EBP synthesis paper can assist in evaluating learners' integration of EBP principles. This kind of paper allows the learner to demonstrate skills gained in writing a clinical question, searching for best evidence, and critically appraising evidence for validity and applicability. Exhibit 17.2 provides an example of criteria that could be used for an EBP synthesis paper.

A project using evidence to generate an outcomes management plan for real-life clinical practice can assist in evaluating the application of evidence to practice. Essential to this evaluation method is application of the evidence, in combination with the clinicians' expertise and families/patients' preferences and values. Exhibit 17.3 provides an example of criteria that could be used for an outcomes management project evaluation.

EXHIBIT 17.2 SAMPLE CRITERIA FOR EBP SYNTHESIS PAPER

10 pages maximum, excluding references and table
Part 1 (90 points)

1. **Describe the background and outline the clinically meaningful question** (5 points).
   Support why ask the question, address each of the PICO (population, intervention, comparison, and outcome) components, provide specific epidemiological data.
2. **Discuss the search process, including sources and results** (5 points).
   Databases, keywords, limits, combinations, number found (per database and final number included), Inclusion/exclusion criteria (DO NOT LIMIT TO FULL TEXT).
3. **Discuss the critical appraisal of evidence, including appropriateness of statistics** (30 points).
   Synthesize information from studies reviewed citing table. Clearly present details of reviewed studies (not background articles) in table with sufficient detail (no sentences, be succinct). Address critical appraisal questions of what are the results, if they are valid results (e.g., strengths & weaknesses of studies), and applicability to the question. Identify statistics (NNT, OR, RRR, ARR, or more traditional tests), give details about them (in table), interpret statistics in text.
   (a) **Evaluation Table** listing each study included in the review, including the (a) author(s) & date of publication, (b) title, (c) conceptual framework, (d) study design, (e) major variables studied, (f) sample description, (g) measurement instruments for each variable, (h) data analysis used, (i) study findings, and (j) study strengths and weaknesses. (DO NOT include these kinds of details in the narrative portion of the paper. Instead refer the reader to the table.)
   (b) **Synthesis Table**(s) that feature data across studies that are common, disparate, connecting or disjointed. Be sure to include only data that tell the story of the evidence. Too much information will make a synthesis table unusable.
4. **State the conclusions (not findings) about evidence** (10 points).
   Flows from evidence, true conclusions about evidence not findings.
5. **Discuss the implications for practice based on the evidence** (from a population standpoint, not personal practice; 10 points).

Identify a **preliminary** plan that flows from evidence, provide specific steps.

6. **Outline the obstacles, facilitators, and challenges to the preliminary plan** (5 points).
   Name or address presence or lack of each, explain how to overcome the ones identified or how to use facilitators.
7. **Discuss the outcomes for preliminary plan** (10 points).
   Name outcomes for evaluation of plan, define how to measure and the time frame for measuring the outcomes, provide definite link to plan for addressing evidence
8. **Describe the contribution of your chosen EBP theory to your preliminary plan** (5 points).
   Briefly explain theory and apply theory to your plan.
9. **Describe the expected benefit of the evidence to *your personal practice*** and include theoretical implications (15 points).
   Speak to your clinical expertise (including ability to interpret research reports) and the assessment data on patient preferences and values.
10. **Reflection: Describe how your evaluation of using the EBP process in writing the paper (from formulating the question to outcome evaluation)** is clear (5 points).

Part 2 (10 points)

1. Argument is clearly and logically presented (8 points).
   Paper builds on each section, connections are clear.
2. APA format is correct (3 points).
   Properly cite in text, properly cite reference list, attend to grammar and punctuation.

EXHIBIT 17.3 SAMPLE ASSESSMENT CRITERIA FOR OUTCOMES MANAGEMENT PROJECT

Evidence base of project is clear (15 points). (Include evidence (external evidence) to support why you need to do this project, i.e., support that there is insufficient or no evidence to fully answer your clinical question; provide evidence that there is an existing problem—baseline data (internal evidence) to support that the

(*continued*)

EXHIBIT 17.3 (*continued*)

problem does indeed exist; evidence of family/patient preferences and values and how influences project; influence of collective group clinical expertise.

Clinically meaningful question is clear (5 points). Use PICO.

Project outcomes are reasonable and clearly identified (5 points). The outcomes flow from the question. All possible outcomes are considered and addressed to answer the question.

Data collection methods (sources & process) are clear (5 points). How obtained approval, collection tool (submission with project is required), who is collecting data, and from whom or what.

Data analysis approach assists in answering the clinical question (5 points). Did you use the right statistical test for the level of data you collected?

Proposed presentation of data is clear (10 points). Graphs are readable on slide/handout, anchors are identified. All data are presented to audience in written form, slide/handout. Data are **synthesized**. Do not provide raw data to audience. Raw data must be submitted with presentation packet for grading.

Implications *for practice changes* based on the data and supporting evidence are clear (10 points). What your data tell you that needs to be different in practice, particularly in light of the existing evidence [internal & external].

Plan for change is clear (5 points). Specific steps for change. Include theoretical framework for change.

Anticipated barriers, facilitators, and challenges *to change* are clear (5 points). These are specific to plan for change.

Outcomes for evaluation *of plan* are clear and measurable including costs (10 points).

Dissemination plan is clear and feasible (5 points). What are you going to do with the information that you gathered in your project?

Lessons learned through the use of the EBP process are clear (2 points). Evaluation of how the project changed based on what you learned while doing it, or what you would have done differently.

EXHIBIT 17.3 (*continued*)

PowerPoint slides and supporting documents enhance presentation (6 points).

1. Group work is evident in the presentation
2. Handouts were helpful to learning
3. PowerPoint presentation was creative
4. Completed presentation within time limit

Overall argument is compelling & worthy of clinician change in practice (10 points).

Packet to be turned in for grading: (2 points)

1. Hard copy of slides in 4-on-a-page format
2. Handout
3. Data collection tool
4. Raw data and summarized data

METHODS OF EDUCATOR EVALUATION

Educators cannot rely solely upon standardized criteria that are gathered centrally and that are applied across all instructors in an organization. Certainly, these learner evaluations can provide important insight into how well the educator is communicating with this group; however, generic evaluations that provide only a number to rate the educator against a set of standardized criteria are not specific enough to provide data for improving teaching skills, especially in relation to EBP. For this level of specificity the educator may have to request data from the learners in a nonstandardized way. Table 17.1 provides an example of the types of questions educators may ask to gather evaluation information to improve teaching, although it is still helpful to quantify data, if appropriate, and have a database set up for data entry. Qualitative information needs to be analyzed appropriately and can provide a rich perspective for educators about their success in communicating EBP principles, particularly learner transfer and results evaluation, as well as program process and outcome evaluation.

Educators need to be cognizant of the impact their teaching style has on learners. Contagion theory when applied to communication indicates that learners' attitudes, values, and behaviors trend from those in their communication network (Carley & Kaufer, 1993). This is evidenced in education when the value an educator places on content they are teaching

TABLE 17.1 Informal Survey to Improve the Course

• What would be changed to make the learning experience for this course better?					
• What was the best part of course?					
• Rate the required tests Mark an X in the appropriate box	Poor	Okay	Not so bad	Pretty good	Excellent
TEXT 1					
TEXT 2					
• Were there any articles especially helpful to the understanding of course content?					
• How can the courses 1 and 2 be more seamless?					
• Suggestions for improving teaching effectiveness?					
• What were benefits of writing the EBP paper?					
• How could the EBP paper be improved as a learning experience?					
• What were the benefits of Outcomes Management project?					
• How could the Outcomes Management project be improved as a learning experience?					
• Other comments about this course or the educator					

is reflected onto learners. Often the best way to evaluate an educator's impact is to ask learners about their perception of how educators valued what they taught and their enthusiasm about the content (Glick, 2002). Other strategies for evaluating educators may include: questioning the educator about self-generated goals, agency goals for programs, and key stakeholders' expectations. Also, evaluation of how an educator creates a culture of data gathering for improving teaching/practice needs to be conducted. For other educators and learners to evaluate, the teachers' enthusiasm for EBP and how it influences evidence-based teaching and/or practice is helpful to understanding program and learner outcomes.

PROGRAM OR OFFERING EVALUATION

In an academic or a clinical setting where there are a series of required courses (e.g., a critical care orientation series), it is imperative that all courses reflect integration of EBP principles. Having only core courses (e.g., an EBP principles course) providing learners with EBP content without application in other areas, particularly clinical courses, reinforces the disconnect that often exists between research and practice. Workshops on EBP can provide a starting point for clinicians where they can gain knowledge and skills; however, educators must provide further opportunities to integrate knowledge and skill in a clinical context. Establishing relevant links between EBP initiatives and patient outcomes is a starting point for evaluating clinical programs that teach EBP.

Gathering evidence from clinicians who are entering, and then upon graduating or completing a clinical program, about the use of EBP principles, is important to program evaluation. Exhibit 17.4 contains examples of questions for those who have completed EBP teaching programs.

EXHIBIT 17.4 EXAMPLES OF QUESTIONS FOR EVALUATING EBP PROGRAM EFFECTIVENESS

Closed Questions:

1. I am confident that critically appraising evidence is an important step in the EBP process.
2. I discussed evidence from a research study with a practice colleague at least three times weekly.
3. The content I learned in ________________ (fill in the blank with the course/program of interest) has helped me to implement EBP principles.

Open Questions:

1. How has your confidence in critically appraising evidence increased since taking ________________ (fill in the blank with the course/program of interest) program?
2. How does discussing evidence with colleagues influence your daily practice?
3. How did attending ________________ (fill in the blank with the course/program of interest) program/course make a difference in how you practiced?

Evaluating integration and application of EBP principles is most important for these clinicians.

INTENTIONAL EVALUATION OF EBP RESULTS IS EXPECTED TO INFLUENCE CHANGES IN HEALTH CARE

Even with the latest advances in EBP measurement, developing a program of evaluation for teaching EBP can sometimes seem daunting. Often there are competing priorities for educators and learners. Intentionality with measurement makes it a primary goal of an educational program. The data gathered through outcome measurement and evaluation are valuable to ongoing planning and processes of the program. Intentional prioritization of what is important for learners to take away from clinical and academic programs can help educators know what is important to evaluate. Unfortunately, it is well established that knowing does not necessarily translate into intentionally gathering meaningful evaluation data that influence how health care professionals are educated, much like knowing EBP principles does not necessarily equal best practice (Davis et al., 1999).

Making a difference in health care requires commitment from educators who intentionally evaluate learner, educator, and program outcomes as part of an ongoing educational plan. These outcome data are internal evidence for educators that enable them to know that their "practice" of education is evidence based as they prepare clinicians who provide best care for health care consumers.

REFERENCES

Aarons, G. A. (2004). Mental health provider attitudes toward adoption of evidence-based practice: The Evidence-Based Practice Attitude Scale (EBPAS). *Mental Health Services Research*, *6*(2), 61–74.

Bakken, L. (2002). An evaluation plan to assess the process and outcomes of a learner-centered training program for clinical research. *Medical Teacher*, *24*(2), 162–168.

Beecroft, P., Kunsman, L., Taylor, S., Gevenis, E., & Guzek, F. (2004). Bridging the gap between school and workplace: Developing a new graduate. *Journal of Nursing Administration*, *34*(8), 338–345.

Benner, P., & Leonard, V. (2005). Patient concerns, choices and clinical judgment in evidence-based practice. In B. M. Melnyk, & E. Fineout-Overholt (Eds.), *Evidence-based practice in nursing and healthcare: A guide to best practice* (pp. 163–182). Philadelphia: Lippincott, Williams & Wilkins.

Bryant-Lukosius, D., & DiCenso, A. (2004). A framework for the introduction and evaluation of advanced practice nursing roles. *Journal of Advanced Nursing*, *48*(5), 530–540.

Carley, K. M., & Kaufer, D. S. (1993). Semantic connectivity: An approach for analyzing symbols in semantic networks. *Communication Theory, 3*, 183–213.

Cole, K., Barker, L., Kolodner, K., Williamson, P., Wright, S., & Kern, D. (2004). Faculty development in teaching skills: An intensive longitudinal model. *Academic Medicine, 79*(5), 469–480.

Coomarasamy, A., & Khan, K. S. (2004) What is the evidence that postgraduate teaching in evidence based medicine changes anything? A systematic review. *British Medical Journal, 329*(7473), 1017–1022.

Davis, D., O'Brien, M., Freemantle, N., Wolf, F., Mazmanian, P., & Taylor-Vaisey, A. (1999). Impact of formal continuing medical education: Do conferences, workshops, rounds, and other traditional continuing education activities change physician behavior or health care outcomes? *JAMA, 282*(9), 867–874.

Fineout-Overholt, E., & Johnston, L. (2005). Teaching EBP: A challenge for educators in the 21st century. *Worldviews on Evidence-based Nursing, 2*(1), 37–39.

Fritsche, L., Greenhalgh, T., Falck-Ytter, Y., Neumayer, H. H., & Kunz, R. (2002). Do short courses in evidence-based medicine improve knowledge and skills? Validation of Berlin Questionnaire and before and after study of courses in evidence-based medicine. *British Medical Journal, 325*, 1338–1341.

Glick, T. (2002). How best to evaluate clinician–educators and teachers for promotion? *Academic Medicine, 77*(5), 392–397.

Gruppen, L., Frohna, A., Anderson, R., & Lowe, K. (2003). Faculty development for educational leadership and scholarship. *Academic Medicine, 78*(2), 137–141.

Hendricson, W. D., Rugh, J. D., Hatch, J. P., Stark, D. L., Deahl, T., & Wallmann, E. R. (2011). Validation of an instrument to assess evidence-based practice knowledge, attitudes, access and confidence in the dental environment. *Journal of Dental Education, 75*(2), 131–144.

Holloway, R., Nesbit, K., Bordley, D., & Noyes, K. (2004). Teaching and evaluating first and second year medical students' practice of evidence-based medicine. *Medical Education, 38*, 868–878.

Horsley, T., Hyde, C., Santesso, N., Parkes, J., Milne, R., & Stewart, R. (2011). Teaching critical appraisal skills in health care settings. *Cochrane Database of Systematic Reviews*, Issue 11. Art. No.: CD001270. DOI: 10.1002/14651858.CD001270.pub2.

Institute of Medicine. (2007). *Evidence-based medicine and the changing nature of health care*. Washington, DC: National Academy of Sciences.

Kessenich, C., Guyatt, G., & DiCenso, A. (1997). Teaching nursing students evidence-based nursing. *Nurse Educator, 22*(6), 25–29.

Kirkpatrick, D. L. (1994). *Evaluating training programs: The four levels.* San Francisco, CA: Berrett-Koehler.

Kiessling, A., Lewitt, M., & Henriksson, P. (2009) Case-based training of evidence-based clinical practice in primary care and decreased mortality in patients with coronary heart disease. *Annals of Family Medicine, 9*(3), 211–218.

Krugman, M. (2003). Evidence-based practice: The role of staff development. *Journal of Staff Development, 19*(6), 279–285.

Levin, R. F., Fineout-Overholt, E., Melnyk, B. M., Barnes, M., & Vetter, M. J. (2011). Fostering evidence-based practice to improve nurse and cost outcomes in a community health setting: A pilot test of the advancing research and clinical practice through close collaboration model. *Nursing Administration Quarterly, 35*(1), 21–33.

Melnyk, B., & Fineout-Overholt, E. (2011). *Evidence-based practice in nursing & health-care: A guide to best practice*. Philadelphia: Lippincott, Williams & Wilkins.

Melnyk, B. M., Fineout-Overholt, E., Feinstein, N., Li, H. S., Small, L., Wilcox, L. et al. (2004). Nurses' perceived knowledge, beliefs, skills, and needs regarding evidence-based practice: Implications for accelerating the paradigm shift. *Worldviews on Evidence-based Nursing, 1*(3), 185–193.

Melnyk, B. M., Fineout-Overholt, E., Giggleman, M., & Cruz, R. (2010). Correlates among cognitive beliefs, EBP implementation, organizational culture, cohesion and job satisfaction in evidence-based practice mentors from a community hospital system. *Nursing Outlook, 58*(6), 301–308.

Munro, N. (2004). Evidence-based assessment: No more pride or prejudice *AACN Clinical Issues, 15*(4), 501–505.

Murad, M. H., Montori, V. M., Kunz, R., Letelier, L. M., Keitz, S. A., Dans, A. L. et al. (2009). How to teach evidence-based medicine to teachers: Reflections from a workshop experience. *Journal of Evaluation in Clinical Practice, 15*, 1205–1207.

Parkes, J., Hyde, C., Deeks, J., & Milne, R. (2004). Teaching critical appraisal skills in health care settings. *The Cochrane Database of Systematic Reviews, 2*.

Pololi, L., Knight, S., Dennis, K., & Frankel, R. (2002). Helping medical school faculty realize their dreams: An innovative, collaborative mentoring program. *Academic Medicine, 77*(5), 377–384.

Ramos, K. D., Schafer, S., & Tracz, S. M. (2003). Validation of the Fresno test of competence in evidence based medicine. *British Medical Journal, 326*(7384), 319–321.

Salbach, N. M., & Jaglal, S. B. (2010). Creation and validation of the evidence-based practice confidence scale for health care professionals. *Journal of Evaluation in Clinical Practice, 17*(4), 794–800.

Sparks-Langer, G., & Colton, A. (1991). Synthesis of research on teachers' reflective thinking. *Educational Leadership, 48*, 37–44.

Wallen, G. R., Mitchell, S. A., Melnyk, B. M., Fineout-Overholt, E., Miller-Davis, C., Yates, J. et al. (2010). Implementing evidence-based practice: Effectiveness of a structured multifaceted mentorship programme. *Journal of Advanced Nursing, 66*(12), 2761–2771.

Part III

Strategies for Creating an Academic Culture for Evidence-Based Practice

In Part III, the focus is on the academic setting. First, there is a look at faculty development issues and programs to prepare faculty to change all levels of academic curricula. The remaining four chapters of this part focus on specific populations of students; in this case, undergraduate, career changer, and doctoral students. We strongly believe that students and nurses at all levels can and should learn to be practitioners who use the best available evidence to guide their practice. If we are to make the kinds of changes that contribute to excellence in patient care, then all who are involved in that care must have an understanding of what works and what does not work according to research. We also, however, need to help nurses and all health care providers understand that EBP is not only about applying high-level, high-quality research findings in practice, but helping our students understand how to take those research findings and use clinical expertise to help patients make informed decisions about their care.

18

Refocusing the Academic Culture

Harriet R. Feldman

Tis education forms the common mind: Just as the twig is bent the tree's inclined.

—Alexander Pope (1688–1744)

Establishing a culture of curriculum change that is responsive to the constant changes in health care is a major challenge for an academic setting. As we educate nurses for tomorrow, this challenge is complicated by being faced with a faculty in transition. According to the American Association of Colleges of Nursing (Nursing Faculty Shortage, 2011), among the factors contributing to the nursing shortage is the average age of nursing faculty (as noted in AACN's 2010–2011 national nursing faculty salary survey): 60.5, 57.1, and 51.1, respectively, for faculty holding the ranks of professor, associate professor, and assistant professor. The report notes, "faculty age continues to climb, narrowing the number of productive years nurse educators can teach." Further, "a wave of faculty retirements is expected across the US over the next decade" (Nursing Faculty Shortage, AACN, 2011, p. 2). So the notion of shifting thinking of nursing faculty in the Lienhard School of Nursing of the College of Health Professions at Pace University to refocus and integrate evidence-based practice (EBP) into all coursework would take time and much effort.

This is the context with which we began our 6-year transition . . . the "Pace" story. The story begins with a grant request in early 2003 to the Hugoton Foundation for its support to "promote the Lienhard School of Nursing as a leader in advancing evidence-based practice (EBP) in New York State, primarily in the downstate area." To get started, we expressed interest in introducing EBP in two different clinical settings, acute care and community-based. A project director was identified to work closely with our research unit to move the project forward. The grant proposal identified a four-prong approach: (1) education/dissemination of knowledge in clinical settings, (2) curriculum development, (3) faculty development, and (4) research. The initiative started with education in the clinical settings, involving research to evaluate the effects of two variations of an intervention program on selected nurse outcomes and patient/family outcomes.

Second, we focused on infusing EBP into the undergraduate and graduate nursing curricula, starting with nursing research courses, including intense faculty development work—an important adjunct to the process. We believed that curriculum change and close alliances with health care delivery systems through strategic partnerships could improve patient care. The need for change was supported by the then-recent IOM report, *Crossing the Quality Chasm: A New Health System for the 21st Century* (2001), which emphasized the need for involving all health practitioners in reinventing the health care system, ensuring that "*Decision making is evidence-based.* Patients should receive care based on the best available scientific knowledge. Care should not vary illogically from clinician to clinician or from place to place" (p. 4).

We identified a project director, Dr. Rona Levin, who had a keen interest in EBP and a long history of working closely with clinical settings to promote nursing research in clinical practice. She and I share a lifelong commitment to nursing practice that is scientifically substantiated. Dr. Levin was already known to the faculty based on a prior grant to bring visiting scholars to the school. In that capacity, she worked with faculty to develop and/or advance their scholarship agendas. In addition, because a key faculty member who taught the research courses was about to go on sabbatical, Dr. Levin agreed to teach those courses, a prime opening for assessing the possibilities for change to an EBP focus. During this same period, she held the position of chair of the New York State Nurses Association (NYSNA) Council on Nursing Research. This Council had developed a Nursing Research Agenda for NY State, which included dissemination of research findings for use in practice and developing an infrastructure to support research utilization. In that role, she began to work with an EBP expert to develop a research proposal that focused on a specific strategy for advancing EBP in the clinical setting. Their work was in collaboration with NYSNA and the Foundation of New York State Nurses, with the Lienhard School of Nursing fast becoming a major player. The stars were beginning to align!

During her time as a visiting scholar, Dr. Levin had an opportunity to teach in the required nursing research courses, so she had a basic understanding of our curriculum. In fact, when teaching the graduate nursing research course, she worked closely with a senior faculty member to begin including EBP content. Further, she engaged faculty in conversations about strategies to incorporate EBP into other courses in both undergraduate and graduate programs. So some groundwork was already laid.

For us to meet the goal of formally infusing EBP into undergraduate and graduate nursing curricula, additional faculty development was needed. We had to expand, and in some cases develop, knowledge about EBP, so that curriculum work could proceed. The business of change had begun, but clearly a more formal approach would move the school forward. A first step was a year-long "scholarship development series" for faculty interested in learning about EBP and pursing a systematic review of literature in a topic of interest.

On the basis of earlier successes with faculty to promote scholarship and some initial acceptance of possible changes to the nursing research courses, the project director first met with the associate dean for academic affairs and the chairs of the respective department (undergraduate and graduate) curriculum committees. These meetings were critical to fully engage the academic leaders and enlist their support in promoting change in the faculty. From these meetings came the following initial plan:

- Gain approval from graduate faculty to adopt a revised graduate nursing research course that uses an EBP framework
- Work with undergraduate faculty to revise the undergraduate nursing research courses in like fashion, both the course for second-career students and the one for traditional 4-year nursing students
- Invite faculty who teach the undergraduate nursing research courses to observe classes in the revised graduate course

By working at the outset with courses most familiar to the project director and, at the same time, revising courses that had the clearest tie into EBP, outcomes would be perceived as credible and effective. Always good to start with a quick win! The next step involved integrating the concepts and processes of EBP throughout curricula at all levels.

Our initial activities led to the first change: revamping and adopting the master's level research course to an EBP framework. To set the stage, faculty was funded to attend local, regional, and national EBP conferences and receive consultation from an EBP expert about integrating EBP into the curriculum. The following semester graduate faculty began to teach the master's research course from an EBP perspective. Student evaluations of the course were positive and they began to see the value of using research and other forms of evidence to guide practice. At curriculum meetings throughout the year, the faculty deliberated many issues related to the amount of research needed in the curriculum and how to further integrate EBP in the graduate research course and others. It was during this period that the School received external funding to move our EBP agenda forward.

Following participation in these conferences, Levin began to mentor the faculty member who principally taught the undergraduate research courses. She was assisted by the senior faculty member that she replaced, who was referred to earlier as on sabbatical. Following this initial work of partnering, the senior faculty member continued to develop existing faculty and those that have followed. This was later extended to include other faculty who were qualified to teach the research course. We followed up with informal faculty presentations at regularly scheduled school-based faculty scholarly colloquia programs and "brown bag" teaching forums where faculty could present to their peers their experiences with teaching EBP. Workshops designed for full-time clinical faculty were introduced and Levin provided guest lectures in various courses, facilitating the design of EBP learning activities in clinical courses. By working closely with undergraduate faculty teaching clinical courses to facilitate integrating an EBP approach, we were able to level and integrate EBP in these courses.

Faculty development activities facilitated integration of EBP concepts and processes into the graduate level first, beginning with the family nurse practitioner program (FNP), and then through the entire curriculum. This was accomplished through the work of the lead FNP faculty member, who with the aid of an external consultant and the visiting scholar initially conducted a review of all FNP clinical courses. Changes to clinical courses were implemented in 2004. In the graduate core courses, students learned about EBP as a decision-making model and practice improvement strategy. Our intent was to enable use of this foundation in clinical courses, where faculty acted as EBP mentors to evaluate evidence and the application of that evidence to clinical practice. The FNP clinical capstone course required students to complete a project where they put evidence into practice. In the spirit of EBP, identifying curriculum outcomes of this innovation became even more essential. We decided to look at changes over time, from when students began their clinical FNP courses, as measured by the EBP Beliefs Scale and the EBP Implementation Scale (Melnyk & Fineout-Overholt, 2008) to program completion. We were greatly encouraged by the data, which showed significant positive gains in FNP students' EBP beliefs and implementation behaviors (Singleton, Levin, & Shortridge-Baggett, 2009).

Building on the master's FNP curriculum, the current Doctor of Nursing Practice (DNP) program was built to reflect the EBP focus, so that the pillars of the program provide a firm foundation in EBP, as well as primary health care and cultural competence (see Chapter 23). With the expertise and guidance of DNP faculty, students are challenged, for example, to consider and address the importance of differences in ethnic and racial factors when looking at patient and provider perspectives in implementing EBP. DNP students also develop an EBP project as a capstone to their program.

The outcomes overall have been quite impressive, including those both planned and unanticipated, as you will see below. The more than 50 external presentations, publications (including a textbook, *Teaching Evidence-Based Practice in Nursing: A Guide for Academic and Clinical Settings* in 2006, as well as the current edition, a regular column in the journal *Research and Theory in Nursing Practice*, and consultations, most notably with the nationally known NYU Hartford Institute for Geriatric Nursing, to revise their literature to reflect EBP) have been most rewarding as EBP information has been disseminated within the field of nursing education and practice. This kind of work and innovation has been sustained over time, with numerous positive outcomes. A few others are listed in Exhibit 18.1. We believe that the shift that faculty was able to make, embracing a new concept and integrating that concept into all courses and curricula is truly a great accomplishment. The EBP work was clearly a catalyst for changes in curriculum, faculty, and our clinical partners, but that was just the beginning. Along the way and subsequent to the changed curricula, many successes were achieved in disseminating the results of our efforts. Further, EBP is now integrated into all curricula, and is being integrated with at least four clinical partners, a true cultural transformation for them and for us.

EXHIBIT 18.1 EXAMPLES OF OUTCOMES OF THE EBP PROJECT OF THE LIENHARD SCHOOL OF NURSING

The Spirit of Planetree Awards (Foundation of New York State Nurses Central New York Nurses Center for Nursing Research 2010 Evidence-Based Practice Award) were created to promote patient-centered care by publicly recognizing individuals who personalize and demystify the health care experience for others, as well as programs and services that support extraordinary achievement in patient-centered care. The initiative helps communicate the character and quality of the caregivers and health care organizations in the Planetree network. The first of these awards went to Northern Westchester Hospital.

Development of an evidence-based protocol at Northern Westchester Hospital (NWH, New York) for the administration of Propofol in the ICU led to a reduction in patients' amount of time on a mechanical ventilator, decreased hospital length of stay, and improved patient outcomes with decreased need for rehab services and increased discharges to home.

American Association of Colleges of Nursing *Innovations in Professional Nursing Education* Award, for projects that promoted curriculum or organizational change, was in place for at least a year and

(*continued*)

EXHIBIT 18.1 *(continued)*

demonstrates outcomes, involved groups of faculty, can be replicated, has potential for dissemination and replication, and advances in nursing education.

International Visitors have come to NWH, through its collaboration with Pace University to observe how we integrate EBP into practice. This includes a proposal for an International Invitational Summit on Developing Academic and Clinical Partnerships for Translating Evidence into Practice. Also, there is interest in partnering among Queensland University of Technology (QUT), Mater Misericordia Health Services and the Nursing Research Centre, Queensland Centre for Evidence Based Nursing & Midwifery, and Pace University, which could lead to the potential to become a Joanna Briggs Institute Collaborating Center and some collaborative research.

Shared appointments of Pace faculty with staff in health care institutions and of staff taking on nursing faculty roles.

REFERENCES

Crossing the quality chasm: A new health system for the 21st century (2001). Washington, DC: The National Academies Press.

Melnyk, B., & Fineout-Overholt, E. (2008). The evidence-based practice beliefs and implementation scales: Psychometric properties of two new instruments. *Worldviews in Evidence-Based Nursing*, 5(4), 208–216.

Nursing Faculty Shortage. (2011, April 14). Retrieved October 16, 2011, from http://www.aacn.nche.edu/media-relations/fact-sheets/nursing-faculty-shortage

Singleton, J. K., Levin, R. F., & Shortridge-Baggett, L. (2009, April). *FNP students' EBP beliefs and implementation*. Poster presented at the Annual Meeting of the National Organization of Nurse Practitioner Faculties, Portland, OR.

PRESENTATIONS ON EBP

Comisky, M., D'Arcy, A., & Misiano, B. (2009, February). *Evidence-based practice: Propofol sedation protocol 11th annual evidence based symposium*. Arizona State University, Glendale, AZ.

Comisky, M., D'Arcy, A., & Misiano, B. (2009, May). *Working together to develop an evidence based practice protocol for Propofol sedation*. Mastery Session, AACN, National Teaching Institute, New Orleans, LA.

Levin, R. F. (2008, March). *Building bridges in academic nursing and health care practice settings: Nurses engaged in evidence-based practice projects*. Lienhard School of Nursing Scholarly Colloquium, Pace University, Pleasantville, NY.

Olney, K., & Carollo, M. (2009, February). *Evidence-based practice: Fall prevention 11th annual evidence based symposium*, Arizona State University, Glendale, AZ.

Wright, F. (2009, October). *Evidence-based practice for performance improvement*. Doctoral Program, Lienhard School of Nursing, Pace University, New York, NY.

19

Teaching Evidence-Based Practice Throughout an Undergraduate Curriculum: Here, There, and Everywhere

Rona F. Levin

A prudent question is one-half of wisdom.

—Francis Bacon

What comes first, the chicken or the egg? In the case of nursing curricula, the question might be rephrased as, "What comes first, research courses or clinical courses?" As with the chicken-or-egg conundrum, there is really no one right answer to the latter question, or the former for that matter. We need to help students learn the information contained in both types of courses, but the order may be irrelevant. There are advantages and disadvantages to either sequence. In the case of offering research prior to clinical courses, students can gain knowledge of the scientific method and concepts of evidence-based practice (EBP), which (we say) they are then able to apply in clinical courses. On the other hand, without knowledge of clinical content, students will find that asking burning clinical questions about practice is quite difficult. This is not to mention that the rich clinical examples of research principles in action, which make a research course palatable for most students, and thus the purported need to base practice on best evidence, will not have meaning. Now the chicken-or-egg question is only a conundrum in baccalaureate and higher degree nursing curricula. Interesting is the case of associate degree nursing (ADN) education in which there is not a research course in the curriculum to grapple with. Yet, are not ADN graduates also expected to base their nursing practice on the best evidence available?

My answer to the above questions is that teaching and learning strategies for helping students to practice nursing from an evidence-based perspective may take place in any course, whether or not students have had a research course first or ever. Under any circumstances, clinical courses need to weave EBP concepts into course content and clinical practica—here, there, and everywhere.

STRATEGIES FOR INTEGRATING EBP CONCEPTS INTO CLINICAL CURRICULA

Should We Throw Out the Textbooks?

According to Sackett, Straus, Richardson, Rosenberg, and Haynes (2000), we should "burn the textbooks" (p. 31). Why? Because they are outdated the moment they are published. Given the increasing rapidity with which new information is disseminated these days, reliance on textbooks for knowledge about clinical practice means that the clinician is not making decisions based on the latest and best evidence. Sackett and colleagues suggest three criteria for deciding on whether or not to use a textbook:

1. The edition has been published within the last year. (Anything older is outdated.)
2. References are plentiful, especially in relation to recommendations for diagnosis and management.
3. Principles of evidence are used by the authors to support their statements. Think about how heavily we all have come to rely on textbooks in the courses we teach. In lieu of throwing them all out, however, perhaps we need to help students to use them critically. One learning activity I have used to accomplish this objective is to have students select any nursing intervention, technique, or protocol from a nursing textbook and determine the evidence the author used to support the recommended practice behavior (see Exhibit 19.1). This activity may be used as an exercise or assignment in an introductory research or EBP course, or in any clinical course in the curriculum. My recommendation would be to use this exercise in the first clinical course in the curriculum.

How Do We Teach Skills for Clinical Inquiry?

Helping students to develop a questioning mind-set is the teacher's most important job. In order to teach this lesson we need to model curiosity, and support the value and necessity of constantly questioning our practice. This strategy can be used in any course, in any setting, at any time there is a teachable moment. When teaching an introductory class on EBP to students at any academic educational level or to practicing nurses, one effective teaching strategy is to provide evidence that suggests a commonly accepted and/or currently used practice has not been supported by evidence. As an

EXHIBIT 19.1 LEARNING ACTIVITY FOR THE CRITICAL EVALUATION OF TEXTBOOKS

Objectives

- Determine whether recommended practices are based on evidence
- Suggest potential problems that may arise from using nonevidence-based textbooks

Directions for Implementation: Have students select a nursing technique or protocol from one of their clinical textbooks and answer the following questions:

1. In what year was the textbook published?
2. Does the author cite any references in the narrative or protocol for the technique or protocol described?
3. Is the citation contained in a reference list or bibliography in the textbook?
4. If the answer to questions 2 or 3 is yes, list the references and identify:
   (a) Whether the reference is a primary or secondary source;
   (b) The type of publication represented (e.g., nursing journal, textbook, clinical practice guideline); and
   (c) The kind of evidence this source represents.

Students either may submit their findings in writing, present them orally in class, or both. Follow-up discussion is recommended. During the discussion, the following questions help students to achieve the learning objectives for this activity:

1. What references, if any, did you find for the selected technique or protocol?
2. If there was no reference to support the recommended technique, what is the author's recommendation based on? How do you know it is valid practice recommendation?
3. What is the value of evidence for nursing practice?

Adapted from Feldman, H. R., & Levin, R. F. (2002). *Instructor's resource manual to accompany nursing research: Methods, critical appraisal, and utilization* (5th ed., pp. 5–7). Philadelphia: Mosby.

example, many faculty teach students that patients who are scheduled for surgery need to remain NPO, that is, not eat or drink anything by mouth after midnight on the day of surgery. This has been a traditional practice for over 40 years. (I can attest to this because I was a practicing nurse 40 years ago.) A recent systematic review of 22 randomized controlled trials (RCTs) (Brady, Kinn, Stuart, & Ness, 2010) comparing the effect of different preoperative fasting regimens revealed that there were no significant differences in perioperative complications or patient well-being between groups that were permitted liquids preoperatively and those who followed a traditional fasting regimen. An important caveat, however, is that these results apply only to patients who are not at risk for complications of anesthesia; that is, for example, pregnant women or patients who are elderly, obese, or have stomach disorders. While this is scientific evidence from research, keep in mind that EBP includes the expertise of the clinician and patient values and preferences in the equation. Thus, the clinician in these cases needs to make the judgment about whether the patient is "at risk" for adverse effects of this new regimen. Yet, such evidence should be presented as part of a class on preoperative preparation of patients, along with a discussion about how to make the best decision for each individual patient. The point of this dialogue with students is to help them understand the need to question their practice, any practice, even what often is thought of as the most routine or assumed to be of benefit to patients. As teachers we need to share with students the evidence that supports the substantive content we include in our courses. As a matter of fact, we may even want to supplement our textbooks with the latest evidence available on a clinical topic, such as the systematic review cited above.

Another strategy to facilitate students' developing a critical, questioning mind-set is to require them to come up with one burning clinical question for every clinical experience. Students may then discuss their questions in a post-conference and determine first if the question is a background or foreground question, and then decide how to proceed in finding the answer. Perhaps students could take turns during a semester to find evidence that bears on their question and then share it with other students during a seminar or post-conference the following week. Another approach would be for all students to agree on trying to answer one of the questions presented in post-conference for the following week. In this case, each student would locate a study or other type of evidence related to that question. It is not necessary that students have had a research course to find a study related to their question. Learning to read studies at a very basic level at this point may, in fact, help students to value research more once they get to take a course in it. In an ADN curriculum, where there is no research or specific EBP course in the curriculum, this type of strategy is essential to incorporate an appreciation and basic understanding of the value of research for practice and the necessity of using the best available evidence to guide practice.

What About Nursing Process Papers?

I would guess that most clinical faculty still require nursing process papers from students. We can use these to develop EBP awareness in our students in every single clinical course. Instead of asking students to provide a purely theoretical rationale for their nursing decisions and actions, or a quote from their textbook to support the practice, ask them to provide a primary source of evidence from the literature for their nursing diagnoses and interventions.

Are Journal Clubs Setting-Specific?

Journal clubs are being used more and more for a strategy to help nurses in the clinical setting to develop critical appraisal skills. Why not use them as an academic strategy to promote students' understanding of research principles and the EBP process? Depending on the number of students in a course, students could work independently or in small groups to assume responsibility for finding a study to answer a specific clinical question and facilitating the discussion about the validity and relevance of the study to their question. In lower-level courses, this question might even be generated by the teacher to make sure the clinical topics in the syllabus are covered. I envision this strategy being used in post-conferences or as a monthly 1-hour session in clinical courses about a topic on the syllabus in lieu of a didactic lecture. (No, we do not have to cover every single item on the NCLEX-RN®. And, yes, there is life after NCLEX-RN®.)

What About EBP Rounds?

In an article on strategies for advancing EBP in clinical settings, Fineout-Overholt, Levin, and Melnyk (2005) discuss rounds as a strategy for introducing EBP in the clinical arena. This is another promising strategy for integrating EBP into clinical courses. Rounds would go something like this:

1. Instructor makes EBP rounds with students during each clinical practicum (or specifically designated practica).
2. Students are asked to come up with at least one clinical question for each patient seen.
3. Select one or two of these questions to serve as a post-conference topic.
4. Have students get together in pairs to search for evidence to answer the clinical question, which they are to present at a post-conference the following week.
5. Facilitate the discussion of how this evidence would be combined with the clinical expertise of the practitioner and the specific patient's values and preferences.
6. Ask students how they might evaluate the introduction of change in practice based on the preceding discussion.

These rounds may be used at any level in any clinical course.

If Not EBP Rounds, What About CATs?

Another clinical strategy suggested by Fineout-Overholt and colleagues (2005) when there may not be enough time for EBP rounds is a technique called CATs (critically appraised topics). An assignment for students in a clinical course would go something like this:

1. Choose a nursing intervention or practice you have discussed in class.
2. Ask students to present (or hand in) a one-page paper, summarizing the evidence on this particular intervention.
3. Depending on the level of the course and whether or not students have had an EBP, statistics, or research course focusing on treatment effectiveness formulas (e.g., NNT, RR), ask students to write a one-page summary (or two if you want double spacing) of the evidence that bears on the nursing intervention and the recommendations for practice that are based on this review.
4. Results of the students' work may be presented to the entire class in a post-conference or class.

SO WHERE ARE WE GOING?

The whole point of this chapter is to get you to think creatively. Stretch your imagination! Take a risk! Go for it! Chances are whatever new teaching and learning strategies you introduce at least will get the students' attention because those strategies are different from the norm. Try it; play with it! That is what makes teaching exciting for us educators, and what makes learning exciting for our students, here, there, and everywhere.

REFERENCES

Brady, M. C., Kinn, S., Stuart, P., & Ness, V. (2010 Update). Preoperative fasting for adults to prevent perioperative complications. *Cochrane Database of Systematic Reviews 2003*, Issue 4, Art. No. CD004423. DOI: 10.1002/14651858.CD004423.

Feldman, H. R., & Levin, R. F. (2002). *Instructor's resource manual to accompany nursing research: Methods, critical appraisal, and utilization* (5th ed.) . Philadelphia: Mosby.

Fineout-Overholt, E., Levin, R. F., & Melnyk, B. M. (fall/winter 2004/2005). Strategies for advancing evidence-based practice in the clinical setting. *Journal of the New York State Nursing Association, 35*(2), 28–32.

Sackett, D. L., Straus, S. E., Richardson, W. S., Rosenberg, W., & Haynes, R. B. (2000). *Evidence-based medicine: How to practice and teach EBM.* London: Churchill Livingstone.

20

"Second" Thoughts on Teaching Evidence-Based Practice to Entry-Level Nursing Students

Jeanne Grace

Any genuine teaching will result, if successful, in someone's knowing how to bring about a better condition of things than existed earlier.

—John Dewey

The traditional approach for introducing nursing research to undergraduate students can best be described as a "research appreciation" course. Much like a music or art appreciation course, the undergraduate nursing research course focuses on developing a vocabulary for discussing research and an appreciation of the researcher's craft. The successful learning experience in a traditional course is characterized by a former student: "I'm not afraid to pick up a research article and read it."

There is, however, a significant difference between appreciating research in the abstract and applying evidence to everyday clinical practice. Evidence-based practice (EBP) strives to provide care that is both effective and efficient. Whereas the skill set for research appreciation emphasizes the ability to recognize and describe the elements of the primary report of a research study, the skill set for EBP is much more pragmatic. Students in an EBP course should learn to

- Identify a clinical problem
- Frame that problem as an answerable question
- Conduct an effective and efficient search for evidence to answer the question
- Determine whether the evidence is valid and applicable
- Apply the evidence to address the clinical problem
- Evaluate the application of evidence in their practice

This skill set explicitly merges clinical expertise (to identify the problem, evaluate the effectiveness/efficiency of the proposed solution, and apply the evidence to the problem) and knowledge of the patient's values with scientific evidence to support clinical decision making.

The paradigm of EBP and the related teaching strategies were initially developed within the discipline of medicine: medical students are traditionally prepared to be individual clinicians with authority and responsibility for making decisions about patients in their care. While this care model may apply for advanced nursing practice, undergraduate nursing students and generalist nurses are more likely to practice in settings where significant aspects of their actions are constrained and prescribed by institutional protocols.

There are two mechanisms through which generalist nurses employed in health care settings can apply evidence to influence practice: institutional and individual. The institutional mechanism typically involves nurses working together to generate evidence-based procedures or protocols, solutions to unit-wide problems, and clinical practice guidelines. The individual mechanism impacts nurses' therapeutic use of self: strengthening empathic understanding (often through application of qualitative research evidence) and promoting one's own physical and mental health. Additionally, the individual mechanism may trigger an awareness of the need for institutional reassessment of existing practices. Health teaching content and strategies may be influenced by either mechanism, depending on the formality of the teaching role. Ideally, the undergraduate EBP course should prepare students for the reality of practicing within these mechanisms. How, then, do we craft authentic EBP experiences for undergraduate students?

Three groups of undergraduate students pose special challenges for teachers of EBP, and each of these groups can be described with the adjective "second." Second-career/-degree students are typically more mature "students in a hurry," who are particularly sensitive to the immediate relevance of their course work. Second-year (or -semester) traditional undergraduates are those with limited clinical exposure, typically taking foundational courses. English-as a-second-language and international students encounter specific barriers to conducting an effective and efficient search for evidence in English-language-centric databases.

SECOND-CAREER STUDENTS

Students seeking nursing education to prepare for a second career often enroll in accelerated baccalaureate programs for non-nurses. Each cohort of students presents with diverse life experiences and prior undergraduate majors; each student expects the accelerated program to expand one's current skill set in ways relevant to enacting professional nursing practice. Given the exceptional demands that an accelerated program makes on their resources—including their time—these students, in my experience, tend to evaluate each learning experience in terms of its apparent contribution to achieving that goal. Clinical courses and experience are valued as most central to their learning goals. Didactic instruction in other areas, including EBP, is valued to the extent that the utility of applying the knowledge in practice is immediately clear.

Close coordination among clinical and didactic instructors is, therefore, particularly important in accelerated programs. For example, students in my application of evidence course read and analyzed summaries of smoking cessation studies at the request of their psychiatric–mental health course coordinator. Medical–surgical and leadership course instructors incorporated the evidence appraisal format taught in the Application of Evidence course into their assignments in concurrent and subsequent courses. The entire accelerated program faculty received a list of the dates after which students in the application of evidence course could be expected to begin applying each EBP skill in other settings.

WHERE TO START?

How do we prioritize the content in an EBP course to facilitate immediate application to clinical practice? The obvious first skill to teach and practice is framing an answerable clinical question. Students are encouraged to look for nursing problems in their clinical practice settings and those problems become the bases for applying the PICO (population, intervention, comparison, outcome) strategy to capture the salient elements of the question. This exercise has the additional benefit, of course, of promoting reflective clinical practice.

Before students can make best use of the electronic resources now available to locate evidence to answer their clinical questions, they must be able to discern the domain (Exhibit 20.1) of the clinical question they are asking. Each domain, moreover, has unique standards for "best evidence" and the critical appraisal of that evidence. Evidence-based medicine identifies four major domains for clinical questions: therapy, harm/etiology, diagnosis, and prognosis (Guyatt & Rennie, 2002). Because nursing concerns are person-centered and not disease-centered, nurses have a unique clinical question domain—human response—and share interest with other disciplines in clinical questions about meaning/context (Grace & Powers, 2009).

It makes sense, then to use the question domains as organizing topics for the EBP course and to provide students with ample practice in first recognizing and then formulating questions in each domain at the beginning of the course.

EXHIBIT 20.1 EBP QUESTION DOMAINS

Domain	Definition	Question Example
Therapy	Cause a desirable change or prevent an undesirable change in a patient's health care situation	*Does patient positioning to avoid tension on the surgical incision reduce the need for pain medications in the immediate post-operative period?*
Harm	Cause an undesirable change or prevent a desirable change in a patient's health care situation: side effects, hazardous exposures	*Do children in households where cigarette smoking occurs have a higher incidence of asthma symptoms?*
Diagnosis	How to determine the individual's health problem	*Is the failure of a new mother to smile at her newborn an accurate indicator of potential for impaired parenting?*
Prognosis	Predicting the future course of the health problem	*How long does it take for a woman to resume her normal activities following transvaginal hysterectomy?*
Human Response	How persons process and manage health issues and health care encounters in their everyday lives	*How do adolescents undergoing cancer treatment deal with chemotherapy-related loss of scalp hair?*
Meaning/ Context	Personal beliefs and values of individuals dealing with health concerns and the contexts that shape them	*What values influence caregivers' decisions to offer or withhold narcotics as an option in acute pain management?*

I suggest therapy as the first clinical question domain to address in class for two reasons. First, the body of evidence for therapy questions is the best developed in both medicine and nursing, both in terms of reports of original studies and forms of knowledge synthesis available. This has implications for teaching search skills and also enhances the likelihood that students will successfully find appropriate evidence to answer their clinical questions. Second, therapeutic interventions are central to students' clinical experience. These students have chosen nursing as a second career because they want to make a positive impact on the condition of their patients, and that is the very essence of therapy.

IN SEARCH OF EVIDENCE

The resources available to enable an effective and efficient search for evidence have developed greatly during the past decade, as have the platforms for making those resources available. Haynes (2007) describes the "5S" model (Exhibit 20.2) of information technology for conducting an evidence search as most appropriate for busy clinicians. Essentially, the strategy involves seeking evidence for practice first in the sources where the evidence has been most "processed," that is, selected, collected, appraised, and combined in clinically useful ways. This approach involves a paradigm shift for those of us who were taught always to consult primary sources as the ultimate authority. For undergraduate students on a steep learning curve and generalist nurse colleagues, however, consulting first the resources that offer the most appraisal help from our scholarly friends makes a great deal of sense. The strongest evidence for practice arises from a body of research studies (quantity) that are appropriately designed to answer the clinical question (quality) and agree in their results (consistency). Undergraduate nursing education is not intended to prepare students with the advanced skills needed to critically appraise or apply

EXHIBIT 20.2 "5S" MODEL FOR EVIDENCE

"5S"	Description	Examples
Expert Systems	Incorporate evidence with patient-specic information	"Smart" electronic records Cardiac risk calculators
Summaries	Frequently updated reviews of the best evidence available to address a clinical problem (often organized by disease diagnosis)	*Up-to-Date* *Clinical Evidence* Evidence-based clinical practice guidelines
Synopses	Critical appraisals of original studies or systematic reviews	*Evidence-Based Nursing* EBP articles in clinical journals
Syntheses	Systematic reviews of a group of original studies addressing a focused clinical question	*Cochrane Library Database of Systematic Reviews* Johanna Briggs Institute
Studies	Original reports of single research projects	Research articles published in peer-reviewed scholarly journals

Source: Haynes, B. (2007). Of studies, syntheses, synopses, summaries, and systems: The "5S" evolution of information services for evidence-based healthcare decisions. *Evidence-Based Nursing, 10*(1), 6–7.

evidence that is preliminary, conflicting, or subject to major validity concerns.

The dilemma in constructing an effective and efficient search strategy for therapy evidence for undergraduate students, however, is the sparse availability of evidence relevant to generalist nursing concerns at the higher levels of information technology. Expert systems and subscription summary products like Clinical Evidence or UpToDate are organized by medical specialty and diagnoses. Where expert systems have been incorporated into patient electronic medical records, students may not have direct access for institutional security reasons. Clinical practice guidelines are widely available online, but not all of them are evidence based. Whereas the search for therapy evidence "should" proceed from expert systems downward, the efficiency of looking for evidence in sources where it is unlikely to exist must also be considered. The specific strategy for conducting a search in any setting benefits from collaboration with a knowledgeable medical librarian.

Depending on the resources available in the setting, a reasonable search strategy for students/generalist nurses begins with consulting one reliable summary source available online. Inspection of the table of contents or index should quickly reveal whether the question of interest is addressed at all. If the nursing clinical problem is not addressed, as is often the case, the next steps involve consulting available electronic databases in an order dictated by the information technology hierarchy and the amount of nursing-relevant content. Where the Cochrane Library databases are available, a search of the Database of Systematic Reviews and Database of Abstracts of Reviews of Effectiveness is a reasonable next step. A current systematic review from either source has a high probability of providing trustworthy clinical guidance on therapies. When no relevant evidence can be found in the Cochrane Library, the search moves on to databases that index summaries, synopses, and syntheses as well as single studies. For nursing concerns, Cumulative Index to Nursing and Allied Health Literature (CINAHL) provides widest coverage of the relevant literature and search tools optimized for EBP. CINAHL is a commercial product available by subscription. Where CINAHL is not an available resource, the National Library of Medicine PubMed provides universal, free access to Medline Plus, the largest index of health care literature. PubMed also incorporates search tools optimized for EBP. For more extensive information on the search process, see Chapter 8.

Knowing how to look for evidence is important, but so is recognizing when to stop looking. If students/generalist nurses have consulted the specified data sources using the identified strategies and have found no relevant evidence, two possibilities exist. It is possible that no strong, practice-ready evidence is available to address the nursing clinical question. It is also possible that the search strategy has run afoul of some quirk in the electronic databases. To rule out the second possibility, I instruct students who have conducted an unproductive literature search to consult a medical librarian immediately for assistance before investing further search time. Even when the literature search is a graded class assignment, seeking assistance from a librarian at this stage has no negative impact on the student's grade.

APPRAISING THE EVIDENCE

Developing effective and efficient search skills in the body of health care literature is often rated by accelerated students as the most valuable content of the evidence application course, but those skills are only a means to the end of better patient care. Although the search strategies maximize the yield of "best evidence," undergraduate students and generalist nurses still need to appraise those results for validity and clinical utility. EBP has evolved a set of "no nonsense" critical appraisal worksheets for evidence to guide this review (Guyatt & Rennie, 2002). Two of the worksheets for appraising therapy evidence are aimed at determining the trustworthiness of summaries (clinical practice guidelines) and syntheses (systematic reviews). Although these worksheets ask the appraiser to consider the quality of the underlying studies on which the guideline or review is based, the appraisals can be completed without detailed knowledge of threats to single study validity. For the same reasons busy clinicians are encouraged to consult pre-appraised and processed evidence products, where available, in preference to single studies, we need to teach the appraisal skills for these products as a "quick start" for students on a steep learning curve.

The critical appraisal worksheets for single studies are specific to each question domain. Each worksheet focuses on the most serious threats to valid findings, given the study design that provides "best evidence." In the context of teaching students how to critically appraise therapy evidence, I introduce some of the concepts also addressed in a research appreciation course, for example, requirements for causality, experimental study design, and statistical analyses for group differences. Because EBP values care that is both effective and efficient, there is an additional emphasis on whether the results are clinically meaningful. Students are presented with "so what" statistics—number needed to treat, weighted mean difference, and confidence intervals—and encouraged to judge whether the evidence suggests a new therapy is worthwhile to incorporate into practice, given the difference it is likely to make in outcomes.

APPLICATION TO PRACTICE

While the critical appraisal worksheets ask the appraiser to consider the "so what" of applying evidence to the care of an individual patient, that consideration is framed in the context of an individual, autonomous care provider. Because undergraduate students and generalist nurses do not often practice in that role, I supplement the generic critical appraisal worksheets with an additional set of application and evaluation questions (Box 20.1).

Care actions may have unintended as well as intended consequences, so I explicitly cue students to think about mitigating risks while applying evidence. I also cue them to consider the institutional mechanism that impacts their care decisions as well as the patient values, which should also impact care. Because nurses in a hurry tend to ignore the final, evaluation step of the nursing process, I cue students on a steep learning curve to plan the evaluation at the same time they are planning the implementation.

Variations on the Theme

Once the basic skills of EBP have been introduced in the context of therapy evidence, the teacher's choice of order for addressing the remaining question domains is flexible. Because evidence for questions of

BOX 20.1 EVIDENCE APPLICATION AND EVALUATION MODEL

- What specific action(s) will I take to apply this evidence to the care of my patient?
- What specific action(s) will I take to reduce the risk of harm to my patient related to applying this evidence?
- How will applying this evidence change my current practice?
- What are the institutional policies/procedures that I need to consider when applying this evidence? Are they in conflict with what the evidence suggests? What institutional resources will I need to apply this evidence?
- How will I incorporate my patient's values into the application of this evidence?
- What outcomes do I need to monitor to evaluate whether the application of this evidence is beneficial?
- What is the time frame for assessing those outcomes?
- What barriers, if any, will prevent me from assessing these outcomes in my practice setting?

harm/etiology and the sources of that evidence have much in common with evidence for therapy questions, it is convenient to address the harm domain immediately after the therapy domain. Accelerated students quickly see the clinical relevance of evidence about therapy side effects and disease risk factors. Once students recognize the limitations of randomized clinical trials as evidence for harm, they are more engaged in learning about quasi-experimental and observational study designs.

An important consideration of any accelerated program is professional role development. For this reason, my personal choices for the next question domains to be addressed are human response and meaning. As a practical matter, the distinctions between these two domains are unimportant, except that questions of human response address the unique scope of nursing practice and the relationships of patients to the health care system. Evidence for questions concerning both domains often arises from qualitative research, providing students with the opportunity to become familiar with this research tradition and the strategies for appraising truth value and utility for practice. (See Grace & Powers [2009] for an appraisal worksheet for these domains.) The effective and efficient search strategy for human response and meaning evidence is modified from that for therapy and harm, because relevant evidence is rarely found in commercial summary products or even syntheses like the Cochrane Library. There is a relevant clinical query for single studies in CINAHL ("qualitative").

Conceptually, the diagnosis and prognosis domains address determining what is happening now and what will happen in the future. Advanced practice nurses are much more likely than generalist nurses to be selecting diagnostic tests for their patients and conveying prognoses, but generalist nurses are involved in patient teaching in both domains. Generalist nurses are also responsible for assuring accurate measurements of vital signs (including pain) in a variety of patients and settings; in this context, evidence about diagnosis questions is extremely relevant to accelerated students in their clinical practice.

Second-Year (or -Semester) Traditional Undergraduate Students

The essential connection between EBP skills and the clinical arena raises issues for the placement of EBP courses in an undergraduate nursing curriculum. If we wish to graduate generalist nurses who are evidence-based practitioners, we need to give students ample opportunity to develop the habits of EBP from their earliest clinical experiences. Conversely, the wisdom and experience needed to incorporate effectiveness and efficiency, as well as patient values, into decisions about clinical actions develops with increased clinical practice and is not fully available to beginning students. One such student noted, "I'm just trying to figure out what to do with my hands, and you're asking me to think about why I'm doing it and whether it is worthwhile!"

When EBP principles are taught as foundational coursework, the unique educational challenge is linking them to practice. Students at this stage of their programs may have limited or no clinical experiences to provide context for asking and answering practice-related questions. It may be possible to link practice of evidence-based skills to the content of their other foundational courses. For example, students could pursue therapy or harm questions based on drugs they are studying in pharmacology or disease states they are studying in pathophysiology. If the foundational curriculum includes a health promotion course with some limited client or community involvement component, the opportunities for applications of evidence increase. There is abundant evidence available, for example, on successful approaches to smoking cessation and increased physical activity in community settings. Alternatively, students can frame and pursue a clinical question based on the prior or current health care experiences of themselves and their families.

AUTHENTIC ASSIGNMENTS

Ideally, the assignments in a foundational EBP course should have the possibility of real-world application and benefits to the student or community (Box 20.2). Some possible assignments are listed below. Where practice is guided by the institutional mechanism, beginning students will, of course, need to collaborate with more experienced clinicians to judge the effectiveness and efficiency of proposed evidence applications. This need for collaboration argues for group projects with active faculty guidance. Where personal or family health promotion is the goal, individual student projects may be more appropriate. Any of the suggested projects would provide an equally suitable learning experience for interdisciplinary courses and students.

Second Language Students

EBP developed in the English-speaking world, and the tools and information technology that support it are English-language centric. Syntheses, synopses, summaries, and expert systems are currently rarely available in any language other than English, and computer-based translations are all too often inaccurate or incomprehensible. Even when single-study evidence is available in the native language of an international student or nurse, the current search tools are not. Thus, a student or generalist nurse who is not fluent in English must make an extraordinary effort to find and apply evidence without the help of English-speaking colleagues.

BOX 20.2 CONTEXTS FOR APPLYING EVIDENCE WHEN CLINICAL EXPOSURE IS LIMITED

- Advice to a friend: Students solicit a health promotion question from non-nursing students and complete the process to supply an evidence-based answer.
- Healthy self: Students identify some healthy change they want to make in their lives and locate evidence on effective ways to achieve that change.
- Family health: Students identify some health challenge for a family member and locate evidence to address that challenge.
- Dorm-based health promotion: Students identify a health promotion opportunity in their student residence and apply evidence to address it.
- Encounter with another: Students identify a patient or family with whom they did not work effectively and seek evidence to increase their empathy and understanding of context.
- EBP clinics: Faculty solicit a problem from a clinical setting and guide a group of students in defining the clinical question, locating evidence to apply to the problem, and making a recommendation for solving the problem.
- Protocol/guidelines update: Students choose an existing protocol or guideline and evaluate whether it is consistent with current evidence.
  - Students identify an area where patient teaching materials are needed and create evidence-based resources.

"Products" of Evidence Application

- Patient teaching material
- Revised protocol
- Revised guideline
- New protocol or procedure
  - Checklist to reinforce "best practices"

SIMPLIFYING THE SEARCH

The evidence search strategy for students with limited English facility depends heavily on the use of subject database headings and clinical queries. Either PubMed (available online at no charge) or the Cochrane Library (freely available in many Third-World countries by national arrangement) has a utility for mapping English language words onto

MeSH (medical subject headings) terms. MeSH headings are a set of comprehensive terms that index all the relevant literature in the database according to topic. Students in possession of the MeSH headings for the salient aspects of their clinical question can be assured of locating all the possible evidence about that question in both the Cochrane and Medline databases, and can also use the MeSH headings to identify the corresponding subject headings in the CINAHL database.

How, then, does an international student find those first English terms to map onto the MeSH headings? On Google! International faculty report that their students frame their clinical questions in their native language, and then enter the PICO terms into Google to identify the English language equivalents. While general purpose Internet search engines cannot be recommended as sources for valid, peer-reviewed health care evidence, they are useful for this limited purpose.

REDUCING THE LANGUAGE BURDEN

Once the body of possible evidence is identified, use of the clinical queries filters reduces the reading burden by eliminating all citations that would not qualify as "best evidence." Students can then review the retained study abstracts to determine whether the evidence merits more comprehensive attention. When the abstract is structured, students can focus on the results section.

Clinical queries are not necessary in the Cochrane Database of Systematic Reviews and the Database of Abstracts of Reviews of Effectiveness, because only "best evidence" syntheses are included. Beyond the abstract, the standard format of a Cochrane systematic review has two sections that ease comprehension for readers with limited English. First, there is a plain-language summary section, which immediately follows the structured abstract. This section, intended for the lay reader, conveys the most important conclusions of the review concisely.

Second, the results of multiple comparable trials in many systematic reviews are presented graphically as forest plots. All evidence users benefit from learning the skills for interpreting these plots, but these skills are especially valuable for second-language or international students. Forest plots convey a maximum amount of information with a minimum amount of text.

INCORPORATING PATIENT VALUES

Patient values are always a component of clinical decision making in EBP, but the incorporation is often implicit. Teaching evidence application to international students provides a wonderful opportunity to make that incorporation explicit. Where individual and societal patient values vary across cultures, so may the evidence-based recommendations for care. Thus, the appraisal of an evidence-based clinical practice guideline for cross-cultural application must include identification of the values, including resource costs, which shaped the original recommendations. Then those values must be compared with the resources, costs, and values in the new setting to determine whether the evidence must be applied in a different way to be effective and efficient.

Because the EBP approach incorporates patient and societal values, as well as evidence into clinical decision making, the result should be care that is culturally competent, effective, and efficient. But there are limits to evidence and research. Within the scope of generalist nursing practice, there are many areas where best evidence is not yet available to guide practice. When there is insufficient evidence to guide a clinical decision, that decision must still be made. We do not have the luxury of deferring care for our patients until unambiguous evidence is available. Like all generalist nurses, students prepared with EBP skills will provide some care justified by expert opinion, tradition, or personal experience. Habitual evidence users, however, should have second thoughts about that care and recognize opportunities for EBP improvement.

REFERENCES

Grace, J., & Powers, B. A. (2009). Claiming our core: Appraising qualitative evidence for nursing questions about human response and meaning. *Nursing Outlook, 57*(1), 27–34.

Guyatt, G. H., & Rennie, D. (2002). *Users' guides to the medical literature: A manual of evidence-based clinical practice.* Chicago: AMA Publications.

Haynes, B. (2007). Of studies, syntheses, synopses, summaries, and systems: The "5S" evolution of information services for evidence-based healthcare decisions. *Evidence-Based Nursing, 10*(1), 6–7.

21

Integrating EBP Into Doctoral Education: Implementing a Post-Master's DNP Nursing Curriculum to Prepare Clinical EBP Leaders: The New York University College of Nursing Experience

Barbara Krainovich-Miller and Judith Haber

The illiterate of the 21st century will not be those who cannot read and write, but those who cannot learn, unlearn, and relearn.

—Alvin Toffler

The momentum in health care to address patient safety and improve the quality of patient care outcomes led by a number of reports by the Institute of Medicine (IOM) and the Quality and Safety Education for Nurses (QSEN) (Cronenwett et al., 2007; IHI, 2011; IOM, 1999, 2001, 2003; The Joint Commission, 2010) through evidence-based practice (EBP) continues to escalate. EBP remains the international mantra of health professionals in nursing (AACN, 2001a, 2001b; ACME, 2006; ACNM, 2007; ANA, 2010a, 2010b, 2011; Cronenwett et al., 2007), medicine (AAMC, 2011; IOM, 2003, 2010), dentistry (ADEA CCIDE, 2009), and other health professionals who have formed the interprofessional educational collaboration named IPEC (2011). There is no question that the key to addressing this mantra requires interprofessional partnerships between and among researchers, practitioners, and educators (IOM, 2003, 2010; IPEC, 2011). There is also little doubt that health care organizations of today and the future will need advanced practice nurse (APN) clinical leaders who are prepared with advanced EBP competencies. Nurse educators are challenged to graduate basic RNs and APNs with core EBP competencies who will use these competencies as a foundation for their respective clinical practice.

Faculty preparing nurse practitioners (NPs) at the Doctor of Nursing Practice (DNP) level are particularly challenged to develop systems level clinical leaders who are experts in using evidence to inform their clinical decision making as well as play a leadership role in creating an organizational EBP culture. A key role for DNP graduates is to implement, inspire others to implement, and lead EBP clinical projects that are focused on quality and safety issues that will improve patient outcomes (Cronenwett et al., 2007; IHI, 2011).

The purpose of this chapter is to present faculty and student barriers to implementing a post-master's (MS) DNP program, and share faculty development and innovative teaching–learning strategies that will help to turn barriers into opportunities for learning for faculty and students, so that faculty will be able to facilitate students' successfully progressing through a post-MS DNP EBP focused curriculum. NYUCN's DNP EBP experience implementing a post-MS DNP curriculum has demonstrated that acquisition of EBP competencies requires that DNP students have repeated, but leveled exposure to EBP concepts that are threaded throughout the curriculum. This overall teaching/learning strategy allows students to develop and perfect the essential EBP competencies (Box 21.1) such as critical appraisal and evidence synthesis (Fulton & Krainovich-Miller, 2010) over time and ensures that they will be able to obtain and demonstrate the DNP program outcomes. Another key ingredient for implementing a DNP curriculum with a strong EBP emphasis is securing the commitment of faculty who will teach in the program that they too will acquire EBP competencies at a proficiency level in order to implement EBP teaching strategies (Krainovich-Miller & Haber, 2006; Youngblut & Brooten, 2001) that will facilitate students' acquiring DNP program outcomes. The final key ingredient for a successful and relevant program is staying true to the tenant of a clinical practice doctorate, which is to graduate DNP APNs who will be prepared to translate existing research, through critical appraisal and synthesis and implementing relevant EBP clinical projects that have the potential for improving patient outcomes (AACN, 2006; ANA, 2011).

RECOGNIZING THE NEED TO PREPARE EBP CLINICAL LEADERS: NYU COLLEGE OF NURSING POST-MASTER'S DNP PROGRAM EXEMPLAR

A needs assessment of partnering health care agencies, NYUCN's current NP and nurse–midwifery students and alumni, and NPs and certified nurse midwives (CNMs) from the tri-state area, indicated that these

BOX 21.1 NYUCN DNP PROGRAM OUTCOMES*

1. Synthesize the "best available" evidence, with clinical expertise, patient preferences, and consideration of resources as it applies to the improvement of clinical practice, systems management, and nursing leadership.
2. Design, implement, manage, and evaluate critical issues within organizational systems.
3. Analyze health care finance data.
4. Manage quality improvement and patient safety initiatives to promote patient-centered care.
5. Lead the initiation, management, and evaluation of interprofessional projects that influence health care outcomes.
6. Demonstrate competencies for influencing public policy to advocate for specified patient populations.
7. Integrate principles of team work, collaboration, and use of informatics to support clinical decision making for quality patient outcomes.
8. Engage in activities that promote professional socialization as scholars.
9. Disseminate orally and in writing, relevant practice outcomes of clinical scholarly projects to the scientific and policy communities.

*NYUCN DNP Program Outcomes approved by NYUCN Curriculum Committee.

constituents desired and supported NYUCN implementing a DNP program. After careful consideration of the pros and cons of implementation (e.g., Dreher, Donnelly, & Naremore, 2005; Loomis, Willard, & Cohen, 2006; Meleis, & Dracup, 2005; Rhodes, 2011; Silva & Ludwick, 2006), consensus among faculty was that the potential positive impact of DNP graduates on improving patient outcomes and the overall health care of society (AACN, 2006) outweighed the concerns not to implement such a program. Therefore, NYUCN made the decision move forward, starting with a Post-MS entry option for those APNs who were NPs or CNMs. Development of the DNP curriculum occurred over a 2-year period and reflected use of *The Essentials of Doctoral Education for Advanced Nursing Practice (DNP Essentials)* (AACN, 2006) numerous other seminal documents (AACN, 2001a, 2001b, 2004; ACNM, 2007; ANA, 2001a, 2001b; IOM, 1999, 2001, 2003, 2010; NONPF, 1995; O'Neil & PWQ, 1998; USDHHS, 2000), and feedback from internal and external stakeholders.

NYUCN had spent the prior 10 years creating an EBP culture for faculty and the undergraduate and graduate programs. There was a long-standing commitment to develop men and women of science, sophisticated research consumers; one of the pillars of the NYUCN strategic plan. Initiatives to advance the NYUCN EBP agenda have included the initial use of McMaster University nursing faculty EBP consultants, one of whom is an internationally known expert, development of an EBP Academy sponsoring faculty development programs that has resulted in a critical mass of NYUCN faculty with EBP competencies, faculty and student EBP journal clubs, and an interprofessional EBP steering committee co-chaired by a nursing faculty member and a dental faculty colleague from NYU College of Dentistry (NYUCD). In the last 5 years, faculty from both colleges have attended over 400 EBP workshop sessions and were working toward becoming a Cochrane Collaboration Center (Cochrane, 2001). Recently, NYUCD and NYUCN became the Cochrane Collaboration's North American Center for Systematic Review Training in Oral Health. A hallmark of this culture change is that graduates of these programs are prepared to be research consumers who use critical appraisal and evidence synthesis, using the PICO (P = patient/population/problem, I = intervention, C = comparison (if available or appropriate), O = outcomes) framework to retrieve all relevant evidence for answerable clinical questions (Flemming, 1998). Further, they use gold standard critical appraisal tools to judge the quality of research evidence for use in practice (Sackett, Straus, Richardson, Rosenberg, & Haynew, 2000).

Box 21.2 indicates the credits, courses and clinical hours, and the major EBP curriculum thread of each course of NYUCN's post-MS DNP curriculum. The strong EBP focus of the curriculum facilitates students' successfully achieving the DNP program outcomes listed in Box 21.1. The post-MS DNP curriculum is 40 credits, representing 11 courses taken over seven consecutive terms, 400 clinical hours, and the approval, implementation, and written and oral defense of a clinical Capstone Project based on an EBP framework. The curriculum is implemented using an Executive Session weekend-format. Based on NYUCN's previous success with using competency-based education outcomes (Lenburg, 1999) to evaluate EBP competencies of its BS and MS programs graduating students, the same approach was used to develop specific DNP program outcomes (see Box 21.1). The EBP framework used for the curriculum provides the interprofessional EBP perspectives of both evidence-based medicine (EBM) (Guyatt & Rennie, 2002; Sackett et al., 2000) and evidence-based nursing (EBN) (Cullum, Ciliska, Haynes, & Marks, 2008). NYUCN's DNP program expects to graduate APNs who are competent consumers of research and EBP clinical leaders who are able to implement EBP clinical projects for their own practices as well as lead EBP initiatives related to organizational patient priorities.

BOX 21.2 NYUCN'S DNP POST-MASTER'S NP OR CNM CURRICULUM AND EBP COURSE FOCUS

Credits	Term 1: Course Name	EBP Concentration
3	Leadership and Organizational Systems Management for Quality Care:	Use of Leadership: focus on Kotter's change model: step 1, create a sense of urgency identifying an agency clinical
3	Integrative Application of EBP I	Use PICO to frame a clinical problem (urgency) from an agency's perspective
6		
Credits	**Term 2: Course Name**	**EBP Concentration**
3	Epidemiology	Cornerstone of more in-depth critical appraisal from population perspective and implication for policy from clinical leader role
3	Improving Health Outcomes Through Quality:	Use of the Clinical Microsystems approach to successfully implement a clinical EBP project —advancing the clinical leaders role—to improve patient outcomes
6		
Credits	**Term 3: Course Name**	**EBP Concentration**
4	Budgeting Concepts	Emphasis on cost-benefit ratio perspective for implementing a clinical project from an inclusive EBP paradigm
3	Integrative Application of EBP II:	Deeper grasp of critical appraisal of best available evidence for identified clinical problem use gold standard tools
7		
Credits	**Term 4: Course Name**	**EBP Concentration**
4	Current Issues in Health Policy:	Developing deeper knowledge of policy implications of EBP projects
3	Genetics and Genomics for Health Care:	Implications for EBP teaching projects
7		
Credits	**Term 5: Course Name**	**EBP Concentration**
3	Capstone Seminar I: Proposal Completion	Determine EBP Capstone Project, synthesis of literature, define implementation process
3		

(continued)

BOX 21.2 (*continued*)

Credits	Term 6: Course Name	EBP Concentration
6	Capstone Seminar & Internship II (200 Clinical Hours)	Secure IRB approval at clinical agency, orally defend and implement EBP Capstone Project
6		
Credits	**Term 7: Course Name**	**EBP Concentration**
5	Capstone Seminar & Internship III (200 Clinical Hours)	Evaluate EBP Capstone Project, complete written scholarly format for Capstone, and defend orally
5		
40	400 hours	

As noted previously, students have seven consecutive semesters to complete their course work and Capstone Project. For students to be successful in acquiring the EBP competencies for completing their Capstone Project (e.g., development of an EBP protocol) in the projected time line, it was deemed essential to start building EBP competencies in the first semester of the DNP program. In this first term, students take a Leadership course along with EBP I that introduces them to theoretical frameworks for guiding change, such as Kotter's (1996) eight-step model, which they might use for implementing an EBP Capstone Project. During their EBP I course they begin to develop an EBP tool kit that assists them in determining a clinical question for their Capstone Project using a PICO format (Khan & Coomarasamy, 2006; Krainovich-Miller & Haber, 2006; Scott & McSherry, 2009). In the second term when they are taking an epidemiology course with an Improving Health Outcomes Through Quality course, which helps students redefine their EBP Capstone Project from a clinical microsystems perspective (Nelson et al., 2008). Many of NYUCN's EBP Capstone Projects are considered quality improvement projects, especially by the health care organization where they are being implemented, as they address patient safety issues such as medication reconciliation as well as improving patient outcomes, such as assessing dental caries and applying fluoride varnish by nondental health care providers (IHI, 2011).

Although Box 21.2 only identifies two courses with an EBP title (EBP I and EBP II), the right-hand column indicates the heavy EBP emphasis of all the nursing courses and EBP linkage to the three non-nursing-taught courses. Two of the three interprofessional courses, budgeting concepts and health policy issues are not taught from a nursing EBP perspective. These courses are part of the graduate curriculum for master of public administration with a focus on health care administration, policy, or finance in the Wagner School of Public Service that expose the DNP students to a rich interprofessional student dialogue and team building, as the students who attend these courses are from multiple business and health disciplines. Such discussions clearly help students link these course outcomes to the EBP paradigm used by NYUCN, as illustrated in Figure 21.1 (DiCenso, Guyatt, & Ciliska, 2005). The third non-nursing course, Epidemiology, is taught by public health faculty in the Steinhardt School of Education, a course that is integral with an EBP-based curriculum. This course reinforces critical appraisal of research from a population perspective.

As noted, NYUCN's post-MS DNP curriculum progression intentionally integrates EBP competencies in each of the nursing courses that occur in the initial four terms, that is, prior to the first Capstone course, which begins in their fifth term. Students are provided with rigorous yet realistic course assignments that enable them to develop the necessary EBP competencies to successfully implement an EBP Capstone Project during their last three consecutive terms. For example, in their first term, as described above, students are introduced in their EBP I course to realistic EBP course learning outcomes and related assignments to measure

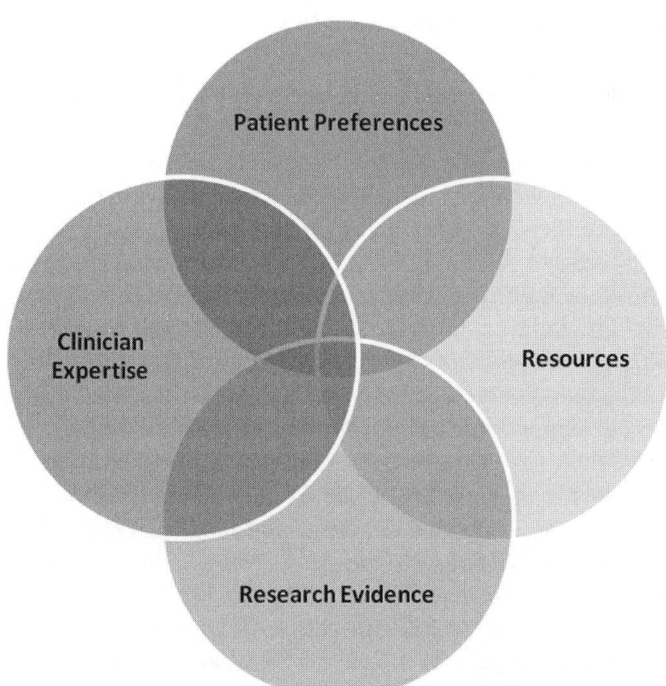

FIGURE 21.1 Evidence-based decisions.

attainment of these learning outcomes. For example, students are expected to: (a) use a clinical agency's quality assurance, risk management, or infectious disease department to ascertain a relevant clinical problem that needs to be addressed; (b) further develop their information literacy skills by meeting with a health science librarian so they can perform more efficient electronic search for the identified clinical problem; and (c) further develop their critical appraisal skills using gold standard clinical evaluation tools for research (e.g., critical appraisal skills program, referred to as the CASP tool, for appraising research evidence) and AGREE Collaboration's (2003) international appraisal instrument for determining the quality of clinical practice guidelines, referred to as the AGREE tool. Also in this term, students are introduced in the Leadership course to develop competency in using a change model and beginning to frame an identified clinical problem to be addressed from the agency's perspective using Kotter's model (1996), which remains relevant today in the clinical microsystems literature (Nelson et al., 2008).

WHAT MAKES IT WORK: FACULTY ACHIEVEMENT OF EBP COMPETENCIES TO FACILITATE STUDENTS' GAINING EBP COMPETENCIES AS CLINICAL LEADERS

NYUCN's DNP EBP curriculum model reflects a paradigm shift for faculty who were familiar with preparing EBP clinicians at the master's level (NPs and CNMs) to use the best available evidence, combined with their clinical judgment and respecting patient preferences and available resources to inform clinical decision making for an individual patient or groups of patients (DiCenso et al., 2005). Faculty was challenged to reconceptualize the EBP product they were preparing. DNP graduates were targeted to be clinical EBP leaders who were guided by the *DNP Essentials* (AACN, 2006). NYUCN faculty conceived of DNP graduates as EBP clinical leaders who would generate systems-level projects, based on the best available evidence, who would lead important changes in their respective institutions, resulting in improved patient outcomes. Graduates would disseminate their Capstone Project as well as future EBP projects locally and nationally. It soon became apparent that faculty, many of whom had experience with MS NP student Capstone Projects, had to reconceptualize performance expectations for DNP students. An assignment such as a PICO project conducted by MS students as a Capstone Project, involve a limited search (e.g., five to 10 studies), critical appraisal and synthesis of this literature in order to make a practice recommendation, and no implementation or evaluation component. In contrast, a PICO project that was a DNP Capstone Project is developed and implemented based on an exhaustive search of the literature, a critical appraisal and synthesis of this literature, conclusions, and recommendations for a project that requires agency and IRB approval prior to implantation, and implementation and evaluation of project outcomes. Examples of completed DNP EBP Capstone Projects are listed in Box 21.3.

It was apparent that the first Cohort of DNPs during their EBP course did not bring to the course the basic DNP competencies of MS-level graduates. Therefore, in order to meet the EBP academic expectation a two-course EBP sequence was initiated for the second DNP cohort (see curriculum in Box 21.2). Thus far, the two-course EBP sequence (EBP I and EBP II) has provided a strong foundation for their epidemiology and quality courses that they take in the second semester; these EBP concepts are reinforced in the EBP II course, which is taken in their third term of the DNP curriculum. Leveling expected program and learning outcomes of the courses was an important exercise for faculty as well. This approach raised expectations of the required faculty to be proficient in EBP competencies. Faculty is expected to be EBP role models for students who themselves are engaged in EBP-related scholarship. Given the intensity of the DNP curriculum, it is critical that faculty have the EBP competencies noted in Box 21.4 to facilitate students' achievement of the DNP-related EBP program learning outcomes listed in Box 21.1.

BOX 21.3 LIST OF EXAMPLES OF NYUCN DNP EBP CAPSTONE PROJECTS

- Psychoeducation for College Students Prescribed Antidepressants
- An EBP Heart Failure Recognition Education Program for Nursing Home Nursing Assistants
- Implementing a Breast Cancer Survivorship Care Plan
- An EBP Education Program for Nursing Home Assistant to Enhance Acute Stroke Symptom Recognition
- Integrating Preventive Dental Care for Non-Dental Health Care Providers in a Pediatric Oncology Clinic
- Stress Reduction in College Students Using Mindfulness Meditation
- Improving Outpatient Prescribing Practices through Medication Reconciliation: A Quality Improvement Project
- Using "Ask-Me-3" Patient/Provider Communication in College Health Setting to Improve Student Consumer Satisfaction

BOX 21.4 FACULTY-REQUIRED EBP COMPETENCIES

Faculty must demonstrate the ability to:

- Formulate PICO clinically relevant questions
- Conduct electronic searches efficiently
- Critically appraise research using gold standard assessment tools
- Discuss the appropriateness of the statistics used in a study
- Evaluate the quantity and quality of the evidence based on the critical appraisal
- Synthesize the evidence to draw conclusions in order to make recommendations for applicability to practice
- Develop appropriate measures for evaluating the EBP project outcomes
- Prepare nonresearch EBP Capstone IRB submissions

OVERCOMING BARRIERS: FACULTY AND STUDENT PERSPECTIVES OF DNP EBP CLINICAL CAPSTONE PROJECTS

Some of the national and international barriers faced by the nursing profession when shifting from research utilization to an EBP model are similar to those faced by faculty who are engaged in implementing a DNP program that has EBP as one of its major threads of the curriculum and requires an EBP Capstone Project be implemented and evaluated in the clinical setting. Barriers noted in Box 21.5 highlight the issues uncovered during the development phase as well as the monthly DNP Workgroup meetings during implementation. It was somewhat surprising during discussions at the Workgroup meetings that many faculty did not have a clear history of the EBP movement, and this may have contributed to other barriers. Another barrier of particular concern related to faculty's lack of understanding regarding what constitutes a DNP EBP Capstone. After multiple discussions it was apparent that some of this misconception relates to: faculty's academic preparation, that is, PhD or DNP; PhD faculty experience teaching in PhD, not DNP programs; PhD and DNP-prepared faculty's lack of experience teaching in a DNP program; and as previously noted, a lack of EBP competency on the part of some faculty, whether PhD or DNP prepared. For example, PhD faculty is by nature prepared in a traditional research paradigm of implementing a program of research and supervising PhD student dissertations. Some of these faculty expressed concern regarding the quality of the DNP EBP Capstone Projects. They did not understand why Capstone Projects students were derived from

BOX 21.5 BARRIERS TO ENGAGING EBP FRAMEWORK FOR DNP PROGRAMS

- Relatively new EBN movement
- Faculty have not been trained in an EBM/EBN framework
- Misconceptions about EBP by nurses
- Multiple models of levels of evidence and grades of recommendations to determine the quality of evidence of EMB and lack of agreement by nursing on the hierarchy of research evidence to use
- Disagreement among nurses about whether EBN is a distinct construct or reflects too much of the medical model
- Misconception that EBN is "cookbook" nursing
- Faculty do not possess expert competency in information literacy
- Lack of training in critical appraisal of research evidence
- Faculty lack of training in conducting efficient electronic searches and use of health science librarian
- Lack of health care agencies' organizational infrastructures to promote EBN practice
- Lack of academic agencies' organizational infrastructure to promote EBN as a framework for faculty development and course development
- Nurse educators not connecting quality patient outcomes to EBN
- Unclear distinctions between and among quality improvement projects, EBN projects, and DNP and research studies.
- Not linking the importance of critical appraisal of research in a master's research course

Source: Adapted from Krainovich-Miller & Haber (2006).

clinical questions versus research questions and why Capstone Projects were not to be called research projects. Faculty expressed concern that DNP students were not required to: (a) use valid and reliable instruments to measure clinical project outcomes, (b) use inferential statistics to determine relationships, (c) address confounding variables, or (d) use larger sample sizes and comparison groups. In addition, faculty did not understand why so much time was spent on determining an answerable clinical question based on the critical appraisal of research, including the strength, quality, and consistency of the evidence to determine what was best available evidence to address a clinical problem. It was apparent that they were confusing DNP EBP Capstone Projects with PhD dissertation studies. During further discussion it was apparent that many only required PhD students' literature reviews to focus on summarizing studies and providing conclusions, which identified a knowledge gap (Fulton & Krainovich-Miller, 2010). Providing and discussing examples of DNP students' literature review analysis and synthesis of the retrieved research related to an identified clinical problem was very helpful in clarifying the differences between the PhD dissertation and a DNP EBP clinical Capstone Project. It was also interesting to note that similar concerns were expressed by faculty who was prepared at the DNP level who attended post-master's DNP programs that admitted nonclinical master's prepared individuals (e.g., administration, education) and/or were from DNP programs that had students "conduct" a study for their DNP project, despite these programs' lack of the appropriate type and number of research courses in their DNP program. Faculty also did not understand why DNP students were not doing "research" instead of an EBP clinical project. Faculty development workshops that focused both on the DNP Essentials and EBP competencies as well as continuing discussion at DNP Workgroup meetings clarified these issues and helped faculty shift to a DNP EBP paradigm.

Another strategy that helped faculty and students see the significance of the EBP Capstone Project was using the PICO approach from the EBP tool kit. Students complete a PICO for their initial EBP assignment. This required that students formulate an answerable clinical question, critically appraising existing research, and determining the quality of the research evidence to make an evidence-informed decision about its applicability for practice for the identified problem/population. It was also evident that some of the faculty who expressed these concerns were new faculty at NYUCN and had not had the benefit of several years of EBP faculty development. Initiating a separate DNP workgroup for those who were teaching in the DNP program allowed these differences to be aired and clarified in a supportive nonjudgmental environment, and created an atmosphere where faculty was motivated to attend EBP faculty development sessions. Thus far, faculty has indicated that both the DNP Workgroups and faculty development workshops were effective in helping them develop new or enhanced EBP competencies, including the use of EBP teaching–learning strategies, such as the PICO format, use of a health science librarian to enable students to search more efficiently, and use of gold standard critical appraisal tools (CASP, AGREE).

Specific critical appraisal faculty development workshops conducted by EBP experts helped faculty gain expertise in critical appraisal so they would be comfortable giving feedback to students. A series of workshops included presentation of: (a) general EBP concepts by local EBP experts; (b) levels or hierarchy of evidence models (Figure 21.2) (LoBiondo-Wood & Haber, 2010); (c) critical EBP concepts, such as quantitative versus qualitative systematic reviews; (d) differences between and among systematic reviews and meta-analyses, metasyntheses, integrative reviews, and

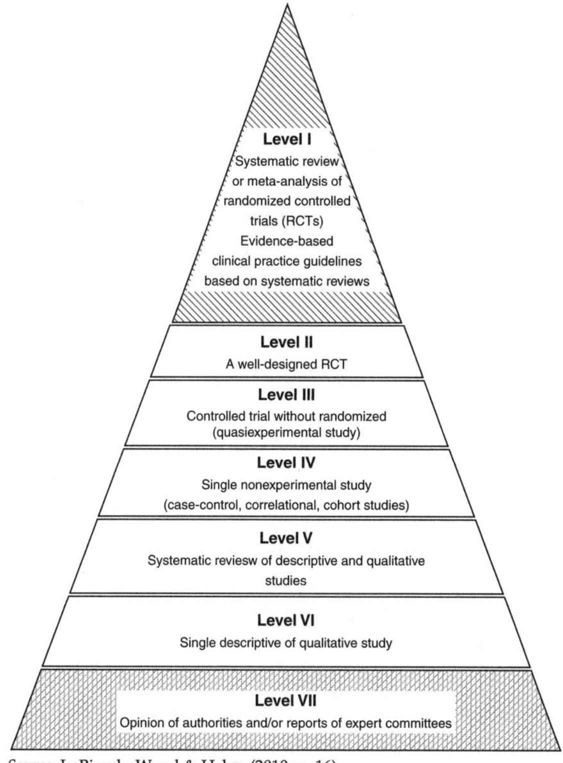

Source: LoBiondo-Wood & Haber (2010, p. 16).

FIGURE 21.2 Levels of evidence.

traditional literature reviews; (e) similarities and differences among the definitions of EBM, EBN, and EBP and relationship to an EBP clinical DNP project; (f) models for rating levels of evidence that judge the strength, quality, and consistency of research evidence) (Figure 21.2); and (g) wearing the lens of internal and external validity when using gold standard clinician evaluation tools such as CASP and AGREE.

POST-MS DNP STUDENTS' EXPECTATIONS AND BARRIERS

Despite clearly stated purposes of NYUCN's DNP program and information sessions, prior to admission, outlining the differences between NYUCN's PhD and DNP programs some students thought, as did some faculty, that they were going to conduct research for their DNP Capstone Project. It was somewhat surprising to hear accomplished clinicians (NP and CNM) indicate that they did not think a clinical EBP project would be valued and/or respected or that one's clinical EBP Capstone Project would not be conducted with one's own patients on a one-to-one basis. Others only wanted to implement a project that they were passionate since they had to "live" with their clinical project for three terms, about a full academic year.

The first step for addressing these barriers (Box 21.5) was similar to what was done with faculty, that is, clarifying the DNP program outcomes and DNP Competencies (AACN, 2006) and continue to listen and clarify over and over again the purpose of a clinical DNP EBP Capstone Project versus a PhD dissertation. In addition, linking the implementation of DNP EBP Capstone Projects to address the critically important issues to which they were being exposed, namely patient safety, quality patient outcomes, and reimbursement (Cronenwett et al., 2007; IOM, 2010; Joint Commission, 2010), helped them to see the importance of their EBP Capstone Project. By the time students were in their Capstone II course (sixth term), the relationship of the curriculum to their achieving the necessary EBP is very evident. At this point they discuss how engaged they are in the practice setting implementing their projects and are increasingly aware of how their clinical leadership is evident to the administration of the institution. It was critical to clarify these issues at the beginning of the students' curriculum. For example, EBP I includes a review of the key EBP history and related concepts (Krainovich-Miller & Haber, 2006) (Box 21.6). Until students saw the linkage between an answerable clinical question and the need to find the evidence upon which to base their Capstone Projects they could not proceed with their Capstone Project. As with faculty, it was interesting to note how many students were not as well versed in the history of EBP and the purpose of the PICO format. Students indicated that repeated explanations were helpful to their being able to embrace the EBP framework and see the clinical importance of DNP EBP Capstone Projects.

Another expected barrier that was critical to address early in the program was students' reaction to faculty's feedback regarding their lack of scholarly writing abilities. Their reaction somewhat surprised faculty as they were well aware of the fact, as noted in the literature (e.g., Granello, 2001; Harris, 2006; Scott, 2001), that graduate students, whether DNP or PhD, who return to school after many years, often have scholarly writing issues. Faculty teaching in the Post-MS DNP program expected DNP students to have similar issues, especially those students who had been out of their MS programs for a number of years. Most of NYUCN's Cohort I and II students had not, as they were busy clinicians, continued to perfect their scholarly writing skills, through publishing, since MS program graduation. Faculty implemented some of the tried and true strategies of requiring that students purchase and use the *Publication Manual of the American Psychological Association* (2010) and to draft and re-draft their papers based on specific faculty feedback. These strategies, over the course of

BOX 21.6 STRATEGY TO OVERCOME SOME BARRIERS: HISTORY EBM/EBP MOVEMENT

- 1972 EBM began in the UK by Dr. Archie Cochrane, an epidemiologist. He severely criticized MDs for their lack of critical appraisal and synthesis of research for use in practice and:
  - Recommended systematic reviews (appraisal and synthesis of like studies) be conducted as they were essential to policy makers, health profession organizations, MDs, and the public
  - Claimed there was a paucity of systematic reviews, which had a negative impact on health care outcomes
  - Recommended a rigorous process be developed for systematically reviewing like studies, in particular RCTs, with periodic updates
  - Charged MDs to use the results of systematic reviews for quality diagnosing and treatment in order for their patients to make an informed decision about whether to accept the diagnosis and treatment plan.
- By 1992 Cochrane's recommendations were formally implemented at Oxford University, and a year later the Cochrane Collaboration was established.
- Currently, the Cochrane Collaboration is considered "the International 'virtual organization'" for systematic, up-to-date reviews of all relevant health care RCTs.
- Although more systematic reviews are produced in the United Kingdom, the United States is gaining momentum primarily due to the managed care movement, shift of clinical decision making from providers to payers, and a change in the medical and legal mind-set from defensive to offensive clinical practice and the safety and quality movement.
- By the early 1990s, physician and nurse colleagues from the United Kingdom and Canada were leading the EBP movement. The actual term "evidence-based medicine" was coined around 1990 by Dr. Gordon Guyatt of McMaster University.
- Scholarly articles and meta-analyses were using or applying terms such as the "strength and quality of the evidence" and "levels of evidence" to refer to a basic framework for categorizing and rating research and then using rigorous criteria to produce systematic reviews.
- Most of the strength and quality of evidence frameworks consider quantitative meta-analyses (quantitative systematic reviews) of

(*continued*)

BOX 21.6 (*continued*)

two or more RCTs, Level I as the gold standard of best available evidence.

- In the United States, work of the Agency for Health Care Policy Research (AHCPR), which generated original evidence-based practice guidelines of the late 1980s and early 1990s, was part of this movement; several guidelines had nurse researchers chairing or functioning as members of guideline review panels.
- McMaster's University developed a leadership position in advancing the evidence-based nursing (EBN) movement through consultation and publications, including the journal *Evidence-Based Nursing*.

Source: Revised from Krainovich-Miller & Haber (2006).

the curriculum, have brought a significant return of their writing skills. Another issue for these students was their presentation skills. They were not used to preparing succinct PowerPoint presentations or delivering their presentations in a time-limited manner. Faculty provided the following strategies, which students' found very helpful: (a) clear guidelines for preparing PowerPoint presentations, including the need to rehearse; (b) specific criteria for presentations guided by an evaluation tool for the students that would be used by faculty and classmates alike; (d) an opportunity for faculty and students to provide students with specific qualitative feedback on each presentation; and, (e) an opportunity for self-evaluation via taping of presentations. They also indicated that holding students to the specified time for the presentation fostered mutual respect for each other.

OUTCOMES AND RECOMMENDATIONS

NYUCN successfully graduated its first Cohort of post-MS DNP graduates ($N = 8$) in 2011. Graduates have already made significant contributions to improving patient outcomes. The list of their EBP projects indicates their clinical relevance and importance to improving patient outcomes. A number of the projects have already been accepted for national presentations at nursing (e.g., ENRS) and interprofessional conferences. They are presenting at their respective institutions to interprofessional teams. The second cohort of students are about to graduate and feedback from them is quite rewarding. They are already being recognized at their institutions as clinical leaders and are being sought after to lead in any number of quality improvement projects. NYUCN is carefully tracking these graduates in terms of dissemination of their clinical projects through presentations and publications.

Our recommendation for successful implementation of a post-MS DNP program is to conduct a needs assessment, include the eternal community when creating the curriculum, adhere to the tenets of the DNP as a clinical practice doctorate, use major documents of AACN, ANA, IOM, make EBP clinical projects the focus of students' Capstone Projects, implement EBP faculty development sessions, and continue to debate the issues during implementation. Further, it is essential to listen carefully to faculty and student feedback and be willing to be flexible, that is, to continue to change aspects of the curriculum as soon as possible after seeing what does not work. This means taking student feedback seriously. DNP education in the 21st century must produce EBP clinical leaders who will make a difference. These graduates will face many challenges, but if they truly understand the value of implanting EBP projects using a clinical microsystems and/or "leadership change" approach, they will be successful in implementing these projects and leading others to implement such projects to improve patient outcomes.

REFERENCES

Accreditation Commission for Midwifery Education (ACME). (2006). *Guidelines for maintaining documentation in nurse-midwifery/midwifery education programs.* MD: Silver Springs.

ADEA Commission on Change and Innovation in Dental Education (CCIDE) & American Dental Education Association. (2009). *Beyond the crossroads: Change and innovation in dental education.* Washington, DC: ADEA.

American Association of Colleges of Nursing (AACN). (2001a). *Hallmarks of scholarly clinical practice.* Washington, DC: AACN.

American Association of Colleges of Nursing (AACN). (2001b). *Indicators of quality in research-focused doctoral programs in nursing* (AACN Position Statement). Washington, DC: AACN. Retrieved on May 8, 2008, from http://www.aacn.nche.edu/Publications/positions/qualityindicators.htm

American Association of Colleges of Nursing (AACN). (2004). *AACN position statement on the practice doctorate in nursing.* Washington, DC: AACN.

American Association of Colleges of Nursing (AACN). (2006). *The essentials of doctoral education for advanced nursing practice.* Washington, DC: AACN.

American Association of Medical College (AAMC). (2011). *The case for strategic talent management in academic medicine.*

American College of Nurse Midwifery (ACNM). (2007). *Revision of core competencies for basic midwifery practice: Highlights and process.*

American Nurses Association. (2010a). *Nursing: Scope and standards of practice.* Washington, DC: ANA.

American Nurses Association. (2010b). *Nursing's social policy statement.* Washington, DC: ANA.

American Nurses Association. (2010c). *Scope and standards of practice for nursing professional development*. Washington, DC: ANA.

American Nurses Association. (2011). *The doctor of nursing practice: Advancing the nursing profession*. Washington, DC: ANA.

American Psychological Association. (2010). *The publication manual of the American Psychological Association* (6th ed.). Washington, DC: Author.

Cochrane Collaboration. (2001). *The Cochrane Collaboration: Preparing, maintaining and promoting the accessibility of systematic reviews of the effects of health care interventions*. Oxford, UK: Cochrane Collaboration.

Cronenwett, L., Sherwood, G., Barnsteiner, J., Disch, J., Johnson, J., Mitchell, P. et al. (2007). Quality and safety education for nurses. *Nursing Outlook, 55*(3), 122–131.

Cullum, N., Ciliska, D., Haynes, B., & Marks, S. (2008) *Evidence-based nursing: An introduction*. Michigan: Blackwell Publishing.

DiCenso, A., Guyatt, G., & Ciliska, D. (2005). *Evidence-based nursing: A guide to clinical practice* (pp. 154–171). St. Louis: Elsevier.

Dreher, H. M., Donnelly, G., & Naremore, R. (2005). Reflections on the DNP and an alternate practice doctorate: The Drexel DrNP. *OJIN: The Online Journal of Issues in Nursing*. *11*(1).

Flemming, K. (1998). Asking answerable questions. *Evidence-Based Nursing, 8*, 68–72.

Fulton, S., & Krainovich-Miller, B. (2010). Review of the literature. In G. LoBiondo-Wood, & J. Haber (Eds.), *Nursing research: Methods and critical appraisal for evidence-based practice* (6th ed., pp. 55–84). Philadelphia: Elsevier.

Granello, D. (2001). Promoting cognitive complexity in graduate written work: Using Bloom's taxonomy as a pedagogical tool to improve literature review. *Counselor Education and Supervision*, *40*(4), 292–307.

Guyatt, G. H., & Rennie, D. (Eds.) (2002). *Users' guides to the medical literature: A manual for evidence-based clinical practice.* Chicago: AMA Press.

Harris, M. J. (2006). Three steps to teaching abstract and critique writing. *International Journal of Teaching and Learning in Higher Education*, *17*(2), 136–146.

Institute for Healthcare Improvement (IHI). (2011). *What's in your toolbox to improve care quality?* Cambridge, MA: IHI.

Institute of Medicine. (1999). *To err is human: Building a safer health system*. Washington, DC: National Academies Press.

Institute of Medicine. (2001). *Crossing the quality chasm: A new health system for the 21st century*. Washington, DC: National Academies Press.

Institute of Medicine. (2003). *Health professions education: A bridge to quality*. Washington, DC: National Academies Press.

Institute of Medicine. (2010). *Future of nursing: leading change, advancing health*. Washington, DC: The National Academies Press.

Interprofessional Education Collaborative (IPEC) Expert Panel. (2011). *Core competencies for interprofessional collaborative practice: Report of an expert panel*. Washington, DC: Interprofessional Education Collaborative.

Khan, K., & Coomarasamy, A. (2006). A hierarchy of effective teaching and learning to acquire competence in evidence-based medicine. *BMC Medical Education*, *6*(59).

Kotter, J. (1996). *Leading change*. Boston, MA: Harvard Business School Press.

Krainovich-Miller, B., & Haber, J. (2006). Transforming a graduate nursing curriculum to incorporate evidence-based practice: The New York University Experience. In R. Levin, & H. Feldman (Eds.), *Teaching evidence-based practice in nursing* (pp. 165–191). New York: Springer.

Lenburg, C. B. (1999). The framework, concepts and methods of the Competency Outcomes and Performance Assessment (COPA) Model. *Online Journal of Issues in Nursing*. Retrieved January 12, 2005, from http://www.ana.org/ojin/topic10/tpc10_2.htm

LoBiondo-Wood, G., & Haber, J. (2010). *Nursing research: Methods and critical appraisal for evidence-based practice* (6th ed., Chapters 3–18). Philadelphia: Elsevier.

Loomis, J., Willard, B., & Cohen, J. (2006). Difficult professional choices: Deciding between the PhD and the DNP in nursing. *OJIN: The Online Journal of Issues in Nursing, 12*(1).

Meleis, A., & Dracup, K. (2005). The case against the DNP: History, timing, substance, and marginalization. *OJIN: The Online Journal of Issues in Nursing. 10*(3).

National Organization of Nurse Practitioner Faculties. (1995). *Advanced nursing practice: Curriculum guidelines and program standards for nurse practitioner education.* Washington, DC: National Organization of Nurse Practitioner Faculties.

Nelson, E., Godfrey, M., Batalden, P., Berry, S., Bothe, A., McKinley, et al. (2008). Clinical microsystems, part 1. The building blocks of health systems. *The Joint Commission Journal on Quality and Patient Safety, 34*(7), 367–378.

O'Neil, E. H., The PEW Health Professions Commission. (1998). *Recreating health professional practice for a new century: The fourth report of the Pew Health Professions Commission.* San Francisco: Pew Health Professions Commission.

Rhodes, M. (2011). Using effects-based reasoning to examine the DNP as the single entry degree for advanced practice nursing. *OJIN: The Online Journal of Issues in Nursing, 16*(3).

Sackett, D. L., Straus, S. E., Richardson, W. S., Rosenberg, W., & Haynes, R. B. (2000). *Evidenced-based medicine: How to teach and practice EBM* (2nd ed.). Edinburgh, Scotland: Churchill Livingstone.

Scott, J. (2001). Using the process approach to improve scholarly writing. *Delta Pi Epsilon Journal, 43*(2), 57–66.

Scott, K., & McSherry, R. (2009). Evidence-based nursing: Clarifying the concepts for nurses in practice. *Journal of Clinical Nursing, 18*, 1085–1095.

Silva, M., & Ludwick, R. (2006). Ethics: Is the doctor of nursing practice ethical? *OJIN: The Online Journal of Issues in Nursing. 11*(2).

The AGREE Collaboration. (2003). Development and validation of an international appraisal instrument for assessing the quality of clinical practice guidelines: The AGREE project. *Quality and Safety in Health Care, 12*, 18–23.

The Joint Commission. (2011). *Improving America's hospitals: The joint commission's annual report on quality and safety.* Washington, DC: The Joint Commission.

United States Department of Health and Human Services. (2000). *Healthy people 2010.* McLean,VA: International Medical Publishing.

Youngblut, J. M., & Brooten, D. (2001). *Evidence-based nursing practice:* Why is it important? *AACN Clinical Issues*, 12, 468–476.

22

Integrating EBP Into DNP Education: The Pace Experience

Joanne K. Singleton, Lillie M. Shortridge-Baggett, Rona F. Levin, Priscilla Sanford Worral, Lucille Ferrara, and the Pace University DNP Faculty Group

. . . the power of forming any correct opinion as to the result must entirely depend upon an enquiry.

—Florence Nightingale

In the first edition of this book a chapter was contributed on behalf of Pace University in which we shared how we revised our master's curriculum, specifically our family nurse practitioner specialty, reframing with an EBP framework (Singleton, Londrigan, & Allan, 2006). That process began in 2001, with full implementation in 2004, and the graduation of the first students for this evidence-based practice (EBP) framed curriculum in 2005. As concluded in that chapter, faculty was moving toward the next challenge after implementation, that being, evaluation of the outcomes of the new curriculum. Although our focus for this chapter is the Doctor of Nursing Practice (DNP) program, it is important to bring the reader up to date on what we have found, as this provided evidence to support the EBP curriculum within the DNP program. In a study to measure students' changes in EBP beliefs and implementation behaviors over time, Singleton, Levin, Shortridge-Baggett, and Londrigan (2009) found that EBP beliefs and EBP implementation, as measured by scales developed by Melnyk and Fineout-Overholt (2003), increased over time in FNP students in the revised curriculum (Singleton, Levin, Shortridge-Baggett, & Londrigan, 2010). The evidence that the integration in the FNP master's curriculum of teaching/learning strategies, which emanate from an EBP framework, improved students' beliefs about EBP and their implementation of EBP practices gave clear direction to faculty in the development of the DNP program and curriculum.

THE CULTURAL CONTEXT FOR THE DNP PROGRAM AT PACE UNIVERSITY

Pace University, with campuses in New York City and Westchester County, has six colleges and schools with over 13,000 students enrolled in undergraduate through graduate education. For over a century Pace University has been known for combining exceptional academics with professional practice experiences.

The Lienhard School of Nursing (LSN; as of 2011, in the College of Health Professions) was founded in 1966. Through its vision the Lienhard School of Nursing strives to "be a leader in innovation and excellence in education, research, and practice in primary health care" (Lienhard School of Nursing 2008). Through its own mission and in support of Pace University's motto, *Opportunitas*, the LSN offers access and opportunity for highly diverse, qualified individuals to begin or advance careers in nursing. "Essential qualities embodied in nursing education at the Lienhard School of Nursing include: the liberal arts and sciences as integral foundations; nursing theory, evidence-based practice, and research as the core body of knowledge; communication, critical thinking, cultural competence, and technological competence as essential skills; and moral and ethical decision making as values to provide society with professionally prepared nurse leaders. The school provides student-centered learning experiences that foster civic, social, and professional responsibility to embrace the challenges of the future. In keeping with the vision, the mission is to continue excellence in teaching, scholarship, practice, and service to prepare graduates to be nursing leaders in health care in the 21st century" (Lienhard School of Nursing, 2008, p. 1).

The DNP program, within LSN's Department of Graduate Studies, at Pace University is grounded in more than 40 years of expertise of the LSN educating primary health care advanced practice family nurse practitioners (FNPs). The DNP program prepares advanced practice nurses to provide dynamic clinical leadership through culturally competent, evidence-based practices and clinical innovations directed at improving health care quality.

The mission of the DNP program is guided by and builds on the strong foundation of the vision and mission of the LSN. Upon this foundation the pillars of the program (see Figure 22.1), primary health care, cultural competence, and EBP, support students as they pursue the program's student learning outcomes, which are also guided by the *Essentials of Doctoral Education for Advanced Nursing Practice* (2006). *Primary health care* as the central pillar represents a philosophical approach to health care intended to promote improved health outcomes for clients. "Primary health care looks beyond primary care and through the collaboration of health professionals, community members, and others working in multiple sectors, emphasizes health promotion, development of healthy policies, and prevention of diseases for all people" (Shoultz & Hatcher, 1997, p. 24). *Cultural competence* is a "... [m]ultidimensional learning process that integrates transcultural nursing skills in all three dimensions of learning (cognitive, practical, and affective), involves transcultural self-efficacy (confidence) as a major influencing factor, and aims to achieve culturally congruent nursing care" (Jeffreys, 2006, p. 25). *Evidence-based practice* is recognized as the process of shared decision making between practitioner, patient, and others significant to them based on research evidence, the patient's experiences and preferences, clinical expertise or know-how, and other available robust sources of information (Rycroft-Malone et al., 2004; Sackett et al., 2000). Student learning outcomes are strengthened and supported throughout the curriculum by the concepts represented by the three pillars (Doctor of Nursing Practice Program, 2011). The DNP model provides a visual representation of the DNP program, which includes the three program pillars as well as themes that are found in program objectives for the DNP.

EVIDENCE-BASED PRACTICE: AN ESSENTIAL PROGRAM PILLAR

Curriculum planning for the DNP program began in 2006. The DNP program is 37 credits, which students complete in a cohort, hybrid, executive format over 3 years (see Exhibit 22.1 for the full DNP curriculum plan). The curriculum plan includes EBP content starting with the first semester, with the students having discrete EBP courses, in the first year second semester, second year first semester, and then across the DNP Mentored Scholarly Project, in which a scholarly evidence-based clinical practice improves.

Graduate faculty who developed the DNP program curriculum clearly recognized that DNP students would need to enhance their knowledge of EBP, and develop a strong skill set to formulate clinical questions, systematically identify the best evidence to answer clinical questions, and translate that evidence into practice. Thus, EBP was identified as an essential program pillar. With a deep understanding of the role of EBP in achieving desired health outcomes and recognizing the importance of EBP articulation with the other two program pillars for students to achieve program outcomes and become clinical leaders, faculty took

EXHIBIT 22.1 DNP PROGRAM STUDENT LEARNING OUTCOMES

For the advanced-standing DNP program the outcomes are as follows:

Within the framework of primary health care and consistent with professional standards, the student will be able to:

1. Synthesize relevant theories from a variety of disciplines to develop frameworks for culturally competent, evidence-based advanced practice nursing in primary health care.
2. Guide the provision of culturally competent, evidence-based primary health care to individuals and populations in a variety of primary care practice settings.
3. Evaluate evidence related to clinical, educational, cultural, and organizational issues, needs and challenges to recommend a course of action for best practices in primary health care.
4. Design mentorship roles in primary health care clinical practice in the development, implementation, and evaluation of culturally competent, evidence-based best practice protocols and projects.
5. Integrate relevant information technology to support culturally competent, evidence-based primary health care delivery.
6. Create change in health policy using the best available evidence with a culturally competent primary health care perspective.
7. Develop collaborations with other disciplines and essential stakeholders to provide culturally competent best practices in primary health care.

up this curricular challenge. In developing the student learning outcomes, each of the three pillars are identified across all student learning outcomes (see Exhibit 22.2). No matter which program pillar may have the central focus, the other two must be in our awareness. We must continually ask how each pillar informs the other, and how each of the pillars is informed by each of the essential DNP content areas. It is the synergy of the program pillars and essential DNP content areas that move us to the program outcomes and enact the program mission. For example, while EBP initiatives are advancing, they are not yet fully where they need to be. Health care continues to struggle with how to ask focused clinical questions in which the multiple dimensions of culture are truly identified, let alone integrated into study sampling and design. Additionally, the research used to generate evidence must be assessed to determine if

EXHIBIT 22.2 DNP PROGRAM CURRICULUM PLAN

Year 1

Fall

Scientific Underpinning for Advanced Practice Nursing
Organizational & Systems Leadership

Spring

EBP Methods & Techniques I
Health Policy for Advanced Practice Nurses

Summer

Teaching and Learning for Advanced Practice Nurses
Ethical and Legal Decision Making for Advanced Practice Nurses

Year 2

Fall

EBP Methods & Techniques II
Health Care Economics & Finance

Spring

Technology and Information Systems for Advanced Practice Nursing
Mentorship I: Doctoral Project I.A
Summer
Doctoral Project work continues

Year 3

Fall

Mentorship I: Doctoral Project I.B

Spring

Mentorship II: Doctoral Project

there was appropriate protection of human subjects and if ethical principles were applied to data collection. An important lesson for students is that applying evidence for clinical practice improvement cannot be applied wholesale, that is, it must be critically assessed to determine for whom the evidence applies. Additionally, we must develop an awareness in students of how study results can be turned into recommendations for future research as well as health policy in regard to cultural and ethnic issues.

The graduate faculty, having been long engaged in EBP education, practice, and research identified EBP as a pillar of the program, which in concert with the other two program pillars—primary health care and cultural competence—was necessary to support students in achieving the program outcomes. In addition to being a program pillar and therefore a thread across the curriculum, faculty determined that there would also be specific EBP methods and techniques courses.

EBP CURRICULUM THREAD

There are seven course objectives for each course in the curriculum. Based on the content focus these objectives address critical appraisal of scientific knowledge for the content focus of the course, and, based on the content of the course, factors that affect best practices, mentorship, meaningful use of technology, health policy, and intra- and interprofessional collaboration.

Course objectives in each and every course across the program address EBP and locate it within the content and context of the course. These building blocks combined with the discrete EBP content in the EBP methods and techniques courses, prepare students to apply the EBP knowledge and skill set they are developing to their DNP Mentored Scholarly Project. In this way students learn to create an environment to support EBP (Institute of Medicine, 2001) and to use evidence as the foundation of decision making (Institute of Medicine, 2003). As the first cohort moved toward their project work, the Joanna Briggs Institute (JBI) for EBP framework was accepted to guide the students in their systematic reviews of evidence related to their projects (Pearson, 2010). Based on almost 10 years of work, the JBI model was developed in 2005. The model provides a framework for considering the major components in the process of evidence-based health care. Pearson (2010) identifies the four major components as: health care evidence generation; evidence synthesis, evidence knowledge transfer; and evidence utilization. The JBI model offers a framework that supports the critical importance of evidence-based information to clinical decision making and improvement.

The first semester courses will be discussed as an example of EBP as a curriculum thread. First semester courses include: Scientific Underpinning for Advanced Practice Nursing, and Organizational, & Systems Leadership. In Scientific Underpinnings for Advanced Practice Nursing, EBP models are introduced, explained, discussed, and applied to clinical practice. EBP and the important role it plays in mentorship and the philosophical issues it presents in the meaningful use of technology are also addressed. In the Organizational & Systems Leadership course leadership evidence is explored, and students participate in gathering evidence of themselves as leaders and gain skill in organizational assessment through which they generate internal evidence to determine how to effectively move a proposed practice change forward. Within their organizational assessment they assess the organization's readiness to support EBP.

EBP METHODS AND TECHNIQUES COURSES

In the second semester of the program (spring of program year 1), students complete the EBP Methods and Techniques I course. This course focuses on the appraisal of evidence from an epidemiologic perspective. Students search and locate clinical practice guidelines and appraise the level and quality of evidence using the AGREE II tool (Brouwers et al., 2010), Healthy People 2020, and the National Health Disparities Report (Centers for Disease Control and Prevention, 2011) to help faculty to select a topic or foci to coach students in learning these appraisals. Additional books used in this course include: Gordis (2009), *Epidemiology* (4th ed.), and Haynes, Sackett, Guyatt, and Tugwell (2006), *Clinical Epidemiology: How to Do Clinical Practice Research* (3rd ed.).

The second EBP course, Methods and Techniques II, is offered in the fall of program year 2. In this course students learn how to conduct an evidence summary. Working as teams directed by Healthy People 2020 and the National Health Disparities Report, students identify clinical questions. The team is coached to address the clinical question through writing an evidence summary by building on the work done in the EBP Methods and Technique I course. They learn about the process of going from the evidence summary to recommending best practices, determining key outcome variables, and planning for small tests of change prior to full implementation.

DNP-MENTORED SCHOLARLY PROJECT

Students begin the DNP Mentored Scholarly Project in the spring of program year 2, and complete the project and program in the spring of program year 3. The first course and clinical is divided into two parts, A and B, with students continuing to work on their projects over the summer. In the first semester of project work students work in teams with a clinical faculty mentor and in partnership with a clinical agency and a clinical agency mentor to identify an area of importance to the agency for practice improvement. The team conducts an organizational assessment to identify the clinical question to be addressed. Based on the question the team develops a systematic review (SR) Protocol to be published by JBI. The team then conducts the full SR, which also is to be published by JBI, and from the evidence identified through the SR the team makes a recommendation to the clinical partner agency for a clinical practice improvement. Each individual member of the team then develops a manuscript to demonstrate their knowledge synthesis based on their project and one of the program pillars or themes that takes their knowledge to an application beyond their project. After meeting the assignment requirements the student then is able to disseminate their knowledge to the larger community of peers through publication of their manuscript.

FROM THE VERY START: ENHANCING STUDENTS' EBP KNOWLEDGE

The program begins with an on-campus orientation to familiarize students with our DNP program model, faculty, support staff, expectations, and program progression. Student access and connectivity to the online program platform is ensured. At the start of the program students are provided with the list of "program books" that they will use in courses across the program. There may also be additional books specific to the courses. When we started the program with our first cohort, faculty selected two books as EBP program books to provide students with foundational concepts, and direction for developing their EBP skill set, including applying the evidence to clinical practice improvement. The selection was based on faculty's academic and clinical practice experience with EBP. Additional books are required in EBP courses to support students in their developing knowledge and skill in EBP specific to course content. Faculty continually assesses program books for subsequent cohorts. With ongoing developments in EBP, revisions of EBP books, and assessment of our DNP student learner needs in this area, EBP program books may be changed or added. Each cohort is provided with the reference for any EBP book used by a previous cohort that is no longer one of the required EBP program books for their cohort. While an EBP program book may be changed, it is possible that it will become a required book for one of the specific EBP courses. Refer to Exhibit 22.3 for the EBP Program books selected for our first four cohorts.

These program books are used to help students prepare for the program and their EBP courses, as well as to address the EBP thread across the curriculum. Additional books are required for the specific EBP courses, and will be identified in the EBP course discussion. DNP faculty use a variety of teaching–learning strategies to ensure that the teaching–learning experiences and learning environments for students facilitate achievement of both individual and overall student learning outcomes. Teaching–learning strategies reinforce the steady acquisition of increasingly complex knowledge at the DNP level. This connects the clinical practice of the advanced standing student to the learning community, where students are asked to use their practice to apply new and developing knowledge in order for students to move their practice to a higher level. As one example, as an assignment in their second EBP Methods course, students

EXHIBIT 22.3 EBP PROGRAM BOOKS FOR COHORTS 1 TO 4

Cohort 1 Fall 2008

Langley, G., Moen, R., Nolan, K., Nolan, T., Norman, C., & Provost, L. (2009). *The improvement guide: A practical approach to enhancing organizational performance* (2nd ed.). Philadelphia, PA: Jossey-Bass.

Melnyk, B. M., & Fineout-Overholt, E. (2005). *Evidence-based practice in nursing and healthcare: A guide to best practice*. Philadelphia, PA: Lippincott Williams & Wilkins.

Cohort 2 Fall 2009

DiCenso, A., Guyatt, G., & Ciliska, D. (2005). *Evidence-based nursing: A guide to clinical practice*. St. Louis, MO: Elsevier Mosby.

Langley, G., Moen, R., Nolan, K., Nolan, T., Norman, C., & Provost, L. (2009). *The improvement guide: A practical approach to enhancing organizational performance* (2nd ed.). Philadelphia, PA: Jossey-Bass.

Melnyk, B. M., & Fineout-Overholt, E. (2005). *Evidence-based practice in nursing and healthcare: A guide to best practice*. Philadelphia, PA: Lippincott Williams & Wilkins.

Cohort 3 Fall 2010

Langley, G., Moen, R., Nolan, K., Nolan, T., Norman, C., & Provost, L. (2009). *The improvement guide: A practical approach to enhancing organizational performance* (2nd ed.). Philadelphia, PA: Jossey-Bass.

Rycroft-Malone, J., & Bucknall, T. (Eds.). (2010). *Models and frameworks for implementing evidence-based practice: Linking evidence to action*. Hoboken, NJ: Wiley-Blackwell.

Cohort 4 Fall 2011

Melnyk, B. M., & Fineout-Overholt, E. (2011). *Evidence-based practice in nursing and healthcare: A guide to best practice* (2nd ed.). Philadelphia, PA: Lippincott Williams & Wilkins.

Polit, D. F., & Beck, C. T. (2012). *Nursing research: Generating and assessing evidence for nursing practice* (9th ed.). Philadelphia, PA: Lippincott Williams & Wilkins.

in cohort 1 conducted interviews with stakeholders in their work environment to determine where these stakeholders believed enhancement in clinical practice was needed. This assignment helped to engender greater collaboration among the nurse practitioner DNP students and the individuals in their organization whom they interviewed. As a result of these interviews and the uncovering of areas where practice could be enhanced, clinical practice improvement initiatives were started.

EBP STUDENT ASSESSMENT AND SUPPORT AT THE START OF THE PROGRAM

Over the past four cohorts we have assessed the needs of students and have implemented several strategies to support students in enhancing their EBP knowledge. We are conducting a longitudinal study of our DNP students from start to completion of our program to assess learning outcomes. EBP Beliefs and Implementation are being measured utilizing the Melnyk and Fineout-Overholt tools that were previously discussed. Our experiences with the first cohort led us to develop eLearning modules on EBP basics. These were put into place with our second cohort to review at the start of the program, and for our first cohort to review as they continued in the program. Over time we have identified the need for students to review basic statistics and research design prior to starting the program, and we have identified and provided them with books selected by faculty. Additionally, we have identified the need for students to develop greater competency and comfort with our library databases and databased searching. Our research librarians have developed two modules, one basic and one more advanced for evidence searching. Students are provided with these links, and starting with our fourth cohort are required to review these modules prior to orientation and to use them as a reference resource throughout the program.

LESSONS LEARNED: STUDENT EVALUATIONS AND FACULTY PERSPECTIVES PROVIDE EVIDENCE FOR FUTURE DIRECTIONS

In general, program evaluations show that DNP students across the program report a developing understanding of the EBP program pillar. Additionally, while this chapter is not reporting on the full EBP Beliefs and Implementation study of our DNP students, across our first three cohorts scores from baseline to end of program year 1, as measured by the EBP Beliefs and EBP Implementation scales, increased. By cohort, results showed, either scores increased from the first measurement to the second in the expected direction, or results approached or reached statistical significance on one or both of the scales.

Students are asked to participate in mid-semester and end-of-semester course evaluations. Mid-semester course evaluations are reviewed by the DNP program director and course faculty and allow for adjustments during the course that are deemed to be appropriate to facilitate student learning. Mid-semester as well as end-of-semester student course evaluations are reviewed at the end of the semester for faculty to consider for course revisions. Course faculty evaluations are also reviewed at mid- and end-of-semester to assess content delivery and strategies employed by faculty to facilitate student learning. Student recommendations for program improvement at the course level for the two EBP courses included: decreasing the number of faculty teaching in the course, and clearly define who the lead faculty is and each faculty's role and expectations for graded assignments; identify for students baseline expectations for EBP prior to the start of the first EBP course so students can close any knowledge gaps in foundational EBP to build on this base. Students engage in teamwork across the program. The intensity of the work grows as the students progress from the EBP courses to the DNP Mentored Scholarly Project. It became clear that students, as well as faculty, needed clearer guidance and development in intraprofessional teamwork. This has resulted in the development of specific detailed teamwork guidelines to assist students and faculty in the intra-/interprofessional teamwork in which they will engage throughout the program. The guidelines require a teamwork charter and expectations for how each team member will complete the work of the project team, how they will collaborate to produce the required deliverables, and tools for ongoing evaluation. The teamwork guidelines are used across the program, and students are oriented to these guidelines through a process approach to teamwork in the first semester of the program. By the end of the third year of the program, and with the graduation of the first DNP cohort, faculty have greater clarity on the knowledge and skillset required for the EBP methods and techniques courses, and the DNP Mentored Scholarly Project. Utilizing the JBI model of evidence-based health care has provided a framework for implementing evidence that is systematic and broad enough to be compatible with any EBP model used in the practice of our clinical partner agencies. Grounded in the JBI framework faculty continue in partnership with our DNP students to meet the challenge of ongoing knowledge and skill development for both faculty and students through the ongoing assessment, enhancement, and refinement of EBP as both discrete content and as an essential program pillar.

REFERENCES

American Association of Colleges of Nursing. (2006). *Essentials of doctoral education for advanced nursing practice*. Washington, DC: American Association of Colleges of Nursing.

Brouwers, M., Kho, M. E., Browman, G. P., Burgers, J. S., Cluzeau, F., Feder, G. et al. (2010). For the AGREE next steps consortium. AGREE II: Advancing guideline development, reporting and evaluation in healthcare. *Canadian Medical Association Journal, 182*, E839–E842. doi: 10.1503/090449.

Centers for Disease Control and Prevention. (2011). National health disparities report. *Morbidity And Mortality Weekly Report, 60*(Suppl). Atlanta, GA: U.S. Department of Health and Human Services.

Doctor of Nursing Practice Program. (2011). *DNP program overview*, New York, NY: Pace University.

Gordis, L. (2009). *Epidemiology*, (4th ed.). Philadelphia: Saunders/Elsevier.

Haynes, R. B., Sackett, D. L., Guyatt, G. H., & Tugwell, P. (2006). *Clinical epidemiology: How to do clinical practice research* (3rd ed.). Philadelphia: Lippincott Williams & Wilkins.

IOM. (2001). *Crossing the quality chasm*, Washington, DC: IOM.

IOM. (2003). *The future of the public's health*, Washington, DC: IOM.

Jeffreys, M. (2006). *Teaching cultural competence in nursing and health care: inquiry, action, and innovation*. Springer, NY: Dover.

Lienhard School of Nursing. (2008). *Mission and vision*, New York: Pace University.

Nightingale, F. (1969). *Notes on nursing: What it is and it is not*, New York: Dover.

Pearson, A. (2010). The Joanna Briggs Institute model of evidence-based health care as a framework for implementing evidence. In Rycroft-Malone & Bucknall (Eds.), *Models and frameworks for implementing evidence-based practice linking evidence to action* (pp. 185–206). New York: Wiley-Blackwell.

Sackett, D., Straus, S. E., Richardson, W. C., Rosenberg, W., & Haynes, R. M. (2000). *Evidence-based medicine: How to practice and teach EBM* (2nd ed.). Edinburgh: Churchill Livingstone.

Shoultz, J., & Hatcher, P. A. (1997). Looking beyond primary care to primary health care: an approach to community-based action. *Nursing Outlook, 45*(1), 23–26.

Singleton, J. K., Levin, R. L., Shortridge-Baggett, L. M., & Londrigan, M. T. (2010). FNP students' EBP beliefs and implementation. *Paper presentation at AACN Master's Education Conference*, New Orleans, LA.

Singleton, J. K., Levin, R. F., Shortridge-Baggett, L. M., & Londrigan, M. T. (2009). FNP students' beliefs and implementation. *Poster presented at the annual meeting of the National Organization of Nurse Practitioner Faculties*, Portland, Oregon.

Singleton, J. K., Londrigan, M., & Allan, J. (2006). Incorporating evidence based practice into clinical education for family nurse practitioners: The Pace University experience. In R. Levin, & H. Feldman (Eds.), *Teaching evidence-based practice in nursing* (pp. 193–204). New York, NY: Springer Publishing.

Part IV

Strategies for Creating a Practice Culture for Evidence-Based Practice

Although students are learning all about evidence-based practice, we also need to educate those in practice. We all need to be on board to effect change. So Part IV looks at different clinical settings, acute care, and community health, to provide exemplars of how these cultures have changed over time. The chapters should also serve as a guide to institutions that do not currently emphasize evidence-based practice. We can all support these efforts and we believe it is the obligation of the education community to facilitate the shift. The individuals who wrote these chapters worked with many academic and clinical partners to make change happen, so readers can benefit from their experiences.

23

Implementing an EBP Council in a Hospital Setting: The Northern Westchester Experience

Fay Wright

If there is no struggle, there is no progress.

—Frederick Douglass

Using evidence to improve clinical practice and thus the quality of patient care is the goal of evidence-based practice (EBP)—yet it is easier said than done. How do organizations make the critical leap from knowing what EBP is all about to implementing best practices on clinical units? Mentoring EBP leaders and coaching clinical champions in the EBP process is the first step to such progress. Translating evidence to clinical practice to improve patient care requires the involvement of direct care nurses in designing, implementing, and evaluating EBP innovations. This chapter presents the experiences of one community hospital's successful empowerment of direct care nurses to implement EBP and to improve patient care through the development of an organizational infrastructure that enabled direct care nurses to engage in EBP. Key components of that infrastructure are shared governance, mentoring, and coaching, all processes that support nurses' professional development and leadership.

SHARED GOVERNANCE

Shared governance is mutual decision making based on the principles of partnership, equity, and accountability for quality patient care (Porter-O'Grady, 1987). In shared governance, all members of the nursing department are empowered to identify ways to improve care and to be creative and inquisitive in their approach to finding solutions and improvements. In order to assume the important leadership role direct care nurses play in shared governance, education, and mentorship are essential, but further infrastructure is also needed to support the work of a direct care nurse in implementing EBP.

At Northern Westchester Hospital (NWH), nursing shared governance practice councils were developed to provide organization to key areas of nursing's influence (see Figure 23.1). The Nurse Executive Council provides overall leadership, developing the strategic plan for the nursing department and coordinating implementation of that strategic plan to meet annual goals. Each patient care unit has a unit council, led by a unit chair who is a direct care nurse, in collaboration with the unit's nurse manager. The unit council chair and the nurse manager are also members of the Nurse Executive Council and the Quality Council. Five additional direct care nurses are elected to represent the patient care unit on each nursing practice council, and lead the specific council initiatives on their unit. The other five practice councils are: (1) Technology and Informatics, (2) Nursing Credential, (3) Professional Development, (4) Scope and Standards, and (5) EBP & Nursing Research (see Figure 23.1). Nursing managers and administrative leaders are also members of the practice councils. Working at the unit level, the unit council coordinates and communicates the strategic plan and works to involve the entire patient care staff in working to meet NWH goals. Coordination and

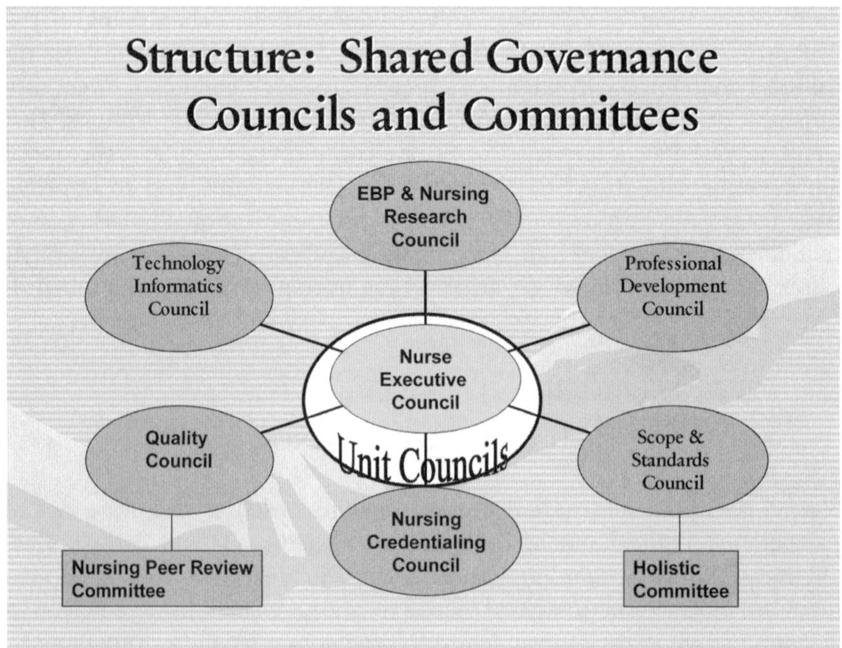

FIGURE 23.1 Northern Westchester Hospital shared governance model.

communication of shared governance work is the role of the unit council members.

When members of the hospital staff have a clinical question or practice concern, they bring it to the unit council. At the unit council meeting there is discussion about the most appropriate way to address the concern, that is, a decision is made as to which practice council is best suited to address the topic. The unit-based representative then brings the issue or question to the specified practice council for further discussion, prioritization, and solutions.

EBP–NRC

Mission and Goals

The mission of the EBP–NRC (Nursing Research Council) is to develop and support EBP initiatives and nursing research projects. The EBP–NRC facilitates the use of EBP to enhance patient outcomes. The EBP also serves as a way to involve and support direct care nurses to translate evidence into practice. The goals of the EBP–NRC are to:

- Promote an environment where nursing practice is based on the best available evidence.
- Develop processes and strategies to implement and sustain EBP.
- Educate and develop EBP clinical champions to support patient care staff in the EBP process.
- Explore and implement nursing research studies when evidence to answer clinical questions is not sufficient.
- Support the development of a culture of inquiry to address clinical questions in order to improve patient outcomes.

At the EBP–NRC meetings, members develop skills in reading and appraising evidence. Through discussions at the EBP–NRC table, the group grows in their collective understanding of how to apply evidence to practice. The EBP–NRC members develop PICO (population, intervention, comparison, outcome) questions and plan the implementation and evaluation of EBP innovations. The EBP–NRC representatives are the unit-based experts for the EBP process, educating and supporting unit staff in their understanding and utilization of EBP.

MEMBERSHIP

EBP–NRC membership includes a direct care nurse from each clinical unit, as well as representatives from nursing management and administration, totaling 15 members. Each unit elects one EBP–NRC representative who serves as a member of the council for 2 years. Members may be re-elected for one additional 2-year term for a total 4 years of membership. When a member no longer serves on the council, one is still involved at the unit level with EBP projects. One-third of the council rotates off every year so there is a constant influx of new members learning the EBP process and spreading knowledge of EBP throughout the organization. An advanced practice nurse serves as the council mentor to support the work of the EBP–NRC. The mentor has a strong knowledge of EBP, group facilitation, organizational process, and educational principles. The mentor facilitates the work of the EBP–NRC through education, coordination of the institutional flow of projects, and directly mentoring the council chair. The mentor is a teacher, role model, and cheerleader for the members of the EBP–NRC. As teacher, the mentor shares her knowledge of research methods, evidence appraisal, and the EBP process. By modeling leadership behaviors and professional communication, the mentor supports group process and EBP–NRC member leadership development. Cheering for learning, and success, the mentor encourages the members, acknowledging their hard work and professional contributions. (See Part I for a detailed discussion of the mentor role.)

The EBP–NRC chair is a direct care nurse who is elected by EBP–NRC council members to work with the mentor to facilitate the work of the EBP–NRC. The chair is the primary clinical champion for EBP, serving as the face of EBP–NRC work at the executive council and as a key person to influence EBP project development and coordination.

The chair works closely with the mentor to coordinate the work of the EBP–NRC. As an EBP clinical champion, the chair influences the work of the council. The chair coaches the EBP–NRC members in their work, coordinating ideas for projects with the council's current workload, hospital initiatives, and priorities. Using experience and knowledge gained from completing successful EBP projects, the chair coaches the members in project development and implementation, providing lessons from her own work to enable others to move their projects forward.

The EBP–NRC chair and mentor meet regularly between council meetings to review project progress and potential obstacles as well as plan council meetings. During the meetings, the mentor provides individualized education about EBP, research, and organizational change theory to support the chair's professional development. Collaborative goals for mutual learning are developed between the mentor and chair. For example, a former chair identified the need for group facilitation skills and wanted to learn to coordinate group discussions, as she had observed the mentor do many times. Based on this learning need, the mentor and chair developed a plan for the chair to develop group facilitation skills through readings, discussions with the mentor, and role-playing group leadership to support the chair's professional development. To support her learning, de-briefing sessions between chair and mentor were held after every EBP–NRC meeting to discuss the chair's group facilitation. Before long, the chair and mentor mutually agreed that the chair was becoming an "expert" group facilitator. The mentor and chair continued to develop learning goals to support the chair's professional development.

EBP PROCESS STANDARDIZATION

To support efficient coordinated work, the EBP–NRC decided to formalize the EBP process at NWH to utilize the Evidence-Based Practice Improvement Model (EBPI) as a method to build expertise in EBP (Levin et al., 2010). The EBPI model provides a simple, clear process to use evidence to improve clinical practice (Levin et al., 2010). Using the "one step at a time approach" (Levin, 2009, p. 124), direct care nurses build confidence in the process of EBP and are able to successfully implement practice improvements based on the best evidence and the most effective processes within the practice setting. The EBP–NRC plans practice innovations as "small tests of change," where one piece of the intended EBP innovation is implemented at a time so that each component can be evaluated before implementing the entire innovation. Small tests of change enable evaluation of the process of innovation to be evaluated, supporting more successful long-term EBP practice improvement (Levin, 2009). Additionally, standardization of the EBP process supports direct care nursing involvement by building their confidence in their leadership in EBP–NRC; they know what to do and how to plan project implementation and evaluation. By utilizing a standardized approach for the work of the EBP–NRC, the members develop confidence and competence in the process so they can focus on the clinical problems and potential evidence-based solutions without having to also keep thinking about what to do next. One staff nurse explains the utility of EBP process standardization: "I know I have to clarify clinical problems with internal and external evidence before a solution can be found. If I don't clarify the problem, I may implement an ineffective solution, not because the solution is ineffective but because it's the wrong solution to the problem or because the solution doesn't work in my unit" (M. Zavros, personal communication, October 30, 2011).

Education about the EBPI model is incorporated into EBP–NRC council member orientation. The orientation class is taught by the EBP–NRC mentor and chair. In addition to education about the EBPI model, the orientation includes clinical scenarios for practice in identifying PICO questions. During the orientation, the hospital librarian provides training about searching the CINAHL and PubMed databases.

Another process standardization developed by the EBP–NRC members is project templates to guide EBP–NRC work. Council members identified that following templates and guidelines makes it easier to organize and implement a project. In addition, when templates are used, all staff involved know the project's goals and work toward those goals. Based on the steps of the EBPI model, council members developed standardized project timelines, tables for evidence review, responsibility charts, and report documents. Standardization ensures the quality of the process, evaluating the work every step of the way for maximal success. All project documents are labeled with the project name and the date the document was edited. This simple norm helps EBP–NRC members stay organized and clarifies communication within the group.

EBP–NRC CLINICAL CHAMPIONS

After completing the orientation, new members are paired with an experienced EBP–NRC unit representative, known as an "EBP clinical champion." The clinical champion serves as an EBP coach to support new members as they develop their knowledge and skills. The EBP clinical champions use their understanding of the EBPI model and their expert knowledge of the practice setting to navigate the complexities of organizational change and to translate evidence into practice improvement (Fineout-Overholt, Levin, & Melnyk, 2005).

Clinical champions developed from the hospital's initial EBP project success. Before the development of shared governance and the EBP–NRC, EBP education and project development were initiated at the hospital. During the EBP educational sessions, Levin (personal communication, May, 2008) discussed the importance of clinical champions as a method of peer support for successful EBP involvement. The first two EBP projects achieved significant improvement in assessment of patient fall risk and sedation assessment. Both projects were submitted and accepted for a national EBP conference (Misiano, Comiskey, D'Arcy, Levin, & Wright, 2009; Olney, Carrolo, Levin, & Wright, 2009). The hospital supported the travel of the five direct care nurses to present at the conference. When they returned, the nurses presented their projects at unit meetings and discussed not only their project successes, but also their feelings of pride in their presentations to the professional audience: "We really improved care with our changes in fall assessment. So many people were impressed by my work! It was worth reading all that evidence!" (K. Olney, personal communication, February 19, 2009). When the nurses shared their pride in their accomplishments, enthusiasm for EBP grew not only as recognition for the EBP improvements in patient care, but also for the recognition of nursing's ability to affect the quality of patient care through evidence.

As clinical champions, the EBP–NRC members enthusiastically lead the hospital staff in EBPI, continuing their personal development while supporting the education of others. The clinical champions are an integral part of the successful EBP program, coordinating unit-based projects and supporting hospital-wide projects with their knowledge and dedication.

The clinical champions also organize an EBP–NRC education binder, with articles about the EBPI model and the council's goals and resources for each clinical unit. The binder serves as an on-the-spot reference for EBPI, database search information, and systematic appraisal of evidence. A list of EBP–NRC council members' emails and projects is included in the binder. The goal for the EBP–NRC clinical champions is to not only support the education of new council members, but to reach out to all hospital staff about EBP.

EBP PROJECT PRIORITIZATION

Enthusiasm for EBP creates a breeding ground for multiple ideas and clinical questions. At times, ideas proliferate like wild flowers. How can ideas be supported without excessive work burden from the competing demands of patient care and EBP project work? Project prioritization is essential to support the EBP–NRC members and to maintain the quality of the EBP project's work.

The EBP–NRC is the gatekeeper of project prioritization, organization, and resource allocation. In collaboration with the nursing executive council, potential projects are prioritized by considering: NWH institutional priorities; clinical questions about patient care, identification by motivated direct care nurses; department-level initiatives; and resources needed to perform the project.

At monthly EBP–NRC meetings, clinical questions are discussed and prioritized based on clinical urgency and current project workload. It is essential to balance project workload for the EBP–NRC council members, specific clinical units, clinical division, and the hospital as a whole. As an example of prioritization, one project on the progressive care unit that was designed to implement an evidence-based guideline for telemetry utilization was placed on hold until a care delivery redesign project that involved the entire clinical division was completed. The demands on the staff to engage in system-wide change and to coordinate an important unit-specific project would have hindered the implementation and success of both projects.

EBP–NRC COUNCIL PROCESS

The EBP–NRC meets monthly for 4 hours. Two of these hours are designed for the clinical champions to discuss current project progress, challenges, and need for support. New clinical questions and project ideas are also identified and prioritized during this part of the meeting. A key agenda item is group discussion of clinical questions and concerns that are potential project ideas.

The second 2 hours of the meeting are spent on individual project work. The clinical champions may meet with the chair or mentor for specific project support, or the project teams may meet on the units to collect data and analyze results. Time is also spent writing project reports and abstracts to submit for presentations and publications.

Clinical Question Identification and Discussion at the EBP–NRC Meetings

Clinical questions are brought forward by the EBP–NRC council members from unit council discussions. The chair brings forward questions from the nurse executive council that consist of divisional or hospital-level concerns. EBP–NRC members work together to clarify each clinical question and to identify the topics of external and internal evidence needed to clarify the question. The internal evidence may include results from chart audits, clinical observation data, or results of process evaluation from a small test of change. External evidence is the literature found from a systematic search of databases.

For example, direct care nurses on the maternity unit at NWH noted that male newborn term infants who were circumcised within the first 24 hours of birth were lethargic trying to breastfeed after circumcision. The infants displayed no feeding cues for an extended period, and often did not feed the prescribed eight times in the first 24 hours. The maternity unit EBP–NRC representative/clinical champion brought the clinical observations to the EBP–NRC after the unit council supported breastfeeding success as a key goal for the unit.

When the maternity unit clinical champion brought the question forward, she believed the answer was going to be postponing circumcision in newborn term infants until their third day of life in order to facilitate successful breastfeeding. With council discussion, the EBP–NRC identified the need to examine internal data to determine the number of term infants demonstrating the problem, timing of the circumcisions, and pain medications currently administered, and to begin a systematic review of the literature to determine what the external evidence might identify as barriers to successful breastfeeding. During council discussions, the EBP–NRC identified the initial PICO question: "Does postponing circumcision in newborn term infants until their third day of life after breastfeeding is established lead to better clinical outcomes than current practice?"

This PICO question guided the initial systematic literature search. The collection of internal data to clarify the problem was also initiated to determine: the timing of circumcision; the time from circumcision procedure to offering the breast to the baby; and what procedures were consistently offered to soothe the baby during the circumcision procedure. The EBP–NRC members advised the maternity clinical champion to look beyond the solution she felt was "right" and look at what the internal evidence would reveal, as well as to see how the external evidence from the systematic search would further clarify the PICO question.

This group discussion consistently proved valuable to project development and outcomes. For the circumcision project, the external evidence revealed: (1) circumcision is a disruption to establishing breastfeeding, regardless of when the procedure is performed; (2) there is an optimal window of opportunity to encourage the infant to nurse post circumcision; (3) this optimal window of time is 30 minutes. The internal evidence identified 75% of the newborn term babies were not brought to their mothers for breastfeeding until 45 to 60 minutes after circumcision. Using the internal and external evidence, the PICO question was revised: In the male newborn, does breastfeeding within 30 minutes after circumcision have a positive effect on breastfeeding, as compared to initiating breastfeeding after this 30-minute window has elapsed?

Discussion of Project Progress at EBP–NRC Meetings

When discussing project progress, the clinical champion discusses what the internal and external evidence is revealing about the project, and presents results from small tests of change. Through discussion of the project progress, the clinical champion benefits from group knowledge and experience to "think through the evidence and its application to the clinical problem." The mentor focuses the discussion on the systematic appraisal of the evidence as a framework for the project, asking, "What does the evidence tell us about the project?" and, "What are the next steps in the process?" This keeps the council focused on translating the evidence into practice and not responding with clinical experience alone. The chair facilitates the discussion, ensuring that any organizational obstacles are assessed and helping the clinical champion identify where project help is needed.

As the breastfeeding project progressed, the next step was to educate the maternity staff on the positive benefits of offering the term infant breastfeeding within 30 minutes of circumcision. The maternity clinical champion, collaborating with the nursery clinical champion, educated the medical and nursing staff on the maternity floor and in the nursery about the evidence. After the education, the nursing staff developed an intervention to minimize the time from circumcision to breastfeeding to 30 or fewer minutes. A small test of change to evaluate the practice was performed with 66 babies who underwent circumcision during 1 month. Baseline and post-intervention data were compared. Results demonstrated that the babies were more successful at breastfeeding after circumcision using the new protocol (90%), compared to baseline or pre- implementation practice (75%). It is now the standard of care that babies are brought to their mother's breast within 30 minutes of circumcision. Through the collaborative effort of the council discussing and refining the problem and synthesizing the evidence, a significant change was made to improve the quality of newborn care. "I was so sure that we needed to change how circumcisions were performed. Through discussing the evidence with the council, I looked beyond my personal beliefs and found an evidence-based solution that really made a difference. The group discussion made all the difference" (K. Mckechnie, personal communication, October 30, 2011).

EBP–NRC SEARCHING AND APPRAISING EVIDENCE

One of the most significant supports for the work of the EBP–NRC is the hospital's medical librarian. Clinical champions independently search for external evidence or work with the hospital medical librarian. The librarian meets with staff members to help with database searches and access electronic copies of articles that are not readily available in full-text form. Helping with finding the most effective search terms and using her expertise to streamline the search process, the contributions of the medical librarian to the effectiveness of the EBP–NRC cannot be underestimated (see Chapter 9). The search results with article abstracts are provided for review, and after the clinical champion identifies the most appropriate articles, the librarian provides electronic copies for analysis.

The initial search results are discussed with the EBP–NRC mentor. This high-level review of the results and abstracts serves as a teachable moment for the clinical champion: not each article found in the search needs to be read. Using a systematic process, the clinical champion and the mentor review the search results to find the highest level of evidence that addresses the clinical question. Many times, the search reveals many interesting articles about the clinical question topic, but ones that do not address the specific question being asked. By reviewing the search results with the mentor, the clinical champion learns how to look at abstracts, focusing on how they apply to the clinical questions with more efficiency. This first review is an organizational method developed by the EBP–NRC to address members' initial feelings of intimidation in reading research-based articles. Discussing the search results with the mentor, the overall number of articles to read can be narrowed and focused for feasibility. Initially, the champions were overwhelmed with the length of the search results and concerned that they had to read all of the articles found in the search. This initial review process decreases the overwhelming nature of systematic search results for clinical practice. With experience, the clinical champion's expertise grows, the initial review becomes more independent, and mentor support is only sought for specific questions about search results.

When articles are chosen for review, the librarian obtains electronic copies of the publications and e-mails them to the project lead, the clinical champion. Articles are then disseminated to the project team working on the specific project. Project teams are composed of clinical champions, other unit staff interested in the project, and members of the EBP–NRC. The mentor also receives copies of all of the articles so that she may serve as a resource to project members. As team members read the articles and have questions, they can e-mail the mentor, who works with the team to understand the content and study methods.

When reading the articles, team members complete a table of evidence (TOE) to synthesize the content of the article for easier discussion (see Table 23.1 for an example).

The TOE is a tool to organize the knowledge found in the evidence into a format that is easily retrievable and applicable to practice, providing a systematic method to appraise and discuss evidence. Completing the TOE demystifies reading evidence for direct care nurses who may not be comfortable with reading research reports. As one direct care nurse noted, "I never thought I could read and understand research. The table of evidence helps me organize how I read the articles, helping me really understand and use the evidence for my practice" (T. Saracelli, personal communication, September 7, 2010).

When a project team member completes a TOE, it is sent to all the members of the project team and to the EBP–NRC via e-mail. Everyone reviews the TOEs, providing feedback by e-mail or at the next council meeting. The TOEs provide the EBP–NRC with accessible evidence to clarify project questions, interventions, and aims. If further external evidence is needed after group discussion, the clinical champion can go to the hospital library during council project work time and perform further searches.

TABLE 23.1 Propofol Infusion Syndrome (PRIS)

Study	Sample	Design/Patient Selection Level/Quality Rating	Findings	Author Conclusions/ Reviewer Comments
Kam and Cardone (2007)	Sixty-one cases of pediatric and adult patients on propofol	Review of literature of case reports highlighting clinical features, pathophysiology, and management of PRIS Electronic search using Ovid database for Medline (1963–2006) and CINAHL and EMBASE databases Level V	Out of 61 cases diagnosed with PRIS, 20 pediatric deaths and 18 adult deaths reported. Association between PRIS and propofol infusions at doses higher than 4 mg/kg/hour for greater than 48 hour duration. An early sign of cardiac instability is a right bundle branch block with convex curved ST segment elevation in precordial leads V1–V3 on ECG. Predisposing factors: young age, severe critical illness of CNS or respiratory origin, exogenous catecholamine or glucocorticoid administration, inadequate carbohydrate intake, and subclinical mitochondrial disease.	AC: PRIS "may be caused by either a direct mitochondrial respiratory chain inhibition or impaired mitochondrial fatty acid metabolism mediated by propofol" RC: Considered in protocol development

EBP–NRC PROJECTS

The EBP–NRC works on large and small projects. The key to a successful project is the leadership of an EBP clinical champion. When a nurse is focused to discover the answer to a clinical question, curiosity to find a better way drives the project to success.

Sample projects include:

- Maintaining Normothermia in the Operating Room
  - Increased compliance with the Surgical Care Improvement (SCIP) (The Joint Commission, 2010) Guidelines to greater than 98%
  - Clinical competency developed to support adherence to the EBP protocol
- Prevention of Opioid Induced Constipation in Oncology Patients
  - Increased staff assessment and documentation of constipation to 100%
  - Increased physician ordering of constipation preventative therapies to greater than 95% for at-risk patients
- Replacing the BRATT Diet (Bezerra, Stathos, Duncan, Gaines, & Udall, 1992) for Acute Gastroenteritis on the Pediatric Unit Evaluating the Effectiveness of Feeding a Pediatric Regular Diet
  - No increase in gastroenteritis symptoms with regular diet
  - Nutrition Care Committee endorsed diet order change
  - Policy revised to reflect EBP
- Replacing Triple Dye for Umbilical Cord Care with dry and clean care
  - Project presented and endorsed by neonatal advisory committee and pediatricians
  - Policy for cord care changed to reflect not using triple dye for cord care
  - No increase in umbilical cord infections
- IV Catheter Gauge Size for Blood Transfusions
  - Policy changed to reflect EBP that RN assesses patient's vein and may determine most appropriate size for nonemergent blood transfusions
  - Decreased multiple IV attempts by 60%

EBP–NRC Support of Shared Governance Councils

The other nursing practice councils consult the EBP council with clinical practice questions that require further information. The council has developed expertise in searching for and synthesizing evidence. Not all clinical questions require a full project. Some are actually process improvement projects that might focus on changing bottlenecks in systems or increasing communication among disciplines. For example, a new fall risk assessment tool and prevention intervention was identified and implemented with an initial 3% reduction in patient falls. The EBP intervention was offering toileting every 2 hours to patients at risk for falls. The intervention, however, required the RN and the patient care assistant (PCA) to collaboratively organize the workload of offering toileting to the fall risk patients. After initial implementation, the fall rate increased to baseline. The EBP–NRC had identified the EBP innovation, but hospital system issues needed to be addressed to support the consistency of the intervention implementation. Based on the evidence, the EBP–NRC recommended that the professional development council provide education about delegation principles and the scope and standards council develop a policy to improve the congruence of the evidence recommendations.

INFRASTRUCTURE SUPPORT FOR EBP

Given the daily demands of nursing practice, infrastructure must be built to support direct care nurses' involvement in EBP. At NWH, one support is the council structure, but other supports are also essential. A supportive infrastructure includes access to database search engines, computer access, copying, financial reimbursement for time spent working on EBP projects, providing mentors, and shared governance.

The chief nursing officer identified the need to have easy access to evidence if the nursing staff was going to be able to implement EBP. Subscriptions to CINAHL, PubMed, and the Cochrane Library were purchased to provide easy access to computerized database search engines. The databases are available through any computer at the hospital and at home through the hospital Internet staff site. This availability enables EBP–NRC members to search for answers to clinical questions even when working the night shift or from home. Additionally, a computer on each unit with word processing, presentation programs, and printing capabilities is dedicated to support shared governance work.

EBP–NRC members are paid for the 4 hours of council meeting time as part of their scheduled work hours. While additional time beyond the monthly 4 hours is often needed for projects, the clinical champions are able to sign up for reimbursement, and when staffing numbers allow and nursing staff are "downsized," they are given first priority to have shared governance paid time off for council work. While each member will attest to their commitment to shared governance and the integrity of the process of EBPI that requires contribution of nonreimbursed professional time, financial reimbursement for their work is essential to reward their commitment to EBP.

EBP–NRC SUCCESS

The EBP–NRC has been remarkably successful. Council projects were recognized by the Foundation of New York State Nurses (Foundation). The Foundation's Board of Trustees recognizes excellence in implementing nursing research in the practice setting by awarding the Evidence-Based Practice Award. This award is given to an individual or group using research-based evidence to make a practice change that results in demonstrated improvement in outcomes for the patient and family, staff, community, or organization. NWH Council members received both the 2010 and 2011 Evidence-Based Practice Award.

The 2010 Award recognized the Intensive Care Unit EBP team—Maureen Comiskey, RN, Alicia D'Arcy, BSN, RN-BC, Barbara Misiano, MS, RN, CCRN—for the project "Implementing an Evidence-Based Protocol for Propofol Administration in Vented ICU Patients: Improving Patient Outcomes and Decreasing Hospital Costs." This project was the first EBP project at NWH. Started before the EBP–NRC was established, the lessons learned from this team's work paved the way for the development of the EBP–NRC structure and future success.

The 2011 Award was given to the Operating Room and Post Anesthesia Care Unit EBP Team—Kathy Pecoraro Pecoraro, BSN, RN, CAPA and Wendy Kopec, RN, CNOR—for the project "Maintaining Perioperative Normothermia: An Evidence Based Practice Approach."

Members of the EBP–NRC have presented completed projects at specialty nursing organization conferences and national EBP conferences. Disseminating the process of EBP at NWH and the EBP–NRC collaborative methods is part of the EBPI process. Successful processes need to be shared so others benefit from our practice improvements. While improvements in the quality of care do reward the hours spent searching and reading evidence, collecting internal data, and evaluating project outcomes, recognition by colleagues at professional conferences is a secondary gain that acknowledges the EBP–NRC members' professionalism and dedication, and motivates them to continue to pursue excellence.

The professionalism and collegiality of the EBP–NRC is inspiring as Lauraine Skekley, the chief nursing officer of NWH states:

> To achieve nursing excellence, registered professional nurses must incorporate science into their practice. The members of the EBP–NRC have learned how to read and evaluate evidence and conscientiously integrate it into improving clinical and operational processes and patient outcomes. I am so very inspired by these professional nurses. I look back on their accomplishments with sheer amazement. I have watched them in their council work and in front of national audiences presenting their projects and I have discovered just how talented and impressive they

really are. I am so very proud to call them my colleagues and to lead them as their CNO. Evidence continues to grow, and the nurses of NWH are participating and contributing through innovation to improve quality of patient care and advance nursing practice. I have seen the excitement grow as their knowledge expands and they become strong leaders and empowered professionals. I encourage all of you to share your knowledge with others; mentor others as you have been mentored; and continue to enhance patients' and families' experiences. (L. Skekley, personal communication, November 30, 2011)

REFERENCES

Bezerra, J. A., Stathos, T. H., Duncan, B., Gaines, J. A., & Udall, J. N. (1992). Treatment of infants with acute diarrhea: What's recommended and what's practiced. *Pediatrics, 90*(1), 1–4.

Fineout-Overholt, E., Levin, R. F., & Melnyk, B. (2005). Strategies for advancing EBP in clinical settings. *Journal of New York State Nurses Association, 35*(2), 28–32.

Levin, R. F. (2009). Implementing practice changes: Walk before your run. *Research and Theory for Nursing Practice: An International Journal, 23*(2), 85–87.

Levin, R. F., Keefer, J. M., Marren, J., Vetter, M., Lauder, B., & Sobolewski, S. (2010). Evidence-based practice: Merging 2 paradigms. *Journal of Nursing Care Quality, 25*(2), 117–126.

Misiano, B., Comiskey, M., D'Arcy, A., Levin, R. F., & Wright, F. (2009, February). Developing an evidence-based protocol for the administration of propofol in the ICU. *Podium presentation at the Arizona State University 10th annual national/international evidence-based practice conference translating research into best practice with vulnerable populations: Innovations in evidence-based practice,* Glendale, AZ.

Olney, K., Carrolo, M. A., Levin, R. F., & Wright, F. (2009, February). Using evidence based practice to develop a falls prevention practice improvement. *Podium presentation at the Arizona State University 10th annual national/international evidence-based practice conference translating research into best practice with vulnerable populations: Innovations in evidence-based practice,* Glendale, AZ.

Porter-O'Grady, T. (1987). Shared governance and new organizational models. *Nursing Economics, 5*(6), 281–286.

The Joint Commission. (2010). *Surgical care improvement project core measure set.* Retrieved October 14, 2010, from http://www.jointcommission.org

24

Establishing a Questioning Practice Community

Mary Jo Vetter, Joan M. Marren, and Seon Lewis-Holman

The art and science of asking questions is the source of all knowledge.

—Thomas Berger

In 2002, after years of a strong leadership tradition of bringing best clinical practices to community health care, the Visiting Nurse Service of New York (VNSNY) was approached by Pace University Lienhard School of Nursing (LSN) to participate in a funded evidence-based practice (EBP) initiative, Advancing Research and Clinical Practice through Close Collaboration (ARCC): A Pilot Test of an Intervention to Improve Evidence-Based Care and Patient Outcomes (Levin, Melnyk, Fineout-Overholt, Barnes, & Vetter, 2010). Achievement of operational buy-in to participate involved overcoming concerns regarding allocation of scarce personnel resources, time away from revenue-producing clinical work and redundancy with ongoing performance improvement (PI) initiatives.

Early on, there was lack of clarity regarding the difference between EBP and performance improvement (PI). Staff was accustomed to being provided with target areas of clinical practice that needed quality enhancement; they were not as familiar with the notion of questioning longstanding practices that may or may not be evidence based. Clinical specialists remained current on best practices in wound, ostomy, and continence care, as well as diabetes and heart failure management. They disseminated this knowledge to staff via workshops and clinician and patient educational material. Rarely was a field nurse asked about a burning interest one had about a clinical problem affecting patients, and researching a topic usually meant reliance on outdated text books or home care periodicals and guide books.

As work began on the pilot study, essential ingredients for success in engaging staff in EBP became apparent. Knowledge of EBP concepts would need to be addressed, access to library resources ensured, and time for staff and managers to work on EBP projects provided. In keeping with the ARCC model of supporting integration of EBP in a practice environment, a mentor was needed to foster adoption of new practices, as didactic education about EBP was not enough to sustain change. The grant project manager, an expert in EBP integration, served in this role. We quickly learned that in order to continually support change in clinical decision-making processes, this mentor needed to be extremely visible and available to clinicians as they shifted to a new way of thinking and acting. Staff needed encouragement and tangible assistance in formulating clinical questions so that the literature could be searched more efficiently and appropriate studies identified. They also needed opportunities to discuss the applicability and strength of the evidence for community-residing populations from related studies of hospitalized patients. They needed help in understanding that sometimes there was no specific evidence available to guide home care practice, and that we needed to utilize best practices while turning our attentions to creating new evidence through tests of change, pilots, and well-designed research studies.

The more we empowered staff to solve clinical problems of interest to them, the more passionate they became about the work, often using their own time to complete project work, keeping up with caseload demands without negative impact on productivity requirements. It became obvious that this undertaking demanded much more than the efforts of a grant-funded academician for this immense practice setting to make strides to integrate EBP among frontline clinicians. An academic/service partnership was therefore conceptualized to advance EBP growth and development at both institutions (Levin, Vetter, Feldman, & Chaya, 2008).

A vacant position in the Clinical Education Department at VNSNY was subsequently converted into a visiting faculty position with the input and assistance from the human resources departments at both VNSNY and Pace. Having no set precedent for the role, much thought went into constructing the multiple responsibilities of the visiting faculty to achieve the objective of EBP integration. In addition to work assignments in the academic setting, the service setting expected the visiting faculty member to:

1. Define and operationalize EBP implementation projects in alignment with VNSNY strategic objectives.
2. Infuse EBP principles in all education and quality activities throughout the organization.
3. Develop scholarly papers for presentation and/or publication based on the work of the partnership; identify opportunities to showcase VNSNY accomplishments in a variety of venues.

4. Conduct practice-relevant research to generate new home care-specific evidence, involving other faculty and students as appropriate.
5. Develop ability of leaders and staff to independently create and disseminate information regarding clinical, educational, and research endeavors.

So the stage was set for VNSNY and LSN staff to work together on improving nursing practice and patient outcomes. Orientation and continuing education curricula were revised and e-learning modules created to make EBP part of the fabric of the clinical practice culture. Teaching strategies were adopted to promote critical thinking about practice patterns. A vendor contract was secured to ensure access to academic search engines with capacity for 30 simultaneous users. Tablet computers, customarily used exclusively for clinical documentation, were enabled to visit key websites for EBP information. Support for scholarly activities included joint faculty, management, and nursing staff presentations at numerous professional meetings (e.g., Levin, Vetter, Foust, & Bowles, 2009; Levin, Vetter, Marc-Charles, Perez-Sandy, & Ifemesia, 2006) and publication of several manuscripts describing the collaborative work (e.g., Levin, Melnyk, Fineout-Overholt, Barnes, & Vetter, 2011; Levin et al., 2010; Levin, Vetter, Feldman, & Chaya, 2008). Senior leadership at both institutions was pleased on multiple levels with the outcomes. At VNSNY, the work contributed to organizational learning about how to implement clinical improvements at the team or microsystem level, especially as it relates to a dispersed, mobile workforce. LSN benefited from the work in being able to make curriculum revisions to include EBP content and processes in order to remain in the forefront of nursing education.

Our efforts led to an important realization at VNSNY: the parallel work of PI staff and those engaged in integrating EBP could be more powerful in combination than each could be individually. EBP provides a systematic framework for defining and focusing a clinical question, gathering evidence and evaluating the strength and relevance of that evidence in the practice setting. As a singular model, it did not seem to provide a practical approach for how to apply the best evidence and sustain improvement. Practice improvement (PI) models provide a well-developed set of tools and strategies for implementing, evaluating, and spreading improvement work with significant emphasis on understanding work processes and systems that either facilitate or create barriers to health care improvements. In comparing EBP and PI models, it was clear that EBP promulgates a systematic method for finding, evaluating, and critically appraising the best available evidence; PI offers strong strategies for designing, testing, implementing, and sustaining improvement using rapid cycle, small tests of change.

It was at this point that a mandate was set forth by the VNSNY chief nursing leader to define a model that leveraged the assets of both approaches and could be used universally across the organization. Stakeholders from VNSNY Quality Management, Clinical Education, and the Research Center along with academic partners from LSN and the University of Pennsylvania School of Nursing collaborated to create a model that encompassed the best of both paradigms.

As recommended by Titler, Steelman, Budreau, Buckwalter, and Goode (2001), to be most effective, the new model for evidence-based practice improvement (EBPI) (Levin et al., 2010) was incorporated into the existing organizational structure that was responsible for PI. (See Chapter 26 for a detailed description of this model.) This department was most knowledgeable about quality management and was also experienced in data acquisition and analysis. They were therefore credible messengers of the added value of EBP. The Quality Management group had already enlisted the clinical directors and managers from each regional office in improvement work. We predicted that by also empowering these frontline advocates with EBPI expertise they could more directly and effectively engage their staff in clinical improvement efforts. Our objective was to identify clinical practice problems that were relevant to field clinicians and important to the organization. We hoped to continue to generate the heightened level of enthusiasm observed in the initial ARCC pilot group across the organization. The next step was to create a cadre of clinical leaders well versed in the EBPI methodology. Thanks to an existing endowment to the VNSNY Research Center, we were able to create the Beatrice Renfield EBPI Fellows program (hereinafter referred to as the Renfield Program), which allowed us to offer an 18-month mentored curriculum to a competitively selected group of nursing leaders at VNSNY. (See Chapters 25 and 26 for a detailed description of this program.)

EBP INTEGRATION STRATEGIES

The success of the Renfield Program led to the integration and hardwiring of EBPI strategies into the organization, particularly in the Quality Management and Clinical Education (QMCE) departments. Examples of EBPI integration strategies include incorporation of assessment and screening tools into the agency's electronic documentation system; updating and creating evidence-based patient education materials; and conducting innovative EBPI workshops and workshops on the standardization of clinical practice protocols, standards, and procedures. Each of these initiatives will be described below.

Incorporation of Assessment and Screening Tools

During the Renfield Program (see Chapter 25 for a full program description), the topics of medication management and pain management were selected based on agency strategic goals and clinical relevance as observed by the Fellows. Two EBPI projects were designed and implemented to address these issues. The projects are briefly discussed below (Chapter 26 describes these projects in detail).

A systematic review of studies conducted by the medication management project team showed adherence, prescribing, and monitoring were common sources of preventable medication-related hospitalizations that are relevant to home care; additionally, an under-detection of cognitive impairment without definitive dementia is a major factor since the cognitively impaired are a vulnerable population (Chodosh et al., 2004; Howard et al., 2007). Findings from this EBPI project lead to the recommendations to integrate the Mini-Cog (Doerflinger & Mary, 2007) and four self-reported adherence questions from the Morisky tool (Morisky, Green, & Levine, 1986) as assessment screens into the electronic documentation system of the organization.

The goal of the second EBPI project was to improve the management of chronic nonmalignant pain in the long-term home health care (LTHHC) population within the agency. Pain relief is a major challenge for patients with chronic pain and the complexity of treatment options for chronic noncancer pain has increased dramatically. EBPI methods guided the collection of internal data to gather baseline data and support the practice problem. The pain team then conducted a gap analysis, developed a focused clinical question, conducted a systematic search for and synthesis of best evidence, and made recommendations for practice improvement. Based on the best evidence, the team designed a protocol for the visiting nurse to use in assessing the appropriateness of a LTHHC patient's pain medication regimen and collaborating with the patient's primary health care provider on pain management. Project implementation consisted of staff education, testing of new practices using PDSA (plan, do, study, act) cycles, and evaluation of outcomes. Project evaluation indicated that the processes used were successful in achieving desired outcomes.

Evidence-Based Patient Education Materials

Other examples of incorporating EBP standards into the organization included updating and creating patient education self-care guides. A process was implemented to search and evaluate current and relevant evidence-based diagnosis and treatment guidelines for chronic conditions such as diabetes, congestive heart failure, hypertension, chronic obstructive pulmonary disease, wound, ostomy, and continence management, including adult learning and self-management principles.

An example of implementing this process involved the 2009 update of the VNSNY Congestive Heart Failure Self-Care Guide. Clinical content experts and educators, one of which was a Faculty-in-Training in the Fellowship program, searched and critically appraised the most relevant best evidence, including protocols, practice guidelines, and guidelines for the diagnosis and management of heart failure from American College of Cardiology, Heart Failure Society of America, New York Heart Association, and American Heart Association. These clinicians were able to integrate the best evidence with their clinical expertise and create a patient education guide that was clinically accurate and relevant, comprehensive, and patient-friendly.

Standardizing the Process of Clinical Protocols/Guidelines/Procedures Development

In an effort to standardize the process for clinical protocols, guidelines, and procedures development, a committee was formed to develop guidelines and incorporate an EBPI approach by searching and analyzing the most relevant evidence (Levin & Lewis-Holman, 2011). The committee also discussed the need for and appropriateness of including the level of evidence (LOE) of a recommendation for clinical practice on any and all protocols, guidelines, and procedures going forward. Because different clinical practice guidelines (CPGs) use different schemas for determining the LOE and/or the quality of evidence presented in a guideline, an attempt was made to standardize the LOE so that VNSNY would use such clinical practice recommendations going forward. After much deliberation, the decision was made to use the Levels of Quantitative Evidence for Effectiveness of Therapy Pyramid (Figure 24.1) (Levin & Lewis-Holman, 2011). The goal of this initiative is that the QMCE staff would become the trainers/mentors/coaches for other VNSNY employees in their respective departments/divisions for developing evidence-based clinical protocols, guidelines, and procedures.

QMCE EBPI Workshops

The aim of the Renfield Program was to appraise and apply the best available evidence to inform practice improvement projects that are aligned with the broader VNSNY quality initiatives and strategic priorities using the EBPI model (Levin et al., 2011). Building on the success of the Renfield Program, a series of workshops on EBPI was conducted for the entire QMCE staff. The EBPI model is an excellent model for practice

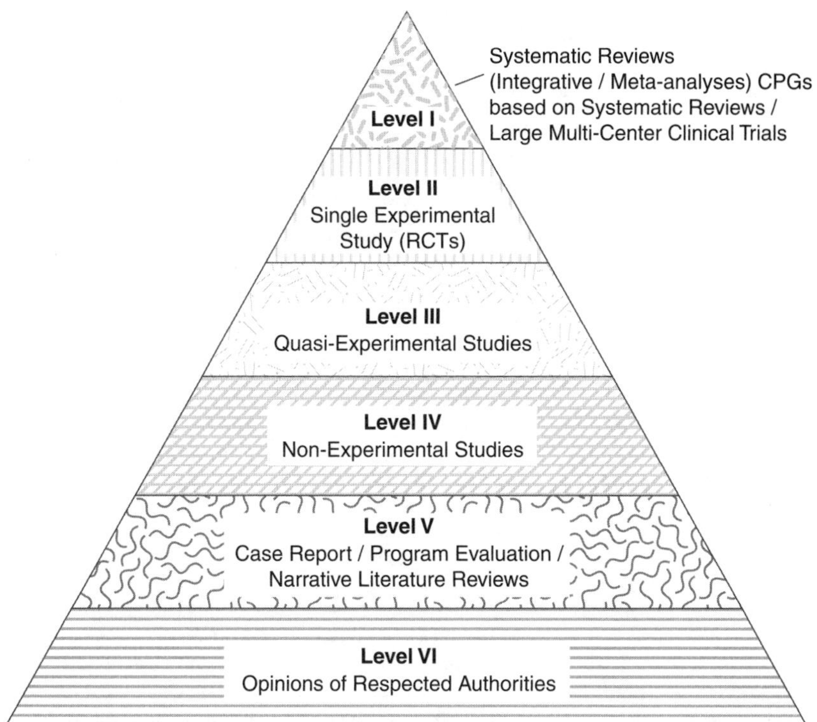

Source: © 2010 by Rona F. Levin and Jeffrey M. Keefer. Adapted from the work of Stetler, Morsi, Rucki, Broughton, Corrigan, Fitzgerald, et al. (1998); Melnyk and Fineout-Overholt (2011); and Levin (2008).

FIGURE 24.1 Levels of quantitative evidence for effectiveness of therapy.

improvement. At VNSNY the goal was that this model would become the framework for practice improvement, as the QMCE department develops evidence-based clinical practices and drives practice improvement for the agency. The QMCE department is well suited to be the driver as we continue to align with existing resources and organizational priorities. The workshops are discussed below.

The spread of EBPI principles to the QMCE department began in the fall of 2009 with the continued collaboration of the visiting faculty from Pace University and University of Pennsylvania developing and offering three interactive workshops. Each workshop included 2 hours of pre-work followed by 3 hours of classroom work to allow time to practice the new skills taught (Exhibit 24.1). In the first workshop, participants learned to describe the EBPI model, develop a focused clinical question, and identify different levels of evidence using abstracts. The participants learned about clinical trials and how to critically appraise the evidence

EXHIBIT 24.1 COURSE DESIGN DOCUMENT (CDD)

I. Scope of the Course/Educational Activity

Course/Educational Activity title:
Evidenced-Based Practice in Quality Management Services

Time allocated for course:
9 hours

Primary contact:

Reviewers:

Type of Staff Development[1]:
[ ] Core Orientation (Phase I)
[ ] Post-Core (Phase II or III)
[ ] In-Service Education
[√] Continuing Education

Modality:
[√] Instructor-Led Training / ILT
[ ] Webinar
[√] Teleconference
[ ] eLearning
[√] Independent Activity

Notes (optional):

Planned first session:
September 22, 2009

Workgroup / Planning Committee:

Approval:

Needs Assessment:
[ ] Learner Request
[√] Management Request
[ ] EBP in the Literature, Health Care, or Law
[ ] Other; please describe:

Evaluation of Learning (80% or greater):
[√] Knowledge Enhancement
[√] Skill Development
[√] Attitude Enhancement
[√] Change in Practice / Performance

Threaded Strands for Content Development provide a unifying theme in staff education. Use them as a frame of reference when developing educational activities and include them in course design where appropriate. Check those that apply:
[ ] Scope and Standards of Practice
[ ] Care Management
[ ] Comprehensive Assessment
[ ] Self-Management
[√] Patient Outcomes
[ ] Reimbursement/ Managed Care/ Fiscal Responsibility
[ ] Regulatory Compliance
[√] Evidence-Based Practice
[ ] Adult Learning Principles
[√] VNSNY Mission, Vision, and Values
[√] Clinical Education Mission and Vision
[ ] VNSNY Policies and Procedures
[ ] PCRS Documentation

II. Purpose Statement

The purpose statement is a general statement of the intended outcome of the course. It should include: (1) Who is this for? (2) What knowledge / skills / attitudes will be addressed? (3) How will this benefit the learner?

Phase I: Quality Management Services staff will develop knowledge of the Evidenced-Based Practice Improvement Model and the skill in accessing and critically appraising evidence.

EXHIBIT 24.1 (*continued*)

III. Development Outline

Objectives[2]	Content Outline	Teaching Methods	Evaluation Measures[3]	Time Frame / Presenter
By the end of this activity, the learner will be able to ... (verbs should be measurable; avoid know or learn)	*Outline key points that will be addressed to support the objective*	*Describe the methods, strategies, materials, resources, and activities for each objective*	*How will you measure the learner has met the objective? List the measures, evaluation, questions, or methods ...*	*State the time frame and presenter for each objective*
Session 1: 9/22/09 9 am–12 noon				
1. Describe the EBPI Model	A. Introduce Phase I objectives, schedule, and approach B. The EBPI Model	Slide Presentation Questions and Answers Group Learning Activity Pre-work: 2 hours. Reading as assigned	Practice critically appraising abstracts and discussing results as a group	
2. Develop a focused, searchable clinical question.	A. Types of questions a. background b. foreground B. Templates for questions of therapy, secondary prevention. prognosis, harm C. Examples of focused, searchable clinical questions.			
3. Identify different levels of evidence using abstracts	A. What are levels of evidence? How do we use them?			
4. Critically appraise evidence for its relevance and validity I: Clinical Trials	A. What are clinical trials? B. How do we assess the validity of a clinical trial? C. What are the treatment effectiveness formulas and how are they used in evaluating outcomes? • Preparation for next session • Evaluation			

(*continued*)

EXHIBIT 24.1 (*continued*)

Session 2: 10/20/09 9 am–12 noon			
1. Critically appraise evidence for its relevance and validity I: Integrative Reviews	1. What are integrative reviews? 2. How do we assess the validity of integrative reveiws? 3. Practice critically appraising clinical integrative reviews in small groups 4. Class review appraisals together • Preparation for next session • Evaluation	Slide Presentation Questions and Answers Group Learning Activity: Interactive review and critique of an intervention review Pre-work : 2 hours: Reading as assigned	Practice critically appraising an integrative review and discussing results at end of session
Session 3: 11/17/09 9 am–12 noon			
1. Critically appraise evidence for its relevance and validity II: Meta-analyses	1. What are meta-analyses? 2. What are the tools I need to understand and critique these types of evidence? 3. Practice critically appraising meta-analyses in small groups 4. Class review appraisals together Evaluation	Slide Presentation Questions and Answers Group Learning Activity Interactive review and critique of a meta-analysis	Practice critically appraise a systematic review and discuss results at end of session

[1]Review the Staff Development Definitions to see if this course qualifies for Continuing Education contact hours.
[2]Refer to the Guide to Approval of Continuing Nursing Education Activities for more information and examples of writing objectives.
[3]eLearning measures include: multiple choice, true/false, fill in the blank, short answer, matching, hotspot, sequence, and Likert scale. ILT can also include case studies, performance checklists, etc.

for its relevance and validity. In the second and third workshops, participants learned about integrative reviews and meta-analyses and how to critically appraise evidence for its relevance and validity. The EBPI workshops continued into the fall of 2010 with two additional offerings, which focused on strategies for searching for evidence to answer a clinical question and appraisal of guidelines for research and evaluation (see Exhibit 24.2).

The overall goal was to fuse EBP-related projects with practice improvement initiatives within the organization in order to spread

EXHIBIT 24.2 COURSE DESIGN DOCUMENT (CDD)

I. Scope of the Course/Educational Activity

Course/Educational Activity title:
Evidence-Based Practice Improvement in Quality Management Services: Part II, Session 2: Searching the Literature

Time allocated for course: 5 hours

Primary contact:

Reviewers:

Type of Staff Development[1]:
[ ] Core Orientation (Phase I)
[ ] Post-Core (Phase II or III)
[ ] In-Service Education
[√] Continuing Education

Modality:
[√] Instructor-Led Training / ILT
[ ] Webinar
[√] Teleconference
[ ] eLearning
[√] Independent Activity

Notes (optional):

Planned first session: September 22, 2010

Workgroup / Planning Committee:

Approval:

Needs Assessment:
[ ] Learner Request
[√] Management Request
[ ] EBP in the Literature, Health Care, or Law
[ ] Other; please describe:

Evaluation of Learning (80% or greater):
[√] Knowledge Enhancement
[√] Skill Development
[√] Attitude Enhancement
[√] Change in Practice / Performance

Threaded Strands for Content Development provide a unifying theme in staff education. Use them as a frame of reference when developing educational activities and include them in course design where appropriate. Check those that apply:
[ ] Scope and Standards of Practice
[ ] Care Management
[ ] Comprehensive Assessment
[ ] Self-Management
[√] Patient Outcomes
[ ] Reimbursement / Managed Care / Fiscal Responsibility
[ ] Regulatory Compliance
[√] Evidence-Based Practice
[ ] Adult Learning Principles
[√] VNSNY Mission, Vision, and Values
[√] Clinical Education Mission and Vision
[ ] VNSNY Policies and Procedures
[ ] PCRS Documentation

II. Purpose Statement

The purpose statement is a general statement of the intended outcome of the course. It should include: (1) Who is this for? (2) What knowledge / skills / attitudes will be addressed? (3) How will this benefit the learner?

Evidence-Based Practice Improvement in Quality Management Services: Part II, Session 2: Searching the Literature

(continued)

EXHIBIT 24.2 (*continued*)

III. Development Outline

Objectives[2]	Content Outline	Teaching Methods	Evaluation Measures[3]	Time Frame/ Presenter
By the end of this activity, the learner will be able to . . . (Verbs should be measurable; avoid know or learn).	*Outline key points that will be addressed to support the objective.*	*Describe the methods, strategies, materials, resources, and activities for each objective*	*How will you measure the learner has met the objective? List the measures, evaluation, questions, or methods. . .*	*State the time frame and presenter for each objective.*
1. Define the clinical question	1. How to identify, clarify and focus a clinical question	Pre-work: 1. Sign-in to Pace Library 2. Complete Video "Searching the Literature: From Case Scenario to Best Evidence, A tutorial on Evidence Based Medicine for the Physician's Assistant and Nursing Program" 3. Think about a clinical question (2 hours) ? Lecture/ Discussion Handouts	Evaluations	
2. Develop strategies and tools for gathering evidence from the literature	1. Determine relevancy of data sources to the clinical question. 2. Present tools to document the search strategy and summarize the evidence	Lecture/ Discussion Handouts Demonstration and Return Demonstration	Evaluation Return Demonstration	

3. Search for relevant evidence to answer the clinical question	1. Search literature. 2. Share and discuss results. Evaluation	Lecture/ Discussion Handouts Demonstration and Return Demonstration	Evaluation Return Demonstration

[1]Review the Staff Development Definitions to see if this course qualifies for Continuing Education contact hours.

[2]Refer to the Guide to Approval of Continuing Nursing Education Activities for more information and examples of writing objectives.

[3]eLearning measures include: multiple choice, true/false, fill in the blank, short answer, matching, hotspot, sequence, and Likert scale. ILT can also include case studies, performance checklists, etc.

implementation of EBPI. Selected projects will be conducted by cross functional teams within the QMCE department who continually interact with staff in multiple programs and departments across the organization. An example of a current project is the research and design of a pediatric risk assessment tool to predict re-hospitalization risk for the pediatric home care population. There are currently no tools in existence that target this specific population in this type of practice setting. Review of the literature reveals a number of characteristics that may be predictive of risks for re-hospitalization, such as gestational age/pre-maturity, comorbidities, chronic conditions, abnormal vital signs, respiratory infections, type of health insurance, and compliance with medical treatment (Camargo et al., 2007; Garelick, Lee, Cronan, Kost, & Palmer, 2001; Morris, Gard, & Kennedy, 2005; Sampalis et al., 2008). A project has been proposed in collaboration with the VNSNY Center for Home Care Policy and Research (the Center) to test a tool initially designed by the Center for the assessment of risk for re-hospitalization in a pediatric population.

The strategy of embedding EBPI subject matter experts within departments, such as Quality and Clinical Education, who regularly intersect with clinical field staff represents a potentially high leverage approach to spreading EBPI across the organization in a consistent and effective manner. The tactic results in EBPI concepts being consistently integrated into and highlighted throughout all training, staff development, and quality assessment and improvement activities. At VNSNY, the goal of creating EBPI subject matter experts throughout the Quality Management and Clinical Education Department will soon be realized. We continue to look for other opportunities to leverage the effective spread of EBPI, and have begun to explore development of subject matter experts within the team leading the design and development of our automated patient care record and clinical information systems. In this way we can move closer to achieving our overall goal of establishing a vibrant questioning practice community by weaving EBPI into the fabric of our organization's clinical and service delivery culture.

REFERENCES

Camargo, C., Ramachandran, S., Ryskina, K., Edelman Lewis, B., & Legoratta, A. (2007). Association between common asthma therapies and recurrent asthma exacerbations in children enrolled in a state Medicaid plan. *American Journal Health System Pharmacists, (64),* 1054–1061.

Chodosh, J., Petitti, D. B., Elliott, M., Hays, R. D., Crooks, V. C., & Reuben, D. (2004). Physician recognition of cognitive impairment: Evaluating the need for improvement. *Journal of the American Geriatric Soiety, 52*(7), 1051–1059.

Doerflinger, C., & Mary, D. (2007). How to try this: The Mini-Cog. *American Journal of Nursing, 107*(12), 62–71.

Garelick, M., Lee, C., Cronan, K., Kost, K., & Palmer, K. (2001). Pediatric emergency assessment tool (PEAT): A risk-adjustment measure for pediatric emergency patients. *Academic Emergency Medicine, (8),* 156–162.

Howard, R. L., Avery, A. J., Slavenburg, S., Royal, S., Pipe, G., & Lucassen, P. (2007).Which drugs cause Preven admissions to hospital? A systematic review. *British Journal of Clinical Pharmacology, 63*(2), 136–147.

Levin, R. F., Keefer, J. M., Marren, J., Vetter, M., Lauder, B., & Sobolewski, S. (2010). Evidence-based practice: Merging two paradigms. *Journal of Nursing Care Quality, 25*(2), 117–126.

Levin, R. F., & Lewis-Holman, S. (2011). Evidence-based practice: Developing guidelines for clinical protocol development. *Research and Theory in Nursing Practice, 25*(4), 233–237.

Levin, R. F., Melnyk, B. M., Fineout-Overholt, E., Barnes, M., & Vetter, M. (2011). Fostering evidence-based practice to improve nurse and cost outcomes in a community health setting: A pilot test of the ARCC model. *Nursing Administration Quarterly, 35*(1), 1–13.

Levin, R. F., Vetter, M., Feldman, H., & Chaya, J. (2008). Building bridges in academic nursing and health care practice settings. *Journal of Professional Nursing, 23*(6), 362–368.

Levin, R. F., Vetter, M., Foust, J. B., & Bowles, K. (2009, March). Building EBP capacity in home care. *Symposium conducted at the meeting of the Eastern Nursing Research Society*, Providence, RI.

Levin, R. F., Vetter, M., Marc-Charles, F., Perez-Sandy, Z., & Ifemesia, I. (2006, July). Implementing EBP in the clinical setting: A focus on process. *Symposium conducted at the meeting of the Sigma Theta Tau International evidence-based practice congress*, Montreal, Quebec, Canada.

Morisky, D. E., Green, L. W., & Levine, D. M. (1986). Concurrent and predictive validity of a self-reported measure of medication adherence. *Medical Care, 24*(1), 67–74.

Morris, B., Gard, C., & Kennedy, K. (2005). Rehospitalization of extremely low birth weight infants: Are there racial/ethnic disparities? *Journal of Perinatology, 25,* 656–663.

Sampalis, J., Langley, J., Carbonell-Estrany, X., Paes, B., O'Brien, K., Allen Mitchell, et al. (2008). Development and validation of a risk scoring tool to predict respiratory syncytial virus hospitalization in premature infants born at 33 through 35 completed weeks of gestation. *Medical Decision Making, (28),* 471–480.

Titler, M., Steelman, V., Budreau, G., Buckwalter, K., & Goode, C. (2001). The Iowa model of evidence-based practice to promote quality care. *Critical Care Nursing Clinics of North America, 13*(4), 497–509.

PRESENTATION REFERENCES

"Advancing Research and Clinical Practice Through Close Collaboration (ARCC): A pilot test of an intervention to improve evidence based care and patient outcomes in a community health setting." *Podium presentation at the 38th biennial convention—Scientific sessions of Sigma Theta Tau International,* Indianapolis, Indiana, October 2005.

"Advancing Research and Clinical Practice Through Close Collaboration (ARCC): A pilot test of an intervention to improve evidence based care and patient outcomes in a community health setting." Podium Presentation at the New York University Research Day, New York, NY, May 2006.

"Partnering to Advance Evidence Based Practice" Symposium presenter July 2006.

"Scheduled Telephone Follow-Up to Improve Patient Outcomes." Poster presentation at Sigma Theta Tau International evidence based practice congress, Montreal, Canada, July 2006.

25

Implementing an EBPI Program in a Community Health Agency: The Visiting Nurse Service of New York Experience (Part I)

Rona F. Levin, Janice B. Foust, Kathryn H. Bowles, Lorraine Ferrara, and Bonnie Lauder

How wonderful it is that nobody need wait a single moment before starting to improve the world

—Anne Frank

This chapter describes in detail a specific program that provided select clinical management and specialist staff at a community health agency, The Visiting Nurse Service of New York (VNSNY), with an opportunity to hone their knowledge and skills related to evidence-based practice (EBP) and practice improvement (PI) in order to serve as EBP champions/coaches to others within the organization. This program, the Renfield Fellows Evidence-Based Practice Improvement (EBPI) Fellows Program (hereinafter referred to as the Renfield Program), is mentioned as one initiative that the VNSNY included in its effort toward establishing a questioning practice community (see Chapter 24). Chapter 25 includes several initiatives that the VNSNY has implemented or is currently implementing to reach its quality improvement goals. Details of the Renfield Program are provided here. Chapter 26 describes specific EBPI projects that were completed as part of the Renfield Program.

The Renfield Program was developed as a collaborative effort among Pace University, University of Pennsylvania, the VNSNY Research Center, and VNSNY Quality Management Services in response to a mandate by VNSNY senior leadership to more fully integrate EBP into the organizational fabric. After realizing the positive influence that an experimental mentored EBP program had on VNSNY staff who participated in the study as part of the experimental group (Levin, Melnyk, Fineout-Overholt, Barnes, & Vetter, 2011), the agency decided to go forward with additional initiatives. The Renfield Program objectives were geared to facilitating participants' ability to improve frontline clinical practice by:

- Identifying focused clinical problems to investigate
- Finding and analyzing the best evidence related to those clinical problems
- Linking EBP and practice PI
- Conducting small tests of change to improve practice
- Spreading best practices throughout the organization

The Renfield Program consisted of an 18-month mentored experience in three phases (see Figure 25.1). Phase I consisted of learning about EBP and PI, understanding how both these paradigms were merged into a new model at VNSNY (Levin et al., 2010), selecting a clinical area for investigation, and honing that area into a focused clinical question. Phase II consisted of evaluating the retrieved evidence related to the focused clinical question. Phase III provided "hands-on" experience to the practice team for developing a protocol for the new innovation and testing the innovation in practice.

As discussed in Chapter 24, agency administrators believed that integrating the EBP approach and methodology with the PI approach currently in use at VNSNY would facilitate program participants' understanding and integration of new knowledge because they were already familiar with the PI paradigm in use at the agency. Thus, the EBPI model (Levin et al., 2010) emerged from the collaboration between the visiting university faculty member and PI proponents at VNSNY (see Figure 25.2). This model served as the guiding framework for the Renfield Program.

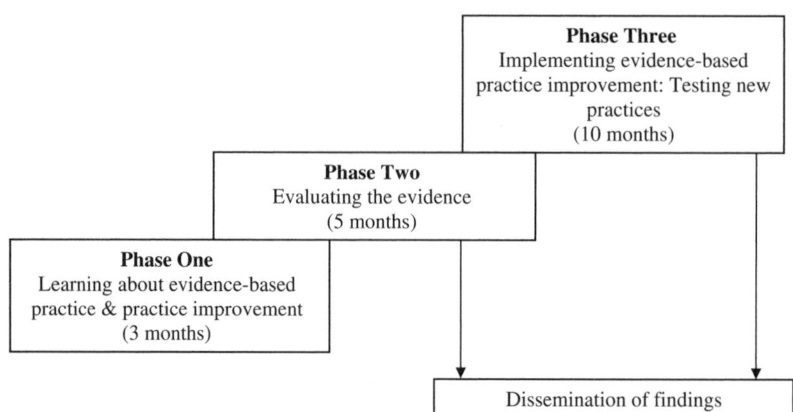

FIGURE 25.1 The Beatrice Renfield EBPI Fellows program structure.

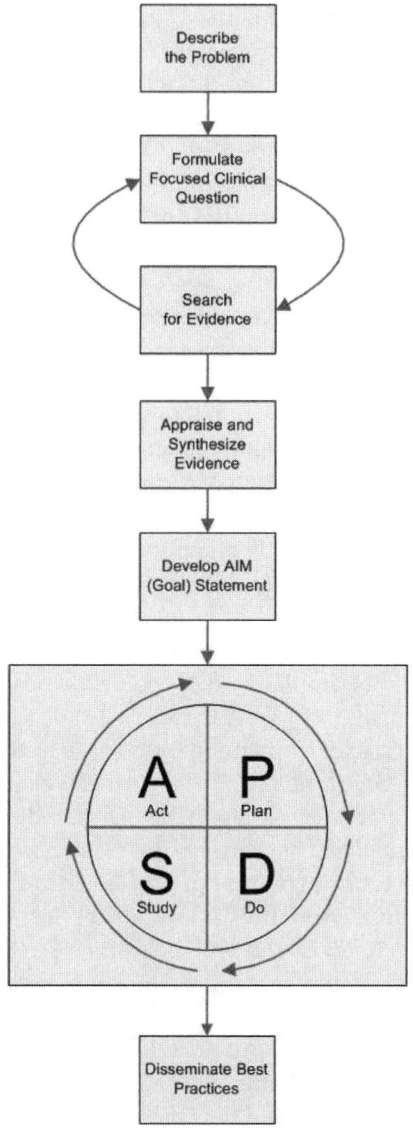

Source: Copyright Rona F. Levin, PhD, RN, and Visiting Nurse Service of New York 2007.

FIGURE 25.2 EBPI model.

THE EBPI MODEL

As depicted in Figure 25.2, the EBPI model (Levin et al., 2010) includes the crucial components of both the EBP and practice or performance improvement paradigms. Those components usually ascribed to the EBP paradigm are the formulation of a focused clinical question and the search for and appraisal of the best evidence to answer that question. The model components taken from the PI paradigm (Langley et al., 2009) are the description of the problem, the development of an aim statement, the PDSA cycle, and the dissemination of best evidence.

The description of the problem is more than a purpose statement. This component of the model focuses on the analysis of internal organizational data and external background literature in order to substantiate the need for improvement in a specified area. Also, the review of the internal and external data often facilitates the narrowing of the problem into a searchable focused clinical question (Levin et al., 2011). Once a question has focus, there is a systematic search for evidence. This type of search is different than the usual literature review on a topic in that it follows a predetermined process in order to find not only evidence, but the best evidence. (See Chapter 12 for a detailed description of the systematic search process.) The review, sorting, and analysis of the retrieved evidence comprise the next component of the model. For this component, project teams summarize the relevant evidence in tables (tables of evidence), analyze the meaning of the evidence, and synthesize their findings into an EBPI project proposal.

Once the new innovation is operationalized for the specific practice setting in which it will be implemented, the next steps are to develop an aim statement and engage in PDSA cycles or small tests of change until the structure and process for implementation of the new innovation is perfected. The "P" in PDSA stands for "plan," or developing a protocol for implementation of the practice change. The "D" stands for "do," or carrying out the plan in a small test of change. The "S" stands for "study" or analyzing the feedback in terms of process or process and outcome results from the small test(s) of change. And, the "A" stands for "act," or using the feedback from the analysis to revise the protocols and/or deal with challenges/issues in the process of implementation. The small test of change step (or steps as more than one PDSA cycle may be needed) is crucial to the success of any EBPI project as it provides for a continuous feedback loop prior to full implementation (Langley et al., 2009; Levin et al., 2010). As an example, one might introduce a new assessment tool for the prediction of falls, which the evidence indicates has better sensitivity and specificity than the assessment tool in current use. The aim of the project might be to decrease the fall rate by 20% within 3 months. The first small test of change might be to test the new tool for interrater reliability among a select group of staff nurses who will perform such assessments. Once interrater reliability is established, the next small test may be to try using the tool on one unit in a hospital or long-term care facility for 1 week with a select group of nurses and nursing assistants to see if there are any challenges in applying the process. Perhaps in this small test one discovers that although the new tool is being used to assess patients risk for falls on admission, the assessment is not revised if and when there is a change in patient status. The next small test would be based on a new protocol for implementation that includes when patients should be reassessed, and so on. Once the process is perfected, then and only then does the team perform a test to measure patient outcomes, or in this example, fall rates, compare outcomes to baseline data, and determine if the goal included in the aim statement was reached.

The final component of the model includes dissemination of the results of the small tests of change to the organizational stakeholders, for example, administrators, managers, and clinical staff involved who were and will be involved in applying the new practice throughout the organization. Dissemination also includes external presentations and publications about the new innovation as a means to share the positive results of implementing improvement using the EBPI approach (Levin et al., 2010).

THE RENFIELD PROGRAM

The primary purpose of the Renfield Program was to prepare clinicians in management positions to evaluate and apply the best available evidence to improve the quality of care. The Renfield Program was built on two notable successful initiatives at the VNSNY. One is a successful educational program (Collaboration for Homecare Advances in Management and Practice [CHAMP]) to improve home health care quality by involving frontline managers in practice change (CHAMP, 2009). The other, mentioned earlier, was a mentored evidence-based program (Levin et al., 2011). Participants from each program were enthusiastic about learning how to use evidence to improve the quality of care. Their feedback along with faculty's experience guided the development of this program. The Renfield Program was designed to capitalize on and create synergy of EBP and quality or PI that would contribute to the fellows' professional development, engage clinical leadership, and improve quality and implementation of best practices.

The Renfield Program was created as an 18-month mentored program with three phases (see Figure 25.1) that focused on: (1) learning about EBP and PI; (2) evaluating the evidence; and, (3) implementing the evidence in practice or EBPI projects. The duration of each phase varied from 3 months (Phase I) to 5 months (Phase II) and concluded with a 10-month Phase III. Rather than all-day sessions, meetings were scheduled every other week for 2 to 4 hours to reinforce the work as an integral part of VNSNY clinical practice. Disseminating findings, both internally and externally, was an important component of the program as a way to share findings that would benefit others and as a professional development opportunity for program participants (herein after referred to as fellows) (Levin, Vetter, Foust, & Bowles, 2009).

Another consideration in designing the program was to identify general topics that were aligned with VNSNY priorities so the organization would benefit as a whole, beyond the specific project teams. Pain management and medication management were selected as common nursing practice issues spanning diverse clinical populations that coincided with several organizational quality initiatives at the time. VNSNY offered continuing education units for each of the phases to recognize fellows' learning and significant commitment to their professional development. In summary, the Renfield Program was designed to assure: (a) relevance to clinical managers' responsibilities; (b) promotion of clinical leadership; (c) integration of EBPI with demands of daily work; (d) engagement of fellows; and (e) program sustainability.

We launched the program with an announcement flyer promoting the Renfield Program as a leadership opportunity for clinical management staff. The flyer provided a brief overview of the program benefits, time frame, expectations, and deadline for application. Interested clinical managers submitted their applications, which asked them to describe their interest in participating in the program and how they would apply this new knowledge in practice. In addition, applicants submitted signed approval letters from their direct supervisors to assure support of the applicants' participation in the program. After the applications were received, two Renfield faculty members conducted brief interviews with each person to learn more about one's interests, answer questions, and clarify expectations of the program. We were very pleased to initially welcome 17 participants who represented diverse positions and programs from within VNSNY. The fellows worked in one of four boroughs of New York City and held positions such as clinical director, patient service manager (frontline manager), clinical nurse specialist, nurse practitioner, and nursing education coordinator. They worked in one of several clinical programs, including acute care, long-term care, pediatrics/maternity, hospice, and Centers of Excellence. To address program sustainability, two fellows participated in the program as "faculty in training" (FIT) and were involved in all aspects of program planning, implementation, and evaluation. Each of the experienced faculty members served as mentors for the FIT.

The program was formally launched by the chief operating officer and vice president and director of the Center for Home Care Policy and Research (CHCPR). They provided the welcome and overview of the program. They introduced the program as one that builds capacity for change, addresses the challenges of applying evidence in practice, and facilitates clinical excellence. Their visible administrative support was energizing and critical to the success of the program.

The content of Phase I included describing EBP and quality improvement as two models that were integrated in the EBPI model (Levin et al., 2010). The fellows identified different levels of evidence schemas and determined which one was most appropriate for program purposes. Fellows gathered and analyzed agency-level data to support the identification of the highest priority clinical problems. Sessions were interactive and the fellows had a chance to apply their knowledge in different assignments and participate in class discussions. By the end of Phase I, each project team had identified a focused clinical question consistent with organizational priorities and supported by internal organizational data. The fellows split into two teams. One team chose to focus on medication management and the other pain management.

The main purpose of Phase II was to search for the best evidence to answer the focused clinical question and develop a summary table of evidence relevant to the clinical question regarding either medication management or pain management. The first step was conducting a thorough review of the best available evidence. A Pace University librarian reviewed how to use systematic approaches for searching the literature, including navigating specific databases and providing insight to using key terms and filters. This information and access to the Pace University Library was critical to the success of the program. Fellows worked collaboratively within their teams to search for and evaluate the best available evidence on their focused clinical questions. Additionally, gap analyses (see Chapter 16) were undertaken to gather internal evidence that would compare current practices to best practices identified in the literature (external evidence). The analysis is essential to support or validate the identified target areas for improvement. Consistent with their job responsibilities, frontline managers accessed internal data and shared their reflections with project teams. Flow charts of internal processes were another strategy to reveal gaps between current nursing practices and identify key areas for improvement. In addition to accessing the evidence, fellows learned how to evaluate and rate the evidence for level and quality. Phase II concluded with interpretation of internal evidence to support a change in practice and external evidence in the form of a summary table of the accessed literature to guide the design of an EBPI project.

Designing and testing the practice change were the major foci of Phase III. During this phase, each project team created and implemented a PI project based on the internal and external evidence relevant to their focused clinical questions. Important to emphasize, once again, is the need to use internal evidence, which provides information about current practice, and external evidence, which provides information about best practices. Both types of information are needed to perform a gap analysis.

Following the EBPI model (Levin et al., 2010), and after performance of the gap analysis, each team developed an aim statement (i.e., goal) to guide implementation of small tests of change. Also, crucial in this phase was the development of two distinct protocols—one to clearly operationalize the evidence-based innovation and one to guide the processes of implementation by VNSNY staff.

As mentioned earlier, the Renfield Program was designed to improve home care quality and provide professional development opportunities for the fellows. The current program was an extension of the Beatrice Renfield lectures, which began as a collaborative partnership with the University of Pennsylvania, School of Nursing to engage frontline clinical leaders in current science and best practice relevant to home health care. In addition, there was a strong commitment among VNSNY administration, Renfield faculty, and fellows to disseminate the findings within the VNSNY and to other professional audiences through presentations and publications. Renfield fellows represented several different geographic regions and positions across a large organization. A critical and practical issue was selecting a clinical team where the practice change would occur. Each Renfield Project team chose a clinical frontline team where at least one fellow had administrative responsibility so they could provide visible leadership needed to introduce and facilitate the practice change process. Administrative support at the clinical frontline level was essential to the success of the projects.

Both projects were approved via expedited review by the Institution Review Board of the VNSNY. Moreover, the projects required educational sessions for the clinical nurses who would administer the new innovation to patients to learn about the evidence-based intervention, the rationale, and aims of the project. At the same time, the project teams emphasized the vital role that the clinical nurses were playing by participating in the practice change—specifically, that clinical nurses who provide direct care have valuable insight into the challenges as well as the barriers to implementing new interventions. Engaging the clinical nurses furthered our program goal to promote a climate of clinical questioning and PI. The clinical nurses' willingness to participate in these projects and their feedback was instrumental in understanding what was working and not working as we started implementing the change. Meetings were scheduled to facilitate open discussion and troubleshoot any issues as they arose. Qualitative and quantitative data were collected that were relevant to each of the specific clinical questions and outcomes, as described later. Each team analyzed its data to determine the effectiveness of the practice change.

The fellows presented at two VNSNY Beatrice Renfield lectures, one at the end of Phase II and again at the conclusion of the program. In Phase II presentations, each project team summarized the available evidence (particularly internal organizational evidence), described insights, and identified general recommendations for practice change. The presentations generated discussion about how the findings might be applied in home care practice and to improvements in organizational processes, such as the computerized patient care record system. The feedback from fellows' peers was encouraging and valuable as the Renfield teams started Phase III.

At the end of the program, the Renfield fellows presented their project findings, including a summary of evidence, the gap analysis, details about the evidence-based interventions, strategies for implementation, and evaluation data. As before, the chief operating officer and vice president and director of the CHCPR led the meeting, which was energizing and created thoughtful discussion about effective strategies to achieve clinical excellence. The fellows were recognized for their work over 18 months and their contributions to improving the quality of care at VNSNY.

METHODS OF PROGRAM EVALUATION

The EBPI faculty devised a mixed-methods approach to program evaluation. Using standardized instruments at baseline and repeating them at 3, 6, and 18 months, coupled with qualitative summaries of formative interviews, the team was able to assess the impact of the program on the participants and this program evaluation was approved by the Institutional Review Board of the VNSNY.

Instruments and Data Collection

Five standardized, valid, and reliable instruments were administered to program participants by the faculty on the first day of the program. Code numbers were assigned to the forms to maintain anonymity and a master list was maintained by one of the faculty to later match subsequent surveys. Outcomes of interest were the fellows' beliefs about EBP, EBP implementation behaviors, group cohesion, job satisfaction, and intention to remain in nursing. The instruments included the following:

The *Evidence-Based Practice Beliefs Scale* (Melnyk, Fineout-Overholt, & Mays, 2008) is a 16-item scale that measures a person's beliefs about the value of EBP on a 5-point Likert scale, 1 = strongly disagree to 5 = strongly agree. Cronbach's alpha was greater than .90 and the scale has a significant positive correlation with educational level and workplace responsibility. Item scores are summed for a range of 16 to 80, with higher scores indicating stronger beliefs.

The *Evidence-Based Practice Implementation Scale* (Melnyk, Fineout-Overholt, & Mays, 2008) is an 18-item scale that measures how often they have performed EBPs in the previous 8 weeks. The item responses range from 0 = not at all to 5 = very often. Cronbach's alpha was greater than .90 and, similar to the Belief's scale, there is a significant positive correlation with educational level and workplace responsibility. Item scores are summed for a range of 0 to 72, with higher scores indicating greater EBP implementation.

Group Cohesion (Good & Nelson, 1973) contains six items in two subscales, attractiveness and cohesion. Measured on a 7-point response scale, lower scores indicate greater cohesion. In studies by nursing systems researchers, internal consistency reliability estimates ranged from 0.73 to 0.83.

Job Satisfaction (Price & Mueller, 1986) measured generalized satisfaction using a 7-item Likert scale, 1 = strongly agree to 5 = strongly disagree on items such as, "I find real enjoyment in my job." Validity and reliability (internal consistency coefficients ranging from .72 to .95) have been established.

The *Nurse Retention Index* (REI) (Cowin, 2001) measured nurses' intentions of remaining in nursing as a career. The scale has six items measured on an 8-point scale ranging from definitely false to definitely true. A higher score is better. Validity and reliability of this instrument are established (Cronbach's alpha = .95 for experienced nurses).

Qualitative assessments were completed after each class/workshop session using a modified version of an open-ended formative assessment tool called the Critical Incident Questionnaire (CIQ) (Brookfield, 1995). The tool allows immediate and anonymous feedback about the most engaging and distancing moments during an educational session. For example, "At what moment in today's class did you feel the most engaged?" The assessment was administered after each class session and completed anonymously.

Finally, a qualitative survey was administered at the end of the program, asking participants to respond to items about their experience in the program; that is, what they thought the program offered in terms of benefits to current practice, benefits to the organization, and opportunity for personal development. Other items asked fellows to describe what they perceived as satisfying about the program and what they perceived as challenging.

Data Management

The data from the quantitative surveys were entered by one of the faculty into SPSS for analysis. The qualitative CIQ responses and qualitative interview notes were reviewed by the team of faculty and comments were summarized under each question.

Data Analysis

Descriptive statistics were used to describe the sample of fellows. The Wilcoxon signed-ranks test for related pairs was used to analyze changes in EBP beliefs, EBP implementation behaviors, group cohesion, job satisfaction, and nurse retention between baseline and 18 months. Content analysis of the qualitative survey was used to glean themes related to the above-mentioned categories.

Results

Fifteen nurses attended the EBP sessions over the 18-month period. Two of the 17 accepted fellows left the organization or did not start the program. Thirteen completed baseline surveys and 13 completed follow-up interviews. At baseline, two were absent and, by the final follow-up two had left the agency. Nursing experience ranged from 6 to 39 years, 89% had a master's degree in nursing, and 87% were female nurses. At baseline, 27% said they did not know much about EBP.

Beliefs about EBP increased from baseline (mean 55.6; SD 2.9) to 12 months (mean 56.2; SD 2.2), but the increase was not significant ($p = .678$). A higher score is better. Experience with implementation of EBP also increased over time from 25.2 (SD 17.4) to 30.7 (SD 13.4) and approached significance ($p = .090$). Group cohesion improved significantly from 18.2 (SD 7.9) at baseline to 14.4 (SD 4.7) at 12 months ($p = .028$). Job satisfaction did not change over time and remained 12.9 (SD 2.8) and 12.9 (SD 3.5), $p = .937$. Finally, career intentions also did not change significantly, and from 45.2 (SD 3.6) to 42.6 (SD 5.9), $p = .283$. Scores for all outcomes from baseline and 3, 6, and 18 months are shown in Table 25.1. The Critical Incident Questionnaire responses were positive throughout the course. Consistently, the nurses valued sessions that were interactive versus lecture.

Fellows' responses to the qualitative survey were consistent. From these responses, the following themes emerged under these survey questions that follow.

TABLE 25.1 Mean and Standard Deviation of Measures Across Time

	Baseline Mean (SD)	Three months Mean (SD)	Six Months Mean (SD)	18 months Mean (SD)
Beliefs About EBP	55.62 (2.98)	56.62 (2.98)	56.50 (3.20)	56.15 (2.23)
Implementation	25.23 (17.35)	26.00 (18.23)	29.42 (15.95)	30.77 (13.45)
Group Cohesion	18.23 (7.91)	16.62 (4.99)	14.08 (5.85)	14.38 (4.77)
Job Satisfaction	12.85 (2.88)	13.62 (3.71)	15.58 (3.70)	12.85 (3.53)
Intention to Stay	45.23 (3.61)	45.50 (6.43)	43.67 (6.04)	42.62 (5.97)

Benefits to Current Practice

Fellows stated that the Renfield Program increased their

- Understanding of EBP and its application to practice
- Awareness of the need to mentor nurses in this process
- Critical thinking about practice problems (e.g., pain assessments)
- Ability to work in a group and come to a consensus

One fellow stated that the program: "Better prepared me in designing, implementing, and disseminating various PI projects and educational endeavors."

Benefits to the Organization

Fellows shared that they believed they could use EBP tools and protocols to:

- Engage in best practices
- Role-model use of evidence
- Disseminate findings
- Standardize practice
- Improve patient outcomes
- Decrease costs
- Revise documentation systems

Opportunity for Personal Development

Fellows' responses indicated that by participating in the Renfield Program they gained the knowledge and ability to challenge current practices, understand and apply level of evidence schemas to the information they reviewed to support current practice or develop new practices, obtain research evidence, and identify solutions to practice problems.

Program Satisfiers

Fellows responded with the themes below when asked what they found most satisfying about the experience:

- Learning the EBPI process
- Using VNSNY data resources
- Understanding clinician practice
- Mentoring by highly skilled faculty
- Interacting with colleagues
- Accessing evidence-based information

Program Challenges

The challenges to integrating EBPI into routine practice that fellows identified are very similar to those identified in the literature as barriers to implementing EBP and research in clinical practice (e.g., Fineout-Overholt, Levin, & Melnyk (2005); Pravikoff, Pierce, & Pierce, 2005):

- Having enough time
- Balancing priorities
- Synthesizing data
- Obtaining internal data
- Identifying clinical questions
- Evaluating and tracking the literature
- Finding relevant studies

Discussion

Small sample sizes precluded having the power to attain statistically significant results across the board, but the trends were in a positive direction for all measures. Despite the small sample size, group cohesion improved significantly from the start of the course to the end. The group members did not all know each other or work together prior to the program, worked well together, and felt more positive about each other after the experience. The project successfully exposed the group members to EBP implementation as evidenced by an approximate 17% increase in the implementation scores. Such a large increase would likely be statistically significant with a larger sample. The small increase in EBP belief scores might be due to fellows' initial belief in the benefits of using an EBP to practice and thus applied to the Renfield Program because of those beliefs. There were no negative effects of the project on nurses' job satisfaction or career intentions. The information from the CIQ each session helped the faculty plan more effective sessions each week, providing rapid response to feedback from the nurses. The qualitative feedback from fellows indicated that the Renfield program helped them to better understand evidence-based PI and use that understanding to improve their own clinical practice as well as provide important feedback to the organization.

SUMMARY AND CONCLUSION

This chapter describes an 18-month mentored learning experience in EBPI, the Beatrice Renfield EBPI Fellows' Program, for individuals at management and clinical specialist levels. During this program, fellows learned the processes of EBP and PI and how to apply those processes to improve clinical practice. Essential to this experience was the development of an EBPI project and the initial implementation of that project with small tests of change to perfect the process of the practice change prior to large-scale implementation. The two projects that emanated from this program provided valuable insights to the VNSNY for process development and practice change. Both quantitative and qualitative approaches were used for program evaluation. Fellow outcomes were all in the positive direction. Larger samples may have attained statistical significance in areas that currently show trends toward improvement. The Renfield faculty strongly recommend pairing qualitative and quantitative evaluation methods of PI projects to gain a rich appraisal of program effectiveness.

ACKNOWLEDGMENTS

The authors would like to thank the Beatrice Renfield Foundation and the Pace University Library for their invaluable support in making the Renfield EBPI Fellows Program a reality. We would also like to acknowledge Ms Shannon Kealey, Instructional Services Librarian, for her invaluable assistance. Finally, we owe a debt of gratitude to the nurses at the VNSNY who participated in the EBPI projects that the fellows' designed and implemented.

REFERENCES

Brookfield, S. (1995). *Becoming a critically reflective teacher*. San Francisco: Jossey-Bass.

Collaboration for homecare advances in management and practice: Advancing home care excellence. (2009). Retrieved from http://www.champ-program.org/ Visiting Nurse Service of New York, Center for Home Care Policy and Research.

Cowin, L. S. (2001). Measuring nurses' self-concept. *Western Journal of Nursing Research*, *23*(3), 313–325.

Fineout-Overholt, E., Levin, R. F., & Melnyk, B. M. (2005). Strategies for advancing evidence-based practice in clinical settings. *Journal of the New York State Nurses Association*, *35*(2), 28–32.

Good, L., & Nelson, D. (1973). Effects of person-group and intragroup attitude similarity of perceived group attractiveness and cohesiveness: II. *Psychological Reports*, *33*, 51–60.

Langley, G. J., Moen, R. D., Nolan, K. M., Nolan, T. W., Norman, C. L., & Provost, L. P. (2009). *The improvement guide*. San Francisco, CA: Jossey-Bass.

Levin, R. F., Melnyk, B. M., Fineout-Overholt, E., Barnes, M., & Vetter, M. (2011). Fostering evidence-based practice to improve nurse and cost outcomes in a community health setting: A pilot test of the ARCC model. *Nursing Administration Quarterly, 35*(1), 1–13.

Levin, R. F., Keefer, J. M., Marren, J., Vetter, M., Lauder, B., & Sobolewski, S. (2010). Evidence-based practice: Merging 2 paradigms. *Journal of Nursing Care Quality, 25*(2), 117–126.

Levin, R. F., Vetter, M., Foust, J., & Bowles, K. (2009). Building EBP capacity in home care. *Symposium conducted at the meeting of the Eastern Nursing Research Society*, Boston, MA.

Melnyk, B. M., Fineout-Overholt, E., & Mays, M. Z. (2008). The evidence-based practice beliefs and implementation scales: Psychometric properties of two new instruments. *Worldviews Evidence Based Nursing, 5*(4), 208–216.

Pravikoff, D. S., Tanner, A. B., & Pierce, S. T. (2005). Readiness of U.S. nurses for evidence-based practice: Many don't understand or value research and have had little or no training to help them find evidence on which to base their practice. *American Journal of Nursing, 105*(9), 40–52.

Price, J. L., & Mueller, C. W. (1986). *Absenteeism and turnover among hospital employees*. Greenwich, CN: JAI Press.

26

Implementing an EBPI Program in a Community Health Agency: The Visiting Nurse Service of New York Experience (Part II)

Lorraine Ferrara, Bonnie Lauder, Rona F. Levin, Janice B. Foust, and Kathryn H. Bowles

Without change there is no innovation, creativity, or incentive for improvement. Those who initiate change will have a better opportunity to manage the change that is inevitable.

—William Pollard

As mentioned in Chapter 25, the Renfield Evidence-Based Practice Improvement Fellows Program (hereinafter referred to as the Renfield Program) facilitated two Evidence-Based Practice Improvement (EBPI) projects: medication management and pain management. This chapter presents a detailed description of each of these projects. The model that project teams used to develop, implement, and evaluate the projects was the EBPI model (Levin et al., 2010). This model, described fully in the previous chapter, was developed at the Visiting Nurse Service of New York (VNSNY) in order to link a practice improvement framework (Langley, Nolan, Nolan, Norman, & Provost, 1996), which was in current use by the organization's Quality Improvement Department, and with which most nurses were familiar, and an evidence-based practice (EBP) approach to achieving best clinical practice. The following two projects were developed and implemented as pilots during The Renfield Program. Both projects were approved by the Institutional Review Board of the VNSNY. Each project, as readers will see, provided valuable information to the VNSNY in order to enhance clinical practice.

FIRST PROJECT: MEDICATION MANAGEMENT

Purpose of Project

The purpose of the first project was to improve medication management among forgetful patients and/or patients who had problems with medication adherence while receiving home care services. To achieve this purpose, we looked at current practices for medication management within the organization, searched for and retrieved evidence on the best available medication management strategies, performed a gap analysis to determine the focus for this project, and developed a plan to bridge the gap.

Description of the Practice Problem

The Outcome and Assessment Information Set (OASIS) is a standardized assessment tool used in home care (www.cms.gov/oasis). The OASIS includes assessment of the patient's ability to adhere to prescribed medications. Yet, clinicians also attend to the patient's willingness to adhere to a treatment regimen as a critical element of care. During early meetings, the EBPI project team noted that home care nurses made very little distinction between *willingness* to adhere versus *ability* to adhere to medication regimens. Renfield fellows reported that nonadherence was most obvious when patients exhibited deficits in decision making or functional limitations that required assistance with routine daily living activities. Consequently, it seemed possible that mild cognitive impairment or medication nonadherence could be overlooked when related to a functional/behavioral deficit. Inconsistencies in practice indicated the need for evidence-based protocols. For example, clinicians routinely reviewed the medication name, dosage, schedule, and side effects with their patients on admission. On subsequent visits, however, clinicians did not consistently verify whether or not a patient was actually taking the medications, especially when the patient appeared to be cognitively intact. Nurses did promptly address medication management issues when patients' exhibited exacerbated disease symptoms. Overall, home care nurses recognized problems with medications as a preventable source of hospital admission and voiced a need for more proactive and time-efficient strategies to address medication adherence as a common practice issue.

Internal Data to Support the Problem

Improvement in medication management is a national benchmark reported to Home Health Compare (www.medicare.gov/homehealthcompare). The Bronx Region of the VNSNY was above the national average in improvement in medication management, but there was variation in results across programs, regions, and nurse teams. The 2007 year-to-date scorecard reported team scores for the percent of patients improving in medication management between admission and discharge, ranging from 21% to 55%, indicating support of the observed variation in care delivered. In addition, medication management was a topic of several VNSNY initiatives where nonadherence was identified as a potential reason for hospitalizations. These findings supported choosing medication management as the focus of an EBPI project. Patient improvement in oral medication management was determined by comparing scores on the OASIS item, described in Exhibit 26.1, at the start and end of home care services.

To further understand current practice, Renfield Fellows conducted a survey and chart audits with the teams with which they worked. Clinicians were asked about their general views and practices of medication management. In addition, patient records were reviewed for specific documentation of medication adherence. The survey of nurses ($n = 6$) revealed how they assessed the patient's knowledge of medication name, frequency,

EXHIBIT 26.1 CENTERS FOR MEDICARE AND MEDICAID SERVICES—OUTCOME AND ASSESSMENT INFORMATION SET (OASIS)

Medication Management

(M2020) Management of Oral Medications: Patient's current ability to prepare and take all oral medications reliably and safely, including administration of the correct dosage at the appropriate times/intervals. **Excludes injectable and IV medications. (NOTE: This refers to ability, not compliance or willingness.)**

0—Able to independently take the correct oral medication(s) and proper dosage(s) at the correct times

1—Able to take medication(s) at the correct times if:

(a) Individual dosages are prepared in advance by another person, OR
(b) Another person develops a drug diary or chart

2—Able to take medication(s) at the correct times if given reminders by another person at the appropriate times

3—Unable to take medication unless administered by another person

NA—No oral medications prescribed

dose, and recognition. The nurses described that they spent less time assessing actual strategies used by patients to manage their medications than assessing knowledge of how to take medications. In addition, the nurses were very concerned with cognitive function, but there was little consistency about how nurses assessed cognitive impairment.

In home care, cognition is routinely assessed on admission with a standardized OASIS question (see Exhibit 26.2). As the nurses stated, however, there is not a clear or consistent approach to applying this question. For the patients who are mildly impaired, there was a tendency to select "zero" as an answer because the patient was oriented to person, place, and time. The important difference in a patient's ability between answers 0 and 3 is whether or not the patient needs assistance under stressful or unfamiliar conditions (answer 1) or specific situations (answer 2), which can be difficult to fully assess during the first encounter.

Involving frontline caregivers as stakeholders in any EBPI project is essential in order to encourage buy-in. In this spirit, home care nurses assisted a Renfield fellow with 10 chart audits to identify how assessment of medication management was documented during subsequent home visits. The patient record audit revealed four patients "always adhered;" one patient required support, and in five instances (50%) medication

EXHIBIT 26.2 CENTERS FOR MEDICARE AND MEDICAID SERVICES—OUTCOME AND ASSESSMENT INFORMATION SET (OASIS)

(M0560) Cognitive Functioning (patient's current level of alertness, orientation, comprehension, concentration, and immediate memory for simple commands):

0—Alert/oriented, able to focus and shift attention, comprehends and recalls task directions independently.
1—Requires prompting (cuing, repetition, reminders) only under stressful or unfamiliar conditions.
2—Requires assistance and some direction in specific situations (e.g., on all tasks involving shifting of attention), or consistently requires low stimulus environment due to distractibility.
3—Requires considerable attention to routine situations. Is not alert and oriented or is unable to shift attention and recall directions more than half the time.
4—Totally dependent due to disturbances such as constant disorientation, coma, persistent vegetative state, or delirium.

adherence was not addressed at all. In the cases where adherence was addressed, there was no indication of how the adherence was assessed. These data revealed deficiencies in the electronic documentation system. The interventions available to clinicians included patient teaching (e.g., doses, frequency), pre-pouring medications, and providing pre-printed education materials, but it did not include the use of medication reminders, a common evidence-based intervention. A free-text section, however, was available for use when clinicians wanted to document additional interventions.

The Focused Clinical Question

With 50% of audited cases not having adherence addressed and data revealing inconsistent strategies to evaluate adherence, the Renfield fellows identified this issue as an important practice problem to address. They also determined that patients with mild cognitive impairment were at risk of not being recognized and, consequently, not having the necessary early interventions and appropriate supports put in place to promote medication adherence. After much discussion and a preliminary literature review, the Renfield team identified the following focused clinical question: *For patients who are nonadherent with medications and/or are cognitively impaired, will the use of evidence-based tools to simplify the medication regimen and promote adherence decrease regimen complexity and improve medication adherence and ability compared to usual care?*

The Evidence

A literature review using the Cochrane Database of Systematic Reviews, Medline, and CINAHL focused on assessment screening tools and medication management interventions revealed several high-level studies that addressed the clinical question. A systematic review identified three common sources of preventable medication-related hospitalizations that are relevant to home care practice including issues related to adherence (33%), prescribing (33%), and monitoring (22%) (Howard et al., 2007). We focused on all three issues. The Renfield team also reviewed several published screening tools and interventions for their ease of use, reliability, appropriateness to home care, and strength of the evidence. These criteria were important to us because we wanted to increase the likelihood of acceptance by the staff, success and, ultimately, long-term sustainability of the protocol throughout VNSNY.

The Medication Management for Older Adult Clients guideline (hereinafter referred to as The Guideline) met these criteria (Bergman-Evans, 2006). The Guideline was created from evidence-based interventions from the literature. The Guideline cited combination interventions as being more effective than any single intervention alone (Bergman-Evans, 2006; Roter, Hall, Merisca, & Nordstrom, 1998). Behavioral interventions to decrease dosing demands and monitoring adherence were other important findings (Kripilani, Yao, & Haynes, 2007) on which we based our protocol.

In addition, the literature confirmed our concern that cognitive impairment is a significant contributor to problems with medication adherence (Gray, Mahoney, & Blough, 1999), or is a risk factor for preventable, medication-related hospitalizations (Leendertse, Egberts, Stoker, & van dem Bemt, 2008). Knowing this, we wanted a brief screening tool to assess cognition, hence, the Mini-Cog (Doerflinger, 2007). We also reviewed medication adherence measures and decided to modify a self-report medication-taking scale to fit our needs (Morisky, Green, & Levine, 1986). Finally, we concluded that behavioral interventions that decrease dosing demands consistently improve adherence (Kripilani et al., 2007).

Project Plan

The Gap Analysis

When we examined the literature and compared it to our current internal data/chart audits and surveys, and the flowchart of current practice, we identified the following gaps in current practice in our agency:

(i) Inconsistent approaches for assessing cognitive functioning;
(ii) Inconsistent approaches for assessing medication adherence and follow-up; and
(iii) No measure of medication regimen complexity.

Measurement Instruments

Four reliable and valid assessment tools were selected to address these gaps in practice and facilitate the measurement of project outcomes. These are:

1. The *Mini-Cog* is a 3-minute instrument to screen for cognitive impairment in older adults. It contains a three-item recall test for memory and a simple clock drawing test. It is easy to administer and is not affected by ethnicity, language, or education. It is useful to detect mild impairment (Doerflinger, 2007).
2. The *Morisky Tool* consists of four self-reported questions about medication taking behaviors such as: "Do they ever forget to take or stop taking their medications?" (Morisky et al., 1986). It is brief and easy to administer.

3. The *Hamdy Tool* was chosen to assist with medication simplification (Hamdy et al., 1995). The Hamdy guides the nurse through five questions about the medication regimen, such as: "Is simplification possible and is the indication for which the original medication prescribed still present?"
4. The *Symptom Bother Scale* was chosen to assist the nurses in monitoring the improvement or decline in the number and status of 13 common symptoms experienced by older adults (Heidrich & Ryff, 1993). For example, the presence of pain or shortness of breath is assessed and, if present, it is rated as to how much it bothers the patient. We believed that adherence to the medication regimen would result in stable or improved symptoms.

Developing the EBPI

Project Aims

Practice improvement projects are guided by aim statements. Aim statements answer the question: "What are we trying to accomplish?" Aim statements place the focused clinical question into measurable terms. For example, one of our Aim statements was: Ninety percent of the mildly cognitively impaired or nonadherent patients will have stable symptom bother scores within 3 months.

Additional goals or desired outcomes of the project were:

1. An increase in the percentage of patients who have a decrease in the number of symptoms, a decline in the amount of bother they report, or no differences in the former two parameters if they remain unchanged in patients assessed with mild cognitive impairment.
2. A decrease in the patient readmission rate by direct care team.
3. A decline in the number of patients identified as being nonadherent.
4. A decline in the number of medications and/or doses of medication per day per patient.
5. An increase in the percentage of patients who improve in medication self-management.

The multifaceted medication management interventions, supported by the evidence, were separated into two areas: (a) reminders and (b) regimen simplification. If the patient was assessed as cognitively impaired or nonadherent, the clinicians would implement reminder and/or simplification interventions. The reminder interventions consisted of: pillboxes with instructions; pill counts used if patient's memory was poor; involvement of caregiver; telephone calls to patients and caregivers; and charts and medication lists. Simplifying medications included having nurses review the drug utilization reports generated by the electronic record system and complete the Hamdy tool (Hamdy et al., 1995).

To be successful, it was very important to integrate the proposed best practice into the current practice. The current practice was illustrated using a flow chart, then that workflow was compared to the practice change protocol. Differences between the two flowcharts were integrated into the current practice flowchart by adding and removing steps as needed. A horizontal deployment flowchart outlined the steps to be taken and presented a timeline with specific visit days (Figure 26.1). The flowchart created a common understanding and agreement on the best-practice protocol, standardization of the process, and guided evaluation of the outcomes.

Process Measures and Tracking Tool

Fidelity to the protocol was monitored by tracking process measures. Team members were given various roles and responsibilities in monitoring the process. The following process measures were tracked:

1. All patients aged 70 and older were assessed for cognition using the Mini-Cog tool and medication adherence using the Morisky tool (Morisky et al., 1986).
2. Nurses administered the Hamdy tool (Hamdy et al., 1995) with all patients found to be cognitively impaired, nonadherent, or with five or more medications.
3. Nurses used reminder and/or simplification interventions for all cognitive impaired and/or nonadherent patients.
4. Nurses assessed cognitively impaired and/or nonadherent patients' symptoms at the start of care and at discharge using the Symptom Bother Scale (Heidrich & Ryff, 1993).

Educational Sessions

Renfield fellows who were also patient service managers (i.e., direct care team managers) conducted a 2-hour education session for their staff. They selected nurses who were interested and willing to participate in the practice improvement project. The education session included an introduction to the project, instruction on how to administer the new assessment tools, suggested evidence-based nursing interventions for addressing assessment findings, and the timeline for the EBPI project.

Project Implementation

Once the project plan and training were complete, the plan, do, study, act (PDSA) cycle or first small test of change begun.

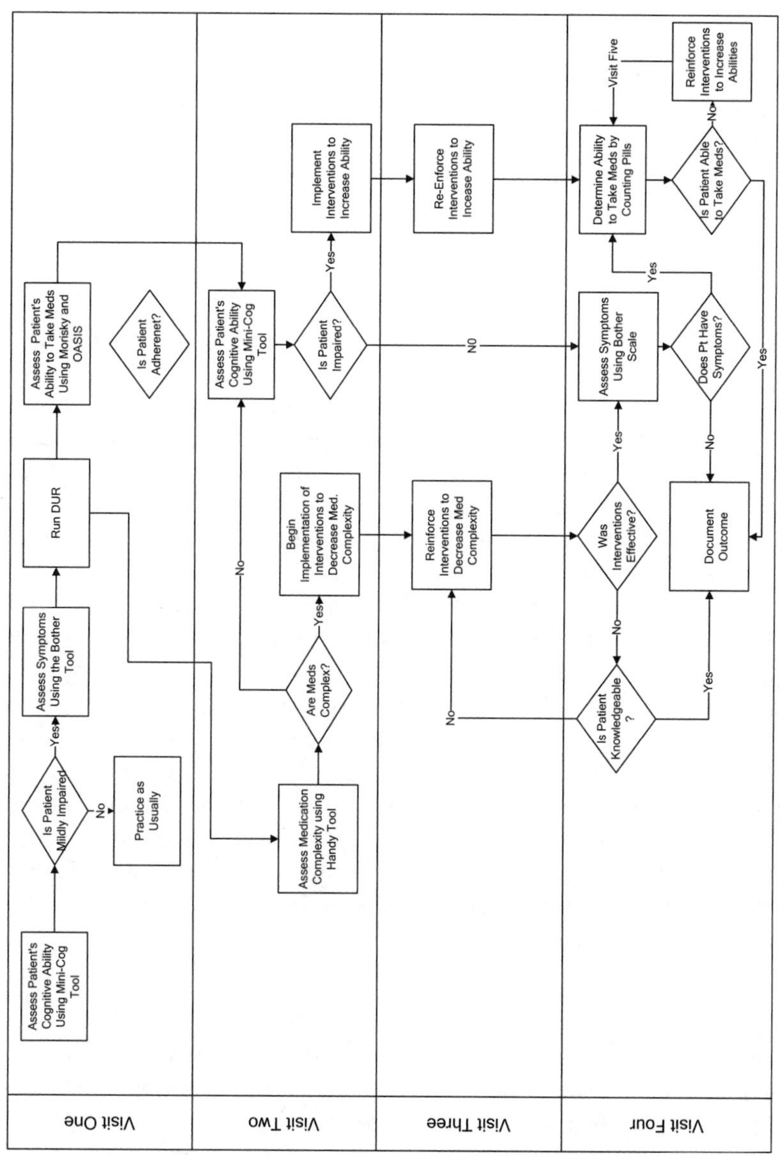

FIGURE 26.1 Flowchart of medication management by nurses.

PDSA Cycle One

Five patient candidates for the study were selected based on age (greater than 70) and their response to the Mini-Cog (Doerflinger, 2007) and four self-reported adherence questions (Morisky et al., 1986). Nurses were given the protocol, paper copies of the four tools, and instructed to document the interventions in the free-text portion of the visit note as appropriate. The completed tools were to be given to the patient service manager, who would forward the documents to team members responsible for tracking the process measures. A second group of people were charged with reviewing the charts of the patients for interventions and clinical outcomes. The "do" component of the first PDSA cycle lasted for 4 weeks.

We learned (study) many lessons during the first PDSA cycle. The two most important lessons at this phase were the need for more oversight and coaching of the clinicians as they piloted this work, and the need to decrease the patients' age to capture more people. We learned that nurses did not follow the protocol in the first five cases. The nurses described how they had difficulty integrating the protocol into practice because there were too many papers and it took too long to use the tools. The clinicians asked for electronic copies of the tools. In addition, they shared that they were not comfortable administrating the tools and they had questions about how they were to be used.

In response to the nurses' feedback (act) and the process monitoring data, we developed additional education about the use and purpose of the protocol and tools, and answered any of the nurses' questions. In addition, we instituted weekly conference calls between the Renfield team and frontline nurses to answer any questions as they worked with the protocol. The clinicians were surprised when their requests were implemented so quickly. One clinician stated, "You are actually listening to what we have to say." The age of the patients evaluated for the protocol was lowered from 70 to 55 years of age because the average age of patients on the clinical team was lower than expected.

PDSA Cycle Two

Twenty-four patients for the second small test of change were elected based on age (greater than 55) and their response to the Mini-Cog (Doerflinger, 2007) and four self-reported adherence questions (Morisky et al., 1986). In order to increase oversight, coaching was incorporated into the process. Patient service managers were given weekly reports by the nurses in the project. The reports included information about the age of patients admitted to ensure all appropriate patients were evaluated. These reports were used during weekly conference calls to follow up with the clinicians about specific patients admitted that week and to track data collection.

Overall, the clinicians stated having the tools and protocol in electronic form made it much easier to implement and sustain the practice change—"It became a matter of habit." The nurses were very surprised at the number of patients who were nonadherent and/or experienced mild cognitive impairment. Figure 26.2 presents examples of clocks drawn by patients who were assessed as alert and oriented on the relevant OASIS item.

For most of the time, the Symptom Bother Scale tool was not implemented at discharge as planned. The nurses viewed this as an "extra" tool that duplicated the current documentation. Therefore, patients hospitalized for nonadherence with medications were used as a proxy to measure the Aim/Outcome. Additional outcomes were identified:

1. In conducting chart reviews, Renfield fellows noted that one out of 24 (4.1%) patients was re-hospitalized due to medications, which compared to an overall team hospitalization rate of 27%.
2. More than 50% of patients were nonadherent most of the time at start of care.
3. Counting the number of medications at start of care and at discharge is not a dependable indicator of medication regimen complexity.
4. The OASIS is not sensitive to capturing improvement in self-managing medications.

Implications and Recommendations for Nursing Practice

On the basis of the results of this pilot EBPI project, there were four implications for nursing practice identified. First, it was beneficial to incorporate

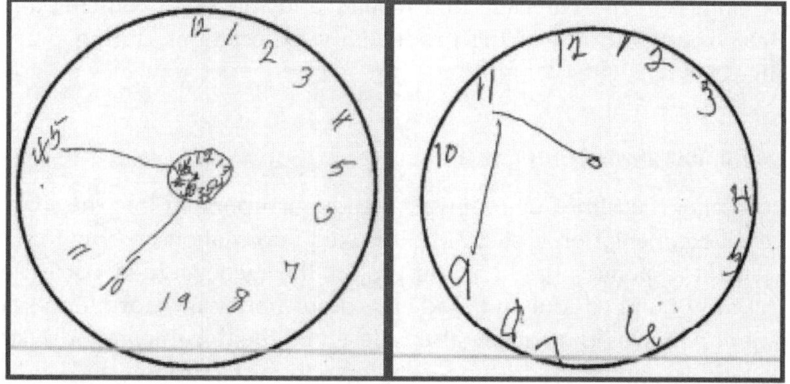

FIGURE 26.2 Abnormal clock drawings (a portion of the Mini-Cog).

evidence-based assessment tools as standard practice. Once integrated into their workflow, the nurses were receptive to better assessment tools and approaches for this common area of practice. The standardized, OASIS assessments and documentation can be more accurate and consistent with the addition of evidence-based tools. Specifically, we found the proper implementation of the Mini-Cog tool was more effective in identifying cognitively impaired patients than the OASIS cognitive assessment item. Second, we needed to enhance medication documentation to include a range of multiple interventions, including the early involvement of caregivers on the first visit. The effective and consistent monitoring of medication adherence can help nurses to identify and justify the need for additional home visits to assist patients with medication adherence. Implementation of the pilot protocol revealed that more than one visit is needed to accurately assess cognitive function and medication adherence. Initial visits are useful to focus on patient assessment and begin medication-related interventions; however, subsequent visits are essential to evaluate whether or not the patient acted on or retained information provided earlier. Third, decreasing the complexity of medication regimens could promote adherence, but more attention is needed to develop and support this intervention, such as involvement of the primary care providers. Last, as might be expected, we found it was crucial to provide support to frontline staff at the team level during practice changes. The benefit of such support is to ensure a standard approach to practice change as well as identify and address problems in a timely manner.

We also learned how important it was to understand and describe current practices before integrating new practices. The flowchart illustrated how the practice change was to be implemented within the context of usual practice. The clinicians reported that the protocol helped them organize their thoughts and actions on the initial visit. Another way to support practice change is to give clinicians time to learn and apply new content outside the classroom and adjust the productivity expectations during practice change cycles.

Plan for Dissemination (Act)

A version of the Mini-Cog tool was already incorporated into the computerized documentation system, but it lacked information on how to score the patient responses. Based on our project, the agency added instructions to the computerized tool and made its completion mandatory for a select group of patients. The agency also redesigned the documentation system to expand the number and types of interventions to support and address medication management.

SECOND PROJECT: PAIN MANAGEMENT

Purpose of Project

The purpose of this project was to improve management of chronic nonmalignant pain in the long-term home health care population (LTHHCP) at the VNSNY. To achieve this purpose we looked at current practices for pain management within the organization, searched for and retrieved evidence on the best available management guidelines for treatment of chronic pain, and developed a plan to bridge the gap.

Description of the Practice Problem

Chronic pain and its management is a consistent problem in our LTHHCP. Direct care visiting nurses identified that patients with chronic pain often were not getting adequate relief. Numerous guidelines and systematic reviews with a high level and quality of evidence support the widespread nature of chronic pain and the importance of addressing assessment and management from an informed stance (AGS Panel, 2002; American Pain Society, 2002; Chou, Clark, & Helfand, 2003; Devulder, Richarz, & Nataraja, 2005; Furlan, Sandoval, Mailis-Gagnon, & Tunks, 2006; Institute of Clinical Systems Improvement, 2007; Registered Nurse Association of Ontario, 2007; Wiffen, McQuay, Edwards, & Moore, 2005). Two major challenges to pain management by both primary care providers and home health care nurses are the complexity of treatment options, the escalating introduction of new analgesic medications, and new analgesic uses for medications currently in use for other health conditions.

Internal Data to Support the Problem

To help us better describe the problem at VNSNY and formulate a focused clinical question, we looked at internal or organizational data. First, we looked at an OASIS question on the initial nursing assessment that measured improvement in pain. OASIS stands for outcome, assessment, information, and set; it is a U.S. national tool that measures patient outcomes in home care. The OASIS item for pain can be seen in Exhibit 26.3.

VNSNY as well as the Centers of Medicare and Medicaid (CMS) use this item to assess whether persons receiving home care show improvement in pain interfering with activity following home care. VNSNY incorporated the outcomes of this item into its LTHHCP's Quality Score Card (Exhibit 26.4). The VNSNY Quality Score Cards provide monthly data on multiple indicators in four domains: Process, Outcomes, Costs, and Satisfaction Measures. Key data elements are highlighted in colors that

EXHIBIT 26.3 CENTERS FOR MEDICARE AND MEDICAID SERVICES—OUTCOME AND ASSESSMENT INFORMATION SET (OASIS)

OASIS Item for Pain
OASIS M0420 Improvement in Pain
(M0420) Frequency of pain interfering with patient's activity or movement:

0—Patient has no pain or pain does not interfere with activity or movement
1—Less often than daily
2—Daily, but not constantly
3—All of the time

demonstrate performance that is: (a) greater than 10% from the VNSNY target in a negative direction (red); (b) between 10% below and the VNSNY target (yellow), and (3) at VNSNY target or better (green). Scorecards are used to provide feedback on organizational performance to staff, and allow the organization to set targets to continually assess and improve performance. We limited our project and report to the outcomes of M0420, Improvement in Pain Interfering with Activity, and included the entire nursing staff, which is divided into several nursing teams in the Brooklyn LTHHCP Region. Report results for January 2007 to October 2007 demonstrated that, as a whole, the LTHHCP was not reaching the target goal for this item, which was that 78% of patients would show an improvement in their pain. The results of the scorecards, therefore, supported the need for a project that focused on enhancing the management of chronic pain in LTHHCP patients.

EXHIBIT 26.4 2007 QUALITY SCORE CARD RESULTS OF M0420 IMPROVEMENT IN PAIN (QUARTERLY) IN ONE REGIONAL OFFICE OF VNSNY

Program Selected: Long-Term Care
Region Selected: K-Brooklyn
Team Selected: All Team

Outcome	Measure	Target	Monthly	Actual YTD
Pain		78%	75% (Yellow)	64.5% (Red)

To better understand current practice regarding the root cause of the problem, we began developing strategies and tools for gathering more internal evidence. A first and common assumption by the organization was that the nurses were not conducting a through pain assessment. A focus group was held with the LTHHCP nurses from the Bronx, New York region of the LTHHCP to test these assumptions. Questions were prepared in advance by the project team (Exhibit 26.5). The focus group was conducted by two project team members; one facilitated the discussion and the other took detailed notes of participants' responses. Results of the focus group showed that the nurses had confidence in their ability to make a thorough pain assessment, but they felt a knowledge deficit regarding new pain medications and their most appropriate use with patients who had differing pain origins. Confusion regarding documentation of pain in our electronic documentation system was another challenge. A frequent area of confusion was the documentation of issues related to pain and its management in a narrative section instead of documenting it under VNSNY *Pain Management Problem*. The *Pain Management Problem* guides the clinician in a thorough assessment, teaching, management,

EXHIBIT 26.5 PAIN MANAGEMENT PROJECT

Focus Group Questions

1. How do you assess pain?
2. If your patient has pain, what do you do to help?
3. How do you document your assessment of pain?
4. How do you document interventions for pain?
5. How do you document whether or not your interventions were successful?
6. Where do you feel you need more knowledge or support for pain assessment?
7. Where do you feel you need more knowledge or support for pain management?
8. Where do you feel you need more knowledge or support with evaluation of the success of your interventions?
9. What do you believe are the most important issues we need to focus on to improve pain management at this agency?
10. Please write down the three most important things that you think we can do at Visiting Nurse Service to improve the practice of pain management. (Participants were told that individual responses were confidential.)

and evaluation of patients' pain using a best-practice approach developed by a group of "pain experts" at VNSNY. Fear of addiction and side effects of pain medication was another common issue among the nurses. Lack of confidence in communicating with the physician about patients' pain management was also a major barrier in achieving optimal patient outcomes with regard to pain. When asked to list the three most important interventions that could be instituted to improve pain management at VNSNY, 100% of the nurses responded that they needed additional educational support as a solution to their gap in knowledge, and requested the availability of an advanced practice nurse who was a pain specialist as a consultant.

Based on the review of the focus group interview themes and best evidence from the literature, the project team developed an audit tool (Exhibit 26.6) to review patient records. This tool was tested by the project team for inter-rater reliability prior to its use in auditing patient records. Criteria for selection of patients for the record audit were: patients in the LTHHCP in the Bronx and Brooklyn with opioid(s) prescribed; and the time frame studied was 10/01/07 to 11/30/07.

At VNSNY pain is measured by patient self-report using a 0–10 scale, with "0" indicating no pain, and "10" indicating the worst possible pain. Of the 66 patient records that were audited, 53% indicated that patients had a pain score of "4" or more (35 patients) and 47% indicated a pain score of less than "4" (31 patients). Results of the audit also showed that the common misconception that nurses were not assessing for pain was not correct. Nurses were consistent in documenting their assessment for pain. Assessment of pain was completed most of the time with 89% of records demonstrating assessment of the presence of pain on each visit. If a pain score was "4" or more, it was found that the *Pain Management Problem* was used on all visits 45% of the time, on some visits 34% of the time, and never 21% of the time. If pain was "4" or more, teaching and evaluation of pain was documented 65% of the time; however, management of the pain or follow-up on unimproved pain was not documented in any of the audited records. Since follow-up was an issue, we examined records more closely and found the following: 48% of the cases ($N = 14$) indicated that follow-up was needed based on the nurse's assessment, yet only 50% of these cases (7) contained documentation that indicated follow-up was needed. Moreover, only 21% of the records indicated that follow-up was done.

Results, using the 0–10 pain scale, showed 48% of the patients' pain improved. Results of the OASIS item (M0420), which measures the frequency of pain interfering with activity, reported 29% "Improved," 14% reported "None," 36% reported "No Change," and 21% reported "Worse." In addition, audits showed insufficient nurse follow-up with physicians for uncontrolled pain and insufficient documentation when follow-up was done. Many patients already taking analgesics continued

EXHIBIT 26.6 AUDIT TOOL FOR PAIN MANAGEMENT PROJECT

Visiting Nurse Service Of New York
We Bring The Caring Home

Renfield Project: Pain Management Team Audit Tool

Reviewer's Name: ______________ **Diagnoses:** ______________
COC________Other________ **Period of Time Reviewed: 10/1/-11/30/2007 Region:** Brooklyn Bronx **Team#:** ______
Time Frame-October 1, 2007- November 30, 2007 (at least four weeks)
Total # of visits in time frame including last and prior OASIS______________
Case#: ______________ **SOC:** ______________ **Case is:** Active Discharged

			Instructions Comments
OASIS Assessment/ Clinical Findings/Pain Management Problem			
1. Presence of pain is assessed on each visit (VNS0337). Include "None" as an assessment.	____Of ___	**NA**	Answer as %. For example "4 of 8" (meaning total number of notes reviewed 4 assessed pain out of 8 charts) 4 of 8
2. Pain was rated 4 or greater. **(Include pain rating in the pain management problem-example,** SN rated pain as 2 under clinical findings but rated pain under "pain management problem as 5 as "worst " since last visit)	____Of ___	**NA**	Answer as %. **If no notes have pain 4 or greater then STOP review at this point**. If "5 of 8" had 4 or greater pain rating then **continue review of the 5 charts only.**
3. If Pain is scored as 4 or greater, were the following additional items completed? a. (VNS0338) Type	____Of ___	**NA**	Answer as %. for each category. For example, of the 5 charts reviewed (with pain 4 or more) "2 of 5" completed the "type" of pain.
b. (VNS0339) Location	____Of ___	**NA**	
c. (VNS0340) Characteristics	____Of ___	**NA**	
d. (VNS0341 Relieved by	____Of ___	**NA**	
e. (VNS0342) Effectiveness	____Of ___	**NA**	
Pain Management Problem			
1. If pain score is 4 or more is there documentation in the Pain Management Problem? **(IF NO DOCUMENTATION ON PAIN MANAGEMENT PROBLEM SKIP TO QUESTION 3)**	____Of ___	**NA**	Answer as %. For example, of the 5 charts reviewed (with pain 4 or more) **"4 of 5"** "documented in the pain management problem".
2. Interventions documented against. a. Assessed	____Of ___	**NA**	Answer as % **only** charts that documented in pain problem. For example, of the 4 charts that document in pain problem 3 documented under assessment. "3 of 4"
Pain Status: Pain symptom rating: worst pain/least pain Frequency of symptoms reported: Pain interferes with: ______________ Aggravating factors: ______________ Alleviating factors: ______________	**Check (✓) what was "assessed" during the time period of review.** (For example, If in all 5 charts reviewed with a pain level of 4 or greater assessed aggravating factors –5 checks should be in front of that assessment.		
b. Taught	____Of ___	**NA**	Answer as %. For example, of the 5 charts reviewed 3 documented under teaching.

Reason for pain **Medication management**: Rationale for around the clock dosing Filling prescriptions in a timely manner Initially causes drowsiness Manage constipation Difference between drug tolerance /drug addiction **Behaviors/ techniques to manage pain:** Engage in activities that distract from pain Exercise, as tolerated Repositioning Immobilization Rest/exercise schedule Imagery Meditation Breathing exercises Develop structured routines Expression of feelings Avoid stressors Manage nausea and vomiting **Symptom/complications to report to care provider:** Increase in pain New pain Constipation Stupor Confusion			**Check (✓) what was "taught" during the time period of review.**
c. **Managed**	____**Of** ___	**NA**	Answer as %. For example, of the 5 charts reviewed 3 documented under managed.
Contact MD for medical consultation, pain regimen ineffective (See Coordination of Care) Referred to other VNS programs: Acute Care, Hospice, LTHHCP, Choice, Infusion Care Referred for additional VNS services: Nursing, SW, PT, OT, SLP, Paraprofessional, Nutritionist Referred to outside healthcare services			**Check (✓) what was "managed" during the time period of review.**
d. **Supported**	____**Of** ___	**NA**	Answer as %. For example, of the 5 charts reviewed 3 documented under supported.
Participation in support groups Acknowledged response to pain			**Check (✓) what was "assessed" during the time period of review.** .
e. Evaluated	____**Of** ___	**NA**	Answer as %. For example, of the 5 charts reviewed 3 documented under evaluated.

Check (✓) what was "evaluated" during the time period of review. (TURN PAGE OVER)		
Patient response to care: Treatment tolerated ✏ Treatment tolerated poorly Clinical Actions: ____ ✏ Patient experienced pain related to treatment Clinical Actions: ____ Treatment observed to be effective ✏ Treatment observed to be ineffective Unable to determine effectiveness -Condition/symptoms unchanged since last visit Condition/symptoms improved since last visit ✏ Condition/symptoms declined/worsened since last visit Clinical Actions: ____	**Patient/Caregiver learning/return demonstration:** Has adequate knowledge Can perform treatment /care without supervision Knowledge inadequate, requires further supervision -✏ Unable to recall information and/or follow detailed instruction Clinical Actions: ____ ✏ Unable to perform Clinical Actions: ____ Requires further supervision	**Patient /Caregiver –Follows suggested Plan:** As often as necessary -✏ More often than necessary Clinical Action Taken ____ -✏ Less than necessary Clinical Action Taken ____ -✏ Rarely or Never Clinical Action Taken ____ **Primary symptom management since last visit** Managed independently Managed with assistance (caregiver, family, HHA) Required intervention of skilled professional Required unplanned /emergent care

Other "Problems" and "Outcomes"			
3. Did the note include documentation on a Pain **Medication** Management Problem (Only pain medications or adjuvant therapy)	**____of ___**	**NA**	
4. Did any other "problems" documented on the note include **specific instruction** in "pain"? *	**____Of ___**	**NA**	*Example, in "OA or HIV Problem check if instructed in pain management, S/S of pain to report etc etc.
5. Did the note include documentation of "outcomes" related to pain? **Include only if documented under outcomes**	**____Of ___**	(Found after evaluation under care plan problem" pain management".	
Coordination of Care (COC): Check under "Problems"- "Managed", "Evaluated" & in "Narrative" (last part of visit note) & in COC Notes			
6. Based on **patient assessment** was F/U indicated?	**Yes or NO**	This is reviewer's conclusion, i.e., pt had pain greater than 6 for 6 week period and nothing was done.	
7. Did the note document F/U was needed? (Check Managed, Evaluated, Narrative or COC.)	**____Of ___**	**NA**	If needed, briefly explain.
8. **If f/u was needed** was it done? (Check "Managed, Evaluated, Narrative or COC.)	**____Of ___**	**NA**	If needed, briefly explain
9. If documented, where? Managed	Evaluated	Narrative	COC
10. If follow up, what was the follow up? **Check ALL that apply.** Contacted MD to change POC related to pain regime Referral to pain clinic F/U tests Change in pain/adjuvant meds Referral PT other, explain notes			
11. During the review time period, did the pain rating improve (Interventions were effective)?	**Yes or NO**	**NA**	(Evidence can be- improvement in pain rating and/ or Improvement 420) If needed explain
12. List all pain medications including adjuvant therapy (Check POC):			
13. Was there a change in pain medications or adjuvant therapy during the time period? (Check POC and dates medications ordered)	**Yes or No**		If yes, briefly explain change

TURN PAGE OVER

14. Was Rehab involved? (Check POC)	**Yes or No**	**NA**	
Episode Outcome			
Frequency of pain interfering w/ activity (M0420)	Score on **Last OASIS =** Date______________	Score on **Prior to Last OASIS=** **Date**______________	
NOTES:			

Pain and Adjuvant Medications

Opioid-Codeine, Codeine and Acetaminophen (Tylenol #3 or #4), Oxycodone (Roxicodone, Percolone), Oxycodone and Acetaminophen (Percocet), Hydrocodone and Acetaminophen (Vicoden, Lorcet, Lortab), Morphine (MS Contin, Oramorph)) , Hydromorphone (Dilaudid), Methadone (Dolohine), Ketobemidone, Fentanyl Transdermal System (Duragesic), Propoxiphene(Darvon), Propoxiphene and acetaminophen (Darvocet),

Non-Opioid/NSAIDS-Acetaminophen, Aspirin, Ibuprofen, Choline Magnesium Trisalicylate (Trilisate), Naproxenl (Naprosyn), Nabumetone (Relfan), Ketorolac (toradol), Celecoxib (Celebrex), Tramadol (Ultram)

Antidepressants-Amitriptyline (Elavil), Nortriptyline (Pamelor), Desipramine (Norpramin), Duloxetine (Cymbalta)

Anticonvulsants-Gabapentin (Neurontin), Carbamazepine (Tegretol), Lamotrigine (Lamictal)

Corticosteroids-Dexamethasone (decadron), Prednisone

Other -Baclofen (Lioresal), Lidoderm Patch (Topical Lidocaine)

to have chronic, unrelieved pain. Inconsistent use of the VNSNY documentation system to document pain management was also found. Instead of using the *Pain Management Problem* section of the document, a narrative section of the note was often used. The narrative notes were also used in instances when the *Coordination of Care Notes* should have been used instead to document follow-up with the primary care provider to coordinate patient care.

The Focused Clinical Question

Following the initial search for the internal evidence and background literature or external evidence, we identified our focused clinical question: Using the PICO (preparation, intervention, comparison, and outcome) format, we arrived at the following focused clinical question:

> In long-term home health patients with chronic non-malignant pain does a nursing assessment regarding the appropriateness of analgesic regimens and collaboration with primary care providers compared with usual care influence patients' perception of pain, quality of life, and daily function?

The Evidence Search

The project team continued to search systematically for, appraise, and synthesize the highest levels of evidence to guide the improvement plan. We sorted through many clinical practice guidelines addressing chronic nonmalignant pain management in the adult. Based on the group's evaluation of existing guidelines using the AGREE tool (The AGREE Collaboration, 2001), we chose four clinical practice guidelines that used the best evidence and addressed our topic (AGS Panel, 2002; APS, 2002; Institute for Clinical Systems Improvement, 2007; Registered Nurses Association of Ontario, 2007). The project team learned how to search the databases and focused on the main three, the Cochrane Library, Medline or PubMed, and CINAHL. Always trying to find the highest level of evidence, we used systematic reviews and clinical practice guidelines based on systematic reviews. Following the collection of the evidence, we used evidence tables to summarize and appraise the evidence. Key findings from the evidence search, which helped to direct our improvement efforts were:

1. Opioids are safe and effective for management of chronic nonmalignant pain (Furlan et al., 2006)
2. Long-term use of opioids can lead to improvement in functional outcomes (Devulder et al., 2005)
3. Gabapentin is effective for neuropathic pain (Wiffen et al., 2005)

4. Effective pain management requires recognition of type of pain: for example, neuropathic or musculoskeletal (Institute of Clinical Systems Improvement, 2007).

Project Plan

Gap Analysis

Following a thorough analysis of the best available evidence to manage chronic pain, we looked at our current practice gathered from our internal organizational data, focus group, and chart audits. We created a flowchart of current practice and best practices identified via the literature review, and then identified the following gaps:

1. Nurses had a knowledge deficit regarding complexity of treatment options for chronic pain by both primary providers and home health nurses.
2. Nurses were not conversant with the plethora of new analgesic medications on the market and new analgesic uses for medications originally developed to treat other health conditions.
3. Nurses' fear of addiction and side effects of analgesics often presented a barrier to appropriate guidance about taking these medications.
4. There was inconsistent documentation about management and follow-up for chronic uncontrolled pain in patient records.
5. Nurses report of lack of confidence in communicating with the primary provider about the treatment regimen for pain.

Developing the EBPI

Project Aims

The next step was to develop an aim (goal) statement. We began by asking the question: "What were we trying to accomplish?" Actually, we wanted to address both process and patient outcome goals. Our patient outcome aims were: (1) There will be a 30% improvement in patient's mean pain rating within 3 months and (2) There will be a 50% improvement in patient's quality of life (QOL) rating within 3 months. Our process aims addressed the documentation issues we uncovered in our initial patient record audits:

1. For 100% of patients, pain will be assessed and documented on every visit
2. For 100% of patients the QOL tool will be completed on first and final visits

3. For 100% of patients the appropriateness of analgesic regimen will be determined and documented
4. For 100% of patients, the effectiveness of analgesic regime will be assessed on each visit
5. For 100% of patients, there will be a note indicating that an assessment was completed for adherence to prescribed regime on each visit
6. For 100% of patients with ineffective pain regimens, the nurse documented contact with the primary care provider and includes recommendations that were made

Process and Outcome Measurement Tools

We adapted the following evidence-based tools to measure our outcome variables so that we could evaluate whether or not we were reaching our project aims that had to do with patient outcomes. The tools selected were based on their established validity and reliability as well as ease of use by patients and clinicians.

1. Pain was measured by self-report using a 0 − 10 visual analog scale
2. Quality of life was measured by the quality of life tool developed by the EuroQol Group (1990)

Process Measures and Supportive Tools

Documentation aims were measured by patient record audit, using the same tool that was used to collect baseline data (Exhibit 26.7). In order to facilitate nurses' implementation of the EBPI protocol, to ensure fidelity of process, and to facilitate nurses' data collection, the project team developed a process tracking tool (see Exhibit 26.8). In addition, the following supportive documents were used to facilitate nurses' implementation of the evidence-based innovation.

Chronic Pain Management Algorithm With a Focus on Pharmacological Management

We chose the Institute of Clinical Systems Improvement (ICSI) practice guideline (2007) algorithm for pain management because it included a focus on identifying the type of pain a patient was experiencing before determining appropriate treatments.

Pain Management: Commonly Used Medications

This one-page, double-sided reference for commonly used medications to treat different types of pain, their dosage, and side effects was adapted as a quick reference to keep the home care nurse informed on current medication options (ICSI, 2007).

EXHIBIT 26.7 PROJECT PROTOCOL FOR SMALL TEST OF CHANGE: PAIN PROJECT

Verify with your PSM the patients to include in the small test of change.
Remember to take the **Quality of Life (QOL)** tool with you and fill it out when you document your notes on the patient.
Review patient's record to determine source or sources of pain and prescribed analgesic regimen.
On each visit to the patients involved:

- Assess for the presence of pain and, if present, pain level (as per patient perception, no matter what that perception is) at that moment and document in clinical findings
- Complete documentation on patient's record for the full pain assessment no matter what the patient's pain level is
- Assess and document in Pain Management problem
- Obtain patient's goals for pain management and document in the Goal Management screen
- Assess the patient's analgesic regimen and determine:
    - Its appropriateness related to the type of pain (source and severity)
    - Whether the patient is adhering to the prescribed regimen
    - Any problem the patient is experiencing in adhering to the regimen
    - The effectiveness of the pain regimen

Make sure you use the narrative note to include information regarding the above items that is not captured in any other part of the patient care plan or clinical findings.
Document in the narrative a rating for MO 420 **Frequency of Pain** interfering with functioning:

0 = Patient has no pain or pain does not interfere with activity or movement
1 = Less often than daily
2 = Daily but not constantly
3 = All of the time

Determine if the patient is on the most effective analgesic regimen for their type of pain. If not, contact the patient's primary care provider to discuss this issue.

Document in the COC screen "PM" (pain management) when communicating with other disciplines about your patient.
Fill out the tracking sheet for the visit

EXHIBIT 26.8 TRACKING TOOL FOR PAIN PROJECT

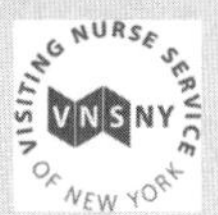

Tracking Tool for Small Test Change

Case Number:

Question	***Response Options/Examples***	***Visit 1***	***Visit 2***	***Visit 3***	***Visit 4***
1. COC #	HK434				
2. ***QOL completed (First and Final visit during small test of change) Please attach when complete test***	X or Blank				
3. Determine Source (s) of Pain	Back				
4. Assess presence/severity of pain ***0-10***	3				
5. Complete documentation of pain in Clinical Findings	Y or N				
6. Documented in Pain Management Problem	Y or N				
7. Is pain regime effective? ***I (Ineffective), E (Effective), M (Moderate) L (Limited)***	M, I, E, or L				
8. Is pt adhering to prescribed regime?	Y or N				
9. If pt is not adhering, briefly describe:					
10. Is analgesic regimen appropriate to pain type and severity?	Y or N				
11. If not on most effective analgesic regime, did you contact the patient's MD to discuss issue?	Y or N				
12. Rate MO 420 ***Frequency of Pain*** interfering with functioning. For each visit (Include score): ***0=no pain, 1= less than daily, 2=daily but not constantly, 3 = all the time***	0, 1, 2, or 3				
13. If the analgesic regime is not effective, did you contact the patient's primary care provider to discuss this issue?	Y, N, or N/A				
14. Did the PCP agree to change the medication regime?	Y, N, or N/A				
15. Was the change consistent with evidenced-based protocols?	Y, N, or N/A				

Beatrice Renfield EBPI Program
Chronic Pain Management

June 2009

EXHIBIT 26.9 SBAR

Renfield EBPI Fellows Program	June 2009
Chronic Pain Management	

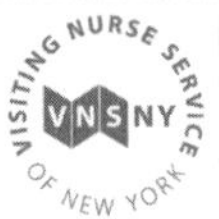

SBAR

Have ALL information AVAILABLE when reporting:
chart, allergies, medication list, code status, vital signs, goals of care
Consider collaboration with PSM, Pain Management Clinic if involved, before calling primary MD

S

SITUATION
State name and role: ("My name is Nurse Nice, with Visiting Nurse Service of New York")
I am calling about______________________________(***patient's name***)
The ***problem*** I am calling about is______________________________
____

B

BACKGROUND
State the ***primary diagnosis &*** pertinent ***medical history***______________
Functional status / changes______________________________
Most recent ***findings***______________________________
Pain: ***Severity rating*** Now_____ Best _____ Worst ______Usual ____ Acceptable___
Location Quality of pain______Response to current tx____________
Mental status____________________ Neuro changes____________________
VS: T_____ BP________________ Pulse rate/rhythm__________ Resp. rate/quality________
Lung sounds_______________ Oxygen______ L/min via___________
GI/GU changes (nausea/vomiting/diarrhea/impaction/hydration)________________
Weight_______ (actual) Loss or Gain Skin color___________ Blood Glucose____________
Wound: site, size, wound bed and margins, drainage type and amt, treatment and frequency
____
DNR Status / pt-family goals of care ______________________________
Prior attempts to treat this problem? ______________________________
____
Other______________________________

A

ASSESSMENT
I think that the patient is______________________________
OR
I am not sure of what the underlying problem is.

R

RECOMMENDATION - I suggest or request:
☐ Medication changes ______________________________
☐ Lab work______________________________
☐ Wound care changes______________________________
☐ Nutrition or fluid restriction changes______________________________
☐ Call physician with______________________________
☐ Other______________________________

CONCLUDE: RE-STATE PLAN/ORDERS, CLARIFY TIME FRAME FOR FOLLOW UP.

Staff Name______________________________ Date & Time______________
Physician's Name______________________________

This material was adapted from material prepared by Quality Insights of Pennsylvania, the Medicare Quality Improvement Organization Support Center for Home Health, under contract with the Centers for Medicare & Medicaid Services (CMS), an agency of the U.S. Department of Health and Human Services. The contents presented do not necessarily reflect CMS policy. Publication number: 8SOW-PA-HHQ07.630. App. 9/07.

SBAR (Situation–Background–Assessment–Recommendation)

SBAR is a technique used to improve efficiency and clarity of communications among health care providers (Boaro, Fancott, Baker, Velji, & Andreoli, 2010). We adapted an extant tool to improve performance and guide the clinician in communicating with the primary care provider (Exhibit 26.9).

Educational Sessions

A 2.5-hour educational session was conducted by two project team members, one an NP with expertise in pain management and the other a VNSNY education coordinator with extensive experience in educating nurses in the organization. The former led the update in pain management and instructed frontline nurse participants in the use of the tools to support best practice; the latter focused on protocol implementation. The educational sessions included case scenarios that were developed from actual cases involving long-term care patients with chronic uncontrolled pain and complicated analgesic regimens. Using these case scenarios, the nurses were introduced to using the *Pain Management Algorithm* to determine the type of pain patients were experiencing and the appropriateness of the medication regime to address the pain. The education coordinator also introduced the one-page document on *Pain Management: Commonly Used Medications* to further guide participating nurses about the indications, dosage, side effects, and any contraindications of the analgesics commonly used for pain.

In addition to the pain management update, nurses received training in how to enhance communication with the primary care provider using the SBAR tool. The nurses practiced communicating recommendations to the primary care provider with the project team members providing support. Following the case scenarios and SBAR practice, the EBPI project protocol was reviewed, instruction in completion of the QOL tool was given, and documentation requirements were reviewed.

Project Implementation

A protocol was developed for implementing the evidence-based innovation (Exhibit 26.7). Key to the success of this pilot project was using PDSA cycles or small tests of change to uncover and rectify process issues that might interfere with achieving project outcomes. Seven patient candidates who had a pain level of "4" or more with opiates prescribed during the 2 months prior to project implementation were selected for the project. Demographics of patients included in the first small test of change included: three male and four female patients aged between 49 and 81 years; a range of 2 to 5 chronic illness (most had 4); most frequent diagnoses were hypertension (5), AIDS (4), DM II (3), osteoarthritis (3). Total medications ranged from 8 to 22 (average =13), and pain medications ranged from 1 to 4 (most had 2).

PDSA Cycle One

The first "Do" cycle was conducted in the Brooklyn LTHHCP, where one of the project team members worked as a clinical director and would be able to provide participating clinicians with the appropriate support for the first small test of change. All participating clinicians attended the educational sessions described above, and were instructed in the project's protocol and data collection tools. This aspect of first small test of change lasted 2 weeks.

The most important lesson learned (Study) during the first small test of change was that clinicians were not implementing the protocol according to design. The most frequent oversights were to forget to complete the QOL assessment on the first visit, and not documenting in the patient record as per the protocol. The project team members and clinicians met to discuss the first small test of change results and how to enhance the process for project implementation. Data collection methods were reviewed. The nurses' stated that the educational sessions were helpful in allowing them to "better assess pain," "educate the client about their pain medications," and "feel comfortable calling the physician" regarding changes to pain regimen. Yet, they needed more guidance on how to monitor protocol implementation and data collection.

The clinicians received additional education on implementation of a revised protocol to include filling out a monitoring sheet for each visit. The addition of the monitoring sheet, a *Nurse Tracking Tool for Small Test of Change* (Exhibit 26.8) prompted the clinician to answer 15 questions to ensure that the protocol was followed. This supplemented anecdotal logs that the project team member at the Brooklyn office maintained following meetings with participating clinicians.

PDSA Cycle Two

Once process issues from the first small test were addressed, the second test of change continued with the same seven patients and seven clinicians to ensure that there was now fidelity of process. Increased oversight and coaching was given by project team members, especially the clinical director of the LTHHP, to the direct care nurses involved in the project.

Project Outcomes

After the process was perfected in the second small test of change, initial patient outcomes were measured in a third small test to see if there was any indication that the new EBPI protocol was able to achieve project aims. After the process was perfected in the second small test of change, initial patient outcomes were measured in a third small test to see if there was any indication that the new EBPI protocol was able to achieve project aims.

Results showed that when pain was rated on a scale of 0–10, the mean pain rating decreased by 1.35 points from 3.85 prior to project implementation to a mean of 2.50 after the third small test of change, a reduction of 35%. This exceeded our target goal of 30% for this project with a very small sample, and thus showed promise for going forward with a larger project in LTHHP. Looking at the quality of life results, although the improvement was only 23% (mean initial score was 47/100 and the mean final score was 58/100) compared to our target goal of 50%, these results are promising enough to encourage implementation of the EBPI innovation on a larger scale. In addition to results related to our aim statement, an increase in the overall QOL score occurred in three of four patients, and an increase of 20 points was seen in two of four patients.

Results of process outcomes showed that patients on appropriate analgesic regimens were initially four out of seven versus the final count of seven out of seven or 100%. All final regimes were consistent with EBP guidelines. Nurses initiated contact with the MD about correcting inappropriate pain regimens in four out of five cases. All nurses now documented both clinical findings and pain problems. Following our second small test of change improvements to the documentation system were made including the incorporation of an assessment for the presence of pain as a required question for all patients at VNSNY.

Implications and Recommendations for Nursing Practice

On the basis of the results of this project the following implications for nursing practice were put forth. Nurses suggested that assessing the type of pain and including specific teaching about managing breakthrough pain be more clearly outlined in the *Pain Management Problem* on the patient electronic records.

Chronic pain and the complicated nature of its treatment require continuing education and updates on pain management to maintain clinical practice based on the best available evidence. Therefore, the Pain Management EBPI Project Team recommended that:

1. Consultative support for clinicians be made available in implementing this EBP throughout the Long-Term Care Division; and

2. Education on new analgesic medications be periodically scheduled to update clinicians on what they need to know to effectively communicate with primary care providers and develop the most effective plan of care for patients.

Plan for Dissemination

The last step in the EBPI process is dissemination of best practice, which is to begin spreading the innovation throughout the organization. First and foremost, the VNSNY administration supported the creation and delivery of recommended educational sessions throughout the organization. Pain Management classes were created and are delivered regularly by an advanced practice nurse and a staff member in Clinical Education to prepare interested VNSNY nurses for certification in pain management.

ACKNOWLEDGMENTS

The authors wish to acknowledge all the VNSNY staff who participated in the Renfield Evidence-Based Practice Improvement Fellows Program and the projects described herein. None of this work would have been possible without their interest in and championing of EBPI within their respective regions/divisions of the organization.

REFERENCES

AGREE Collaboration. (2001). *Appraisal of Guidelines for Research & Evaluation (AGREE) Instrument*. Retrieved from http://www.agreecollaboration.org

AGS Panel on Persistent Pain in Older Persons. (2002). The management of persistent pain in older persons. *Journal of the American Geriatric Society*, *50*(6 Suppl), 205–224.

American Pain Society (APS). (2002). *Pain in osteoarthritis, rheumatoid arthritis and juvenile chronic arthritis* (2nd ed.) Glenview, IL: American Pain Society (APS).

Bergman-Evans, B. (2006). Evidence-based guideline. Improving medication management for older adult clients. *Journal of Gerontology and Nursing*, *32*(7), 6–14.

Boaro, N., Fancott, C., Baker, R., Velji, K., & Andreoli, A. (2010). Using SBAR to improve communication in interprofessional rehabilitation teams. *Journal of Interprofessional Care*, *24*(1), 111–114.

Centers for Medicare & Medicaid Services. OASIS. (2007).Retrieved from http://www.cms.gov/oasis

Chou, R., Clark, E., & Helfand, M. (2003). Comparative efficacy and safety of long-acting oral opioids for chronic non-cancer pain: A systematic review. *Journal of Pain Symptom and Management, 26*(5), 1026–1048.

Devulder, J., Richarz, U., & Nataraja, S. H. (2005). Impact of long-term use of opioids on quality of life in patients with chronic, non-malignant pain. *Current Medical Research Opinion, 21*(10), 1555–1568.

Doerflinger, D. M. (2007). How to try this: The mini-cog. *American Journal of Nursing, 107*(12), 62–71.

EuroQol Group. (1990). EuroQol—A new facility for the measurement of health-related quality of life. Appendix J EQ-5D. *Health Policy, 16*, 199–2008.

Furlan, A. D., Sandoval, J. A., Mailis-Gagnon, A., & Tunks, E. (2006). Opioids for chronic noncancer pain: A meta-analysis of effectiveness and side effects. *Canadian Medical Association Journal, 174*(11), 1589–1594.

Gray, S. L., Mahoney, J. E., & Blough, D. K. (1999). Adverse drug events in elderly patients receiving home health services following hospital discharge. *Annals of Pharmacotherapy, 33*, 1147–1153.

Hamdy, R. C., Moore, S. W., Whalen, K., Donnelly, J. P., Compton, R., Testerman, F. et al. (1995). Reducing polypharmacy in extended care. *Southern Medical Journal, 88*(5), 534–538.

Heidrich, S. M., & Ryff, C. D. (1993). Physical and mental health in later life: The self-system as mediator. *Psychology and Aging, 8*(3), 327–338.

Howard, R. L., Avery, A. J., Slavenburg, S., Royal, S., Pipe, G., Lucassen, P. et al. (2006). Which drugs cause preventable readmissions to the hospital? A systematic review. *British Journal of Clinical Pharmacology, 63*(2), 136–147.

Institute for Clinical Systems Improvement. (2007, March). *Assessment and management of chronic pain* (2nd ed.). Retrieved from http://www.icsi.org/pain__chronic__assessment_and_management_of_14399/pain__chronic__assessment_and_management_of__guideline_.html

Kripalani, S., Yao, X., & Haynes, R. B. (2007). Interventions to enhance medication adherence in chronic medical conditions: A systematic review. *Archives of Internal Medicine, 167*(6), 540–550.

Langley, G. J., Nolan, K. M., Nolan, T. W., Norman, C. L., & Provost, L. P. (1996). *The improvement guide: A practical approach to enhancing organizational performance.* San Francisco: Jossey-Bass Publishers.

Leendertse, A. J., Egberts, A. C., Stoker, L. J., van den Bemt, P. M. HARM Study Group. (2008). Frequency of and risk factors for preventable medication-related hospital admissions in the Netherlands. *Archives of Internal Medicine, 168*(17), 1890–1896.

Levin, R. F., Keefer, J. M., Marren, J., Vetter, M., Lauder, B., & Sobolewski, S. (2010). Evidence-based practice improvement: Merging 2 paradigms. *Journal of Nursing Care Quality, 25*(2), 117–126.

Morisky, D. E., Green, L. W., & Levine, D. M. (1986). Concurrent and predictive validity of a self-reported measure of medication adherence. *Medical Care, 24*(1), 67–74.

Official U.S. Government Site for Medicare Home Health Compare. (2008). Retrieved from http://www.medicare.gov/homehealthcompare

Registered Nurses Association of Ontario. (2007). *Assessment and management of pain, supplement.* Retrieved from http://rnao.ca/sites/rnao-ca/files/Assessment_and_Management_of_Pain.pdf

Roter, D. L., Hall, J. A., Merisca, R., Nordstrom, B., Cretin, D., & Svarstad, B. (1998). Effectiveness of interventions to improve patient compliance: A meta-analysis. *Medical Care, 36*(8), 1138–1161.

Wiffen, P. J., McQuay, H. J., Edwards, J. E., & Moore, R. A. (2005). Gabapentin for acute and chronic pain. *Cochrane Database Systematic Review, (3),* CD005452. http://info.vnsny.org/sites/renfield/Phase%20III/Pain%20Management/Pain%20Protocol/Appendix%20J%20EQ%20-%205D%20REVISED[1].pdf

Part V

Strategies for Crafting Creative Collaborations for Evidence-Based Practice

The final set of chapters that form Part V move us outside of individual settings to look at ways to partner with other institutions. The first of these chapters is about how to set up an alliance, and includes very practical steps for moving forward this kind of initiative. For example, there is a section that focuses on how to engage key players in a statewide effort, as well as how to create a vision, mission, objectives, and structure. The second chapter in Part V moves us to a broader level and crosses state and national lines to establish global partnerships. By involving faculty and students in this initiative, project goals were met.

27

Establishing an EBP Alliance: Come Together Right Now

Ellen R. Rich and Patricia Lavin

Coming together is a beginning; keeping together is progress; working together is success.

—Henry Ford

An evidence-based practice (EBP) alliance provides the ability to harness the expertise of a broad range of clinicians, academics, nursing leaders, and students, freeing nurses from their institutional silos and preventing the need to "reinvent the wheel." An alliance is comprised of individuals working together to promote nursing research and the use of the best available evidence in order to assure the provision of excellent care. This chapter will outline the steps for creating an EBP alliance, including strategies, lessons learned, and examples of some alliance-based projects.

BENEFITS OF AN EBP ALLIANCE

The principal benefit of an EBP and research alliance is access to resources from the membership. Based on the conceptualization of these alliances as member exchanges, resources are generally free or available at reduced cost.

An EBP alliance unites institutions with various levels of expertise in EBP and nursing research. Those beginning on the path can be enriched by others that are further along by engaging in programs and initiatives that have been successful at the other institutions. For example, a quality improvement initiative that has lowered urinary tract infection rates at one hospital or home care agency may be attempted at another. The experience gained by the initial adopters can help guide those at the other institution(s). Such best-practice projects can be embraced at the regional level, providing even greater impact on patient care outcomes. Educational programs to promote EBP skills among bedside nurses or students may be shared among member institutions either in a face to face or electronic media format. Not having to design and offer basic educational coursework frees up local nursing educational manpower and can provide time to design more diverse offerings that can be coordinated between agencies. Additionally, the quality of access to library resources varies greatly between institutions. Online databases are quite costly and extensive access may be limited in smaller institutions. An alliance member or subcommittee with a special project that has limited library resources can ask a fellow member with more expansive library access to generate a literature search and supply electronic versions or articles. Conference and meeting space may be exchanged between alliance members. The alliance can pool resources to host a regional EBP/research conference.

Other helpful resources that can be shared are experience-based lessons, such as how to bring research projects to an IRB or even how to launch an IRB if one is not already in place. One institution may have poster-making equipment that can be made available to other members at reduced cost.

Member institutions that are more advanced in the pursuit of EBP and research can also benefit from a regional alliance. In addition to the benefits mentioned above, a regional alliance can provide access to research subjects beyond one's own setting, thus enhancing a project's sample size and power. Students from member academic institutions can participate in real-world EBP and research projects to fulfill their academic needs while providing needed assistance for nurses whose time for research and EBP is often limited due to day-to-day patient care responsibilities. Students at member academic institutions who are in need of subjects for master's or DNP projects or doctoral-level research may be able to obtain them from fellow alliance member agencies.

Perhaps the most valuable benefit of a regional alliance is access to a broad range of clinicians, researchers, academic faculty, and their students. Nurses at member agencies have expertise and in-depth knowledge that can be shared beyond the borders of their individual institutions, enriching larger numbers of colleagues.

For those on the Magnet journey, a regional alliance offers the opportunity to participate in a broader range of activities that can strengthen the evidence of the institution's readiness. For all, the outcomes of participation in an EBP/research alliance benefit the patients cared for and the students that we teach.

ESTABLISHING THE NEED AND GETTING STARTED

The first step in forming an EBP alliance is to assess what already exists in your region. Your work will be simple if an alliance has been developed in your area. A web or literature search using the key words "nursing research" or "evidence-based nursing practice," "alliance," "group," "council," "collaborative," or "consortium" may reveal the existence of an alliance in your area. You can follow the lead from there, contacting any existing groups and expanding your search as needed.

Once you have determined what groups have been formed you may need to define your geographic region. For example, if there is a nearby alliance that does not currently include your area, you can opt to inquire about the possibility of expanding that alliance to encompass your region. This decision will be based on geographic and population characteristics, with the goal of having sufficient potential member organizations within the region.

Another strategy is to check with your state nurses' association. In our case, the statewide nurses association had formed a research council that designed and promoted a statewide nursing research agenda. To operationalize this program, the organization supported the creation of regional alliances. At the time of our inquiry, there were three alliances in our state of which none were in our geographic area. Once we established our local need, we organized a conference call with leaders of the existing alliances in our state. This call provided us with helpful information about workable strategies and potential challenges. Take advantage of connecting with experienced alliance members, whether close by or in another area of the country, keeping in mind that there may be unique issues based on regional location.

IDENTIFYING AND INVOLVING CONSTITUENT GROUPS

Ideally, there will be a diversity of member organizations in your alliance to ensure a rich exchange of expertise. A combination of academic, hospital, home care, and community organizations provides an avenue for evaluation and implementation of best practices and nursing research projects across settings.

Once a need has been identified, it is helpful to enlist the support of a few colleagues who are enthused about the idea of a regional EBP and research alliance. This group can create talking points outlining the benefits of a research/EBP consortium to present at regional research and EBP conferences and at professional gatherings such as deans' councils, nurse executive groups, community and home care nursing forums, and honor society chapter meetings.

The American Nurses Credentialing Center's Magnet designation program provides motivation for organizational involvement in evidence-based nursing practice and research activities. Recruitment discussions should emphasize the opportunities for growth in these areas that might otherwise not be available to an individual institution.

You will likely find that organizations are at different levels in terms of research and EBP activities. When starting our alliance, we sent potential members a simple online survey to assess their organization's involvement in EBP and research. We found that some institutions had active EBP and research programs while other constituents completely lacked such structures. Marketing the alliance can be targeted to the institution's level of EBP and research mastery. Benefits for those with the least expertise are the clearest—they can be mentored by members of the more mature organizations. However, the opportunity for expansion of initiatives and research projects to multiple sites may be attractive to organizations that are further along in research and EBP activities.

ENGAGING THE KEY PLAYERS WITHIN ORGANIZATIONS

Once we identified a structure and process for our regional alliance we set out to find out if organizations within the region would be interested in participating. We identified potential members by utilizing our contact list from our state-wide organization of nurse executives and from our regional nurse educator's professional organization. A letter of inquiry was formulated seeking the level of interest among our regional health care organizations in participating in a regional alliance. The letter was sent to schools of nursing, home care agencies, community hospitals, and academic medical centers.

Once the letter was sent, a core group of nurses from various organizations committed to creating the regional alliance by participating in monthly meetings and sharing resources such as meeting space and time invested in regional initiatives. Members of this core group were driven by interest and commitment, and through word of mouth and continued electronic contact with organizational leaders, membership increased.

Members of the alliance are chief nursing officers, nurse researchers, nurse educators, nurse executives, clinical nurse specialists, advanced practice nurses, direct-care nurses, and faculty members from our regional schools of nursing. Individual nurses represent community hospitals, academic medical centers, home care agencies, and schools of nursing.

As the regional alliance continues to evolve, our intent is to have commitment to organizational participation. At this point in our history, our membership is based on interest as well as commitment from the chief nursing officer, who typically nominates either a nurse educator or the nurse researcher to participate. These representatives have access to clinical experts within their agencies when their expertise is needed for special projects. In addition some organizations have elected to have their direct care nurses as well as their clinical specialists participate in our clinical taskforces. The diversity of our membership helps to bring varying clinical and operational expertise to the table for program development and decision making.

COMING TOGETHER

Unless your region's geographic area is small, you will likely be faced with challenges related to face-to-face meetings. In-person meetings are optimal for building initial enthusiasm about an alliance, but over time attrition may result due to travel time and expense. Our alliance spans a high-density city and an expansive suburban area. Initially we alternated meeting sites to accommodate both location extremes, which resulted in attendance significantly higher for those nearest the meeting location and lower for those at a distance. Ultimately a virtual meeting format, which allowed both voice and online computer access proved to be much more accessible for members. One disadvantage is that social cues that are present during face-to-face meetings and team-building activities are missed. Often our membership meets face to face only during our annual conferences.

One organization does need to have access to a virtual meeting provider account that accommodates access by the appropriate number of potential members (some plans limit the number of participants). Some of your member organizations may already have access to virtual meeting applications, which your alliance can use without incurring additional expense.

Virtual meeting technology has not only facilitated general, subcommittee, and working group alliance meetings, but it has allowed members to hear presentations and engage with EBP experts from distant locations. As another modality, the online survey can easily be created to poll members about topics such as EBP and research priorities, changes to bylaws, future agenda items, and special projects. Additionally a listserv can connect your members and provide a forum for discussion and resource identification. Members can receive updated information and the alliance can market itself and any programs it offers through the creation and use of a website. With such a rich array of technological options you can find a combination that works best for your alliance members.

CREATING VISION, MISSION, OBJECTIVES, AND STRUCTURE FOR YOUR ALLIANCE

Once you have a core group of committed members you need to establish the guiding statements, goals, and structure for your alliance. The business literature is an excellent source of information on developing these. We gathered the core group of members in a face-to-face meeting and an experienced colleague moderated the brainstorming process.

A vision statement outlines what is possible for your alliance in the future and what you want to accomplish. The mission statement delineates how you wish to accomplish that vision. Objectives help divide the mission into attainable and measurable pieces. You may wish to craft a values statement as well. All of these components should be congruent, realistic, and reflective of the desires and capabilities of the membership.

The creation of bylaws and a committee structure will also need to be addressed. Bylaws should provide structure without being overly prescriptive. Again the business literature or resources related to parliamentary procedure will assist in bylaws development. Committees to be included will flow from the alliance's objectives. Smaller working groups are often most effective for special projects, especially when diverse and geographically separated institutions are the norm. The bylaws should allow for creation and dissolution of committees as needed.

FISCAL VIABILITY

The fiscal needs of an alliance are dependent upon the magnitude of its objectives. An alliance with a strong pool of volunteers can operate initially with little expense and later expand its breadth. Costs for items such as website development, conference venues, speakers, and meeting software should be anticipated when planning for funding. Some resources may be available through member organizations. For example, an alliance research conference may be co-sponsored by a member hospital, with the potential for free meeting space and covered speaker fees. Information technology or informatics students at a member academic institution may be able to facilitate website development and instruction for website maintenance.

Funding options may include a dues structure, grants, and possibly seed money from the state nurses association or another professional organization. If determining a dues structure, set one that will cover costs and provide some extra funds to avoid the need to raise dues in subsequent years. You will need to provide documentation describing benefits of membership to justify the request for dues.

An alliance can apply as a 501C3 organization to the IRS to be classified as a nonprofit and therefore exempt from federal taxes and possibly state corporate taxes. This status classifies your organization as a charitable one which has been established under the category of scientific or educational endeavors.

DO NOT REINVENT THE WHEEL

An EBP and research collaborative provides access to power in numbers and a variety of resources. The search for answers to clinical questions does not need to reside in one particular institution, but can be addressed more completely within a larger milieu. Alliance-wide special projects can be designed according to member needs and addressed from various angles based on the natures of the involved organizations. To illustrate this concept an example of such a project is described here.

Spurred by payment guidelines issued by the Center for Medicare and Medicaid Services, our alliance was surveyed and members chose to focus on the topic of pressure ulcer prevention. Objectives of the project were to (1) Ascertain the state of the science, (2) Identify national and/or professional organizational guidelines, (3) Appraise those guidelines, (4) Enumerate key evidence-based strategies to be included in organization policies and procedures, and (5) Review existing member organization policies and procedures related to pressure ulcer prevention for evidence documentation and inclusion of key strategies.

Alliance members who were interested in a Pressure Ulcer Taskforce volunteered to participate. Three wound care experts from member institutions were identified as clinical leaders for this project. As the topic of pressure ulcer prevention is broad, following a review of the literature taskforce members selected three important pressure ulcer prevention foci: nutrition, support surfaces, and turning and positioning. One of the clinical experts was identified for each of these areas, and workgroups were formed. Alliance members affiliated with the groups to create subcommittees representing their areas of interest and each group had an identified facilitator.

A partnership was forged with a faculty member from one of the alliance's academic institutions. Students taking her EBP and research course used the three pressure ulcer prevention foci as topics for required assignments. Groups of students selected one of the three areas and performed literature searches, critiqued the evidence, identified existing clinical guidelines, and evaluated them using a standard appraisal tool. Students' information was then shared with the clinical experts and members of each focus area, who then determined the best fit between the existing evidence and the clinical setting. The clinicians were then charged with assessing the transferability of elements of the evidence to the practice arena.

On the basis of evidence gained from the students' work, key strategies for pressure ulcer prevention were identified by the clinical experts for each of the three areas. The next step was to assess whether these strategies were included in member organizations' policies and procedures. Clinical institutional alliance members were asked to voluntarily submit their policy and procedure documents for pressure ulcer prevention to one facilitator. Once received, institution names were removed from the policy documents. A crosswalk table was created for each of the three areas, listing the key strategies in rows and the policy numbers in columns. Fifteen policy/procedure documents were received. Members of each subcommittee divided the policies and completed the crosswalk table, noting which strategies were included. Strategies for turning and positioning, nutrition and support surfaces, and crosswalk results were shared with alliance member institutions with the goal of inclusion of best practices at all participating institutions. This project illustrates outcomes that may be achieved through collaboration between clinical and academic partners facilitated by an EBP practice alliance.

DISSEMINATING OUTCOMES

For change to be implemented at the bedside, outcomes of research and EBP projects need to be disseminated both within and outside of the alliance. Several modalities can be employed for internal dissemination. PowerPoint presentations or executive summaries may be shared through e-mail or at virtual meetings. Members can then further disseminate the information to key personnel within their organizations. If an alliance website exists, outcome data may be housed there and shared with colleagues using links. An alliance e-newsletter can refer members to important data and documents.

An alliance research/EBP conference provides an arena to share outcomes with other members and external colleagues. Often individual health care agencies host their own conferences, which may lead to date conflicts, repetition of presentations, and diminished attendance. The involvement of multiple institutions in a larger conference can help prevent these issues.

Dissemination to a larger audience includes presentations at regional, national, and international conferences as well as publication. The expertise of faculty and nurse researchers from member institutions can be employed to help nurses develop abstracts, posters, and presentation materials. Other areas of expert assistance that can be tapped include coaching for scholarly presentations, editing, and writing for publication.

SUSTAINING INVOLVEMENT

As with many organizations, sustaining member involvement in a regional alliance can be challenging. Clinicians, administrators, and faculty generally have a heavy load of competing responsibilities. Alliance involvement is voluntary and may be seen as an add-on that could be viewed as dispensable when other demands become overwhelming.

Strategies for sustaining involvement include assuring that the work is divided in a way that is fair and manageable. The responsibilities of officers and board members should be clearly outlined and not over inclusive. Task-oriented workgroups with clearly defined goals and timelines make participation more attractive. Rotation of duties is also recommended and the work of committee members and officers recognized. Outcomes of projects and benefits of alliance membership should be emphasized on a regular basis to keep the positive accomplishments in view.

LESSONS LEARNED

It is important to initiate your alliance with a team of committed members. In our case, one visionary individual conceived of and implemented the alliance during the first years of its existence. Competing responsibilities had the potential to divert her energies from the group. Identify and assign roles or elect to offices early in the process.

It is to be expected that clinicians and faculty members may change work settings over time. It is helpful to ask organizational members to inform alliance leadership if they plan to leave their organization or assume a new role that precludes representation of their agency in the alliance. A request should be made for a new contact person within the agency. Since so much communication is virtual, it is imperative that electronic address lists be current and accurate.

Creating meeting structures that meet the needs of all levels of nurses and faculty is imperative. The schedule of meetings is made well in advance so our membership can manage their time and prioritize attendance at our meetings. The meetings were initially held weekly, on the same week day, at the same time. Agendas are sent out in advance and agenda items are requested. When the monthly meetings became a challenge for our membership, we transitioned to a quarterly schedule and manage any other issues that arise via e-mail communication.

Finally, communication within organizations is a perennial challenge. It important that alliance members who represent their institutions create mechanisms for communication to fellow nurses within their organizations. Outcomes of alliance work can be shared and clinical questions that are generated can be brought from the bedside to a diverse group with pooled resources.

28

Global Partnerships for EBP: Crossing State and National Boundaries

Rona F. Levin, Lillie M. Shortridge-Baggett, Susan W. Salmond, and Cheryl Holly

Coming together is a beginning; keeping together is progress; working together is success.

—Henry Ford

We often meet people in life at different junctures of time and place, thinking the encounters are coincidences; yet the meetings are really part of synchronistic plan that is destined (Redfield, 1993). This is the first of nine principles enumerated in the Celestine Prophecy, a novel about a journey that changes the perspectives and thus lives of its characters. One of the chapters focuses on how the meeting of characters in the novel had meaning beyond the initial encounters. And so this chapter is about how the authors' encounters in different circles led to an amazing partnership that benefited all concerned.

The story begins many years ago when one of the authors (Levin) worked as a dean in New Jersey where the current dean of the University of Medicine and Dentistry of New Jersey (UMDNJ) (Salmond) was a faculty member at Kean College and then head of that nursing program (encounter 1). Two of the authors (Levin and Shortridge-Baggett) originally met through the New York State Nurses Association when they served together on the Nursing Research Council of that organization and worked together on research and publications (encounter 2). Many years later they became faculty colleagues at Pace University, taught courses together, and served on the committee to develop Pace's DNP program (encounter 3). The fourth encounter, however brief, was a casual meeting at a New York hospital research conference where the fourth author (Holly) served as director of research (encounter 4). The next encounter occurred at an AACN Doctor of Nursing Practice Conference several years later where Levin and Holly had a brief conversation about UMDNJ having become a Joanna Briggs

Institute Collaborating Center, that Holly served as its director, and perhaps Pace and UMDNJ could work together (encounter 5). Shortridge-Baggett and Levin had been discussing how to establish a collaborating relationship with the Joanna Briggs Institute (JBI) and Pace University. One of the challenges to Pace's becoming a collaborating center was the resources necessary to meet the criteria for such status, for example, having to develop and publish a certain number of systematic reviews annually. Also, individuals who would become directors of the center needed to take JBI training courses for conducting systematic reviews. Given that the JBI was in Australia and, at the time, Levin and Shortridge-Baggett did not know that collaborating centers with trained faculty could also provide training, the option of Pace's developing a collaborating center did not seem to be an option without traveling to Australia for the training.

Also, at this time both UMDNJ and Pace University's Schools of Nursing were in the initial stages of implementing their DNP programs. A major focus of both institutions' DNP projects was on systematic reviews of evidence to guide nursing practice albeit each institution had different approaches. Levin shared with Shortridge-Baggett that UMDNJ was already a JBI Collaborating Center and that perhaps Pace could be an Evidence Synthesis Group of that Center and work with UMDNJ. We both agreed that this was the way to go and then began dialogue with Salmond and Holly about a partnership. The development, implementation, and initial outcomes of that partnership is the story that follows. But first we need to familiarize readers with JBI, its mission, and its organizational structure.

THE JOANNA BRIGGS INSTITUTE

The JBI was developed in 1996 in Adelaide, Australia, to promote evidence-based practice (EBP) to improve global health. Health professionals from over 40 countries collaborate to promote evidence synthesis and the translation, transfer, and utilization of knowledge for nursing practice (JBI, 2012). This work is guided by the JBI Model, which includes evidence generation, evidence synthesis, evidence/knowledge transfer, and evidence utilization (JBI, 2012; Pearson, 2010; Pearson, Wiechula, Court, & Lockwood, 2005). See Figure 28.1 for The JBI Model of Evidence-Based Health Care.

In the center of the model is EBP, which includes the actual evidence, the context or practice situation, client preference, and the clinical judgment of the health care professional. The overall goal of the Model is global health. To achieve this lofty goal, evidence upon which to base health

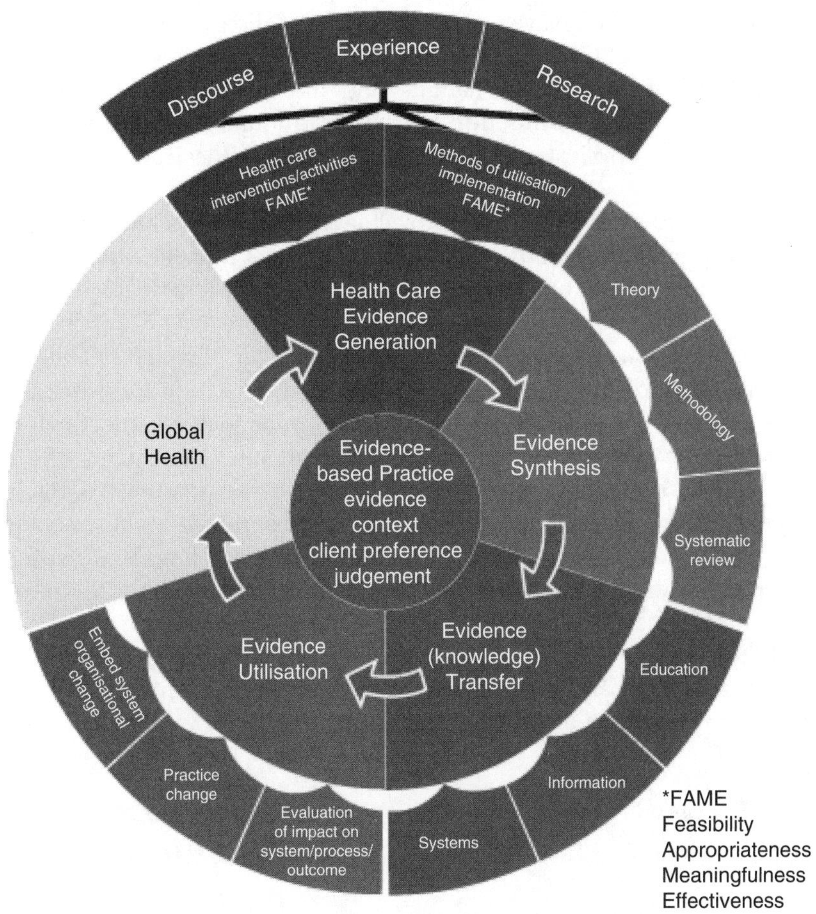

Source: http://www.joannabriggs.edu.au/About%20Us/JBI%20Approach. Reprinted with permission.

FIGURE 28.1 The JBI model of evidence-based health care.

care decisions needs to be generated. This evidence comes from discourse, experience, and research. The evidence is appraised using the FAME appraisal guide of feasibility, appropriateness, meaningfulness, and effectiveness.

The next critical step in the process of achieving the ultimate goal of improving health care is synthesizing the existing evidence, that is, conducting a systematic review on the focused clinical question of interest. The process of being trained to conduct systematic reviews is the focus of this chapter. Another important aspect of the model is evidence (knowledge) transfer. This is done via education and provision of information as well as assisting with system changes. The final part of the model is the actual utilization of the evidence. This includes evaluation of current practice, implementing practice changes, and then embedding the practice change in the care systems through organizational change. The careful and systematic application of this model is hypothesized to result in global health.

A major strategy that JBI uses to achieve the synthesis and dissemination of best evidence about global health issues is through collaborating and affiliating centers. One of these centers is the New Jersey Collaborating Center for Evidence-Based Practice located at the UMDNJ School of Nursing. The collaborating centers achieve their goals through establishing different network groups. These network groups include Evidence Synthesis Groups (ESGs), Evidence Appraisal Groups (EAGs), and Evidence Utilization Groups (EUGs). Extensive programs have been developed by JBI for each of these with software and training manuals. Ongoing support is provided to the centers by JBI. These supports include conventions, colloquia, publications, and regular communications. If you or your institution is not a current member, you can access the JBI website to obtain information on membership and all the ways you can participate. The JBI provides an opportunity to advance EBP through global collaboration of academic and practice institutions. The involvement can be for educational purposes or provision of care.

DEVELOPMENT OF A PARTNERSHIP

Initial meetings at Pace University focused on garnering support from stakeholders for the partnership. These stakeholders included the director of the DNP Program, the DNP faculty, and key administrators in the Lienhard School of Nursing. Important to these discussions was a cost analysis of the different participation levels in the JBI. A partnership between Pace University's LSN and the UMDNJ Collaborating Center with Pace becoming an Evidence Synthesis Group (ESG) was a much less expensive option than the LSN becoming a JBI Collaborating Center on its own. In addition it would provide an opportunity for Pace's LSN group to become more expert in carrying out systematic reviews and then determining if it wanted to commit further resources toward becoming a full center. Becoming an ESG, however, would entail naming a director (released time at least), providing staff support, and developing faculty and students to gain skill in conducting systematic reviews at the very least. We received administrative support and a promise of resources to provide for DNP faculty training in conducting systematic reviews of evidence.

An additional requirement of becoming an Evidence Synthesis Group besides naming a director was having at least two people complete the JBI Training Program for conducting systematic reviews. This training program included an introduction to JBI, their software package designed to assist health and other researchers and practitioners to conduct systematic reviews with evidence, and the software of quantitative, qualitative, economic, and narrative data (see Exhibit 28.1 for a list of necessary training sessions). Levin and Shortridge-Baggett worked on the initial application and realized they needed to discuss the provision of training with UMDNJ. Since UMDNJ was a Collaborating Center, they were certified

EXHIBIT 28.1 THE JOANNA BRIGGS TRAINING PROGRAM FOR COMPREHENSIVE SYSTEMATIC REVIEW

The comprehensive systematic review training include an introduction to JBI and Comprehensive Systematic Review using SUMARI, a software package designed to assist health and other researchers and practitioners to conduct systematic reviews with evidence. There are five modules covering the different software programs for different types of evidence.

Module 1: RevMan (Review Manager)—Used for preparing and maintaining Cochrane reviews.

Module 2: JBI-MAStARI (Meta-Analysis of Statistics, Assessment and Review Instrument)—Designed to manage, appraises, extract, and analyze quantitative data as part of a systematic review of evidence.

Module 3: JBI-QARI (Qualitative Assessment and Review Instrument)—Designed to manage, appraise, extract, and synthesize qualitative data as part of a systematic review of evidence.

Module 4: JBI-ACTUARI (Analysis of Cost, Technology, and Utilization and Review Instrument)—Designed to manage, appraise, extract, and analyze economic data as part of a systematic review of evidence.

Module 5: Module is JBI-NOTARI (Narrative, Opinion, Text Assessment, and Review Instrument)—Designed to manage, appraise, extract, and synthesize data as part of a systematic review of evidence arising out of expert opinion texts and reports.

Source: http://www.joannabriggs.edu.au/Appraise%20Evidence/JBI%20SUMARI%20(systematic%20review%20software)%20FREE as trainers. The next step was to negotiate training for Pace faculty by UMDNJ certified JBI trainers. This could be a win-win partnership for all concerned.

One of the goals of the Pace faculty were to be certified by JBI, which would permit them to be able to conduct and publish systematic reviews. This required at least a 5-day training program including the introduction to JBI, its management software, and three of its analytical software programs: JBI-MAStARI, which is for quantitative studies; JBI-QARI, which is for qualitative studies; and, RevMan, which is the Cochrane software used for quantitative studies. This training can cost around $1,500 per person. Part of the negotiations between Pace and UMDNJ was to have the training sessions spread over time rather than one intensive program and to have the Pace faculty take the training courses at UMDNJ with the faculty and students at UMDNJ and their clinical partners who were already scheduled to take the course modules. This permitted all program participants to meet and interact with each other and to have a lower cost for the program.

IMPLEMENTATION OF A PARTNERSHIP

Important to note here is that students in Pace's DNP Program were required to develop a clinical EBP project for their capstone (see description of this program in Chapter 22). This necessarily would entail a systematic review of evidence on their clinical question. After further discussion with the DNP Program director and faculty of the DNP Program at Pace, a decision was made to include those LSN faculty who were guiding students' EBP projects in the systematic review training. Additionally, DNP faculty agreed that the Pace DNP students should also be exposed to at least the first two training sessions in order to gain skill in that aspect of their project development.

The timing of the partnership agreement was perfect; that is, the faculty would receive training in the systematic review modules in the spring of 2010 in time to work with their first cohort of DNP students on the systematic reviews of evidence for their projects in the summer of 2010. Students would receive preliminary training on one module in June of 2010 and would at least gain familiarity with the JBI approach to conducting these reviews and gain initial skill in using the software to be used for developing the reviews. The module selected for the students to learn was JBI-MAStARI, which is designed to manage, appraise, extract, and analyze quantitative data as part of a systematic review of evidence. The focused clinical questions the students were asking were best answered by review of quantitative research data.

Because of the academic collaboration and potential JBI partnership, UMDNJ offered Pace discounted rates for faculty attendance at the training sessions. In addition, faculty brought one student representative from the first DNP cohort and one librarian to experience this process and receive all training sessions. The student, a graduate assistant, could then assist faculty with the training sessions to be held for all other Cohort 1 students in June. Having the faculty, student, and librarian assist the students in conducting their systematic reviews was very valuable. Having an ongoing relationship with UMDNJ's Collaborating Center was important too during this learning process. Moreover, UMDNJ faculty trainers reviewed systematic protocols of some Pace DNP student groups prior to submitting to JBI for review. This was extremely helpful as the UMDNJ faculty/students had already completed several JBI systematic reviews. Other ways that UMDNJ faculty facilitated Pace's DNP students' work was to provide answers to, for example, software questions, and with whom to communicate at JBI for assistance.

OUTCOMES OF A PARTNERSHIP

This global partnership has resulted in several successful outcomes. The initial goal of providing training for faculty and staff in the conduct of comprehensive systematic reviews was achieved. Four faculty members, one librarian, and one graduate assistant completed the training. An additional faculty member received the training this past summer. One of these faculty was able to then complete the Train-the-Trainer Program held proceeding the seventh Joanna Briggs Institute International Colloquium, Chicago, Illinois, in the fall of 2010. Faculty from both UMDNJ and Pace University presented a symposium on the value of academic and clinical partnerships for advancing global health at the first JBI Colloquium held in North America (Shortridge, Salmond, Holly, Singleton, & Levin, 2010). Some faculty presented a symposium at the Eastern Nursing Research Society (ENRS) on A Primer in the Systematic Review: A Presentation of the Systematic Review/Knowledge Translation Research Interest Group (Holly et al., 2012).

Five Pace DNP student teams were successful in conducting and publishing their systematic reviews as part of their doctoral studies. The training process has been continued for subsequent Pace University DNP cohorts with Cohort 2 publishing their systematic review protocols and just completing their systematic reviews as this chapter is written. There are now systematic reviews being planned in which faculty from the two Schools of Nursing and clinical partners will be coauthors. This is an important accomplishment.

CONCLUSION

Academic and clinical partnerships are important for many reasons, including the ability to share resources. Their value in advancing EBP, too, has been discussed here, especially in training for and conducting systematic reviews of evidence to guide clinical practice. Having this synthesis of the research evidence is critical for provision of the best available health care. No longer can we conduct a literature review and feel comfortable changing practice based on a nonsystematic review evidence. Not all evidence is created equal. Likewise doctoral students cannot feel comfortable that they have identified a gap in knowledge for which research should be conducted if they have not done a systematic review of the evidence on their question.

Through this global collaboration goals for faculty and student training at Pace and for building capacity at UMDNJ were achieved. The collaboration permitted the Pace students to be mentored successfully on their clinical projects and conduct and publish their systematic reviews. These have been shared with Pace's clinical agency partners to provide evidence and recommendations for their ongoing practice improvements. For UMDNJ the partnership facilitated its goal of building capacity and infrastructure for the conduct of systematic reviews to advance nursing science and, ultimately, to improve patient care.

ACKNOWLEDGMENTS

We wish to acknowledge the JBI, especially Alan Pearson, AM, professor of Evidence Based Healthcare and executive director, the JBI, located at the Faculty of Health Sciences, the University of Adelaide, South Australia, for the excellent resources of JBI and ongoing support for facilitating EBP globally.

We also want to thank the faculty, staff, students, and clinical partners at UMDNJ and Pace University who have participated in the partnership. We also want to thank the administration of both schools of nursing for their support of this partnership.

REFERENCES

Holly, C. (2010). Systematic reviews as a capstone project. Presentation at building academic and practice partnerships for evidence-based practice. *7th Joanna Briggs Institute International Colloquium*, Chicago, IL, USA, September 13–15, 2010.

Holly, C., Salmond, S. W., Shortridge-Baggett, L. M., Worral, P., Singleton, J. K., & Slyer, J. T. (2012). A primer in the systematic review: A presentation of the systematic review/knowledge translation research interest group. *Symposium at the 24th Eastern Nursing Research Society*, New Haven, CT, March 28–30, 2012.

Joanna Briggs Institute. (2012). *Joanna Briggs collaboration*. Retrieved from http://www.joannabriggs.edu.au

Pearson, A. (2010). The Joanna Briggs Institute model of evidence-based health care as a framework for implementing evidence. In J. Rycroft-Malone & T. Bucknall (Eds.), *Models and frameworks for implementing evidence-based practice: Linking evidence to action* (pp. 185–205). NJ: Wiley-Blackwell.

Pearson, A., Wiechula, R., Court, A., & Lockwood, C. (2005). The JBI model of evidence-based health care. *International Journal of Evidence Based Healthcare, 3*, 207–215.

Redfield, J. (1993). *Celestine prophecy*. MA: Wheeler.

Shortridge-Baggett, L. M., Salmond, S. W., Holly, C., Singleton, J. K., & Levin, R. F. (2010). Building academic and practice partnerships for evidence-based practice. *Symposium at* 7th *Joanna Briggs Institute International Colloquium*, Chicago, IL, USA, September 13–15, 2010.

GLOSSARY[1]

Audit and Feedback Audit and feedback is monitoring of critical indicators of practice (e.g., meperidine use) and providing the data/information back to those responsible for patient care (Davis, Thomson, Oxman, & Haynes, 1995; Oxman, Thomson, Davis, & Haynes, 1995; Schoenbaum et al., 1995). Audit and feedback is an ongoing process that is done periodically (e.g., every 3 months) during the implementation, evaluation, and sustainability phases of translating evidence into practice. Feedback reports can use data aggregated at different levels, such as the individual provider, patient care unit, service line, organization, or health system. It is helpful to provide data that compares indicators over time to demonstrate improvements (or lack thereof) in the evidence-based practices (Jamtvedt, Young, Kristoffersen, Thomson O'Brien, & Oxman, 2004).

Bayes Theorem Bayes Theorem is used to estimate the probability of a particular condition in a group of people with specific characteristics to the likelihood of that condition occurring; post-test odds = pre-test odds × likeliness ratio.

Change Champions Practitioners from the local peer group who continually promote evidence-based practice (EBP). They impart information about the EBP, encourage peers to align their practice with the evidence, demonstrate skills and knowledge necessary to carry out the EBP, and teach new and existing personnel about the EBP (Titler & Everett, 2001).

Clinical Practice Guideline A systematically developed statement designed to assist the practitioner and patient make decisions about appropriate health care for specific clinical circumstances (NHS Research and Development: Centre for Evidence-Based Medicine [NHS], 2001).

[1] *Note:* Contributed, in part, by Marita Titler, PhD, RN, FAAN.

Clinical Significance A judgment about the interpretation of the statistical results (that the difference or relationship has meaning for patient care) (Mateo & Kirchhoff, 1999).

Confidence Interval (CI) Quantifies the uncertainty in measurement. It is usually reported as a 95% CI, which is the range of values within which we can be 95% sure that the true value of an effect for a whole population lies within a range. For example, for a number needed to treat (NNT) of 10 with a 95% CI of 5 to 15, we would have 95% confidence that the true NNT value lies between 5 and 15 (Mount Sinai Hospital-University Health Network: Centre for Evidence-Based Medicine, 2001).

Cost-Effectiveness Analysis Converts effects into health terms and describes the costs for some additional health gain (e.g., cost per additional MI prevented) (NHS, 2001).

Effect Size A statistic that indicates the efficacy of a treatment or intervention. For example, when a study employs a correlational analysis, the correlation coefficient is informative of the effect size. When employing a *t* test, Cohen's *d* (a derivative of standardized and unstandardized mean differences) is the pertinent index of effect size. Other statistics used to determine an effect for dichotomous variables are relative risk and odds ratio (see definitions below).

Effectiveness Effectiveness is determining if an intervention or treatment works in the real world without controls of an efficacy study.

Efficacy Efficacy describes research that is designed to test interventions under tightly controlled conditions (e.g., dedicated person to deliver the intervention in a controlled clinical setting) with a homogenous patient population (e.g., women 65 to 80 years of age with osteoporosis). Efficacy studies are done prior to application of the intervention in the real world (Brown, 2002).

Evidence-Based Guideline A written guide of evidence-based health care practices/actions. The recommendations for practice should be referenced and identify the strength of the evidence for each of the practice recommendations. Component parts of evidence-based guidelines vary but usually include a brief description of the practice topic (e.g., acute pain), the types of patients for whom the guideline can be used (e.g., elders, hospitalized elders, children, or adults), the assessment and interventions used to carry out the EBPs and the risk/benefits of the EBP.

Forest Plot A graphic representation of effects of individual studies included in a meta-analysis as well as the overall effect across those studies, providing a visual display of heterogeneity as well as whether the overall effect favors the experimental or control condition.

Macrosystem This term is used interchangeably with organizational context to convey the organization or health system "at large" in which the EBP is being implemented. Macrosystems are composed of multiple microsystems.

Meta-analysis An overview that uses quantitative methods to summarize results *or* a mathematical summary of results of several studies (Mateo & Kirchhoff, 1999; NHS, 2001).

Meta-synthesis A method of summarizing qualitative findings so that they may be viewed in a larger interpretive context and presented in an accessible and usable form for practicing nurses (Sandelowski, Docherty, & Emden, 1997).

Microsystem Microsystem is used to convey the patient care unit(s), ambulatory clinic(s), or other specific patient-care areas within the macrosystem in which the EBP is implemented. For example, an EBP on acute pain management may be first implemented in two or three patient care units or microsystems prior to being "rolled out" across the entire organization or macrosystem. Microsystems are composed of the unit culture, leadership, nature of the personnel, manner in which people in the unit relate to one another in delivery of services/ patient care, and routine monitoring of performance within the specified patient care unit.

Number Needed to Treat (NNT) The number of patients who need to be treated to prevent one bad outcome. It is the inverse of the absolute relative risk (ARR): NNT = 1/ ARR (NHS, 2001).

Odds Ratio An effect size statistic that compares two groups in terms of the relative odds of a status of an event (e.g., death, illness, successful outcome, receipt of treatment, gender, or exposure to a toxin). The dependent variables are inherently dichotomous (e.g., good outcome or bad outcome).

Opinion Leaders Opinion leaders are informal leaders from the local health care setting who are viewed as important and respected sources of influence among their peer group (e.g., nurses, physicians). A key characteristic of opinion leaders is that they are trusted to evaluate new information in the context of group norms. Opinion leaders are evaluators who are trusted to judge the fit between a technology or new practice and the local situation (Titler & Everett, 2001).

Organizational Context The organizational context is the health system environment in which the proposed EBP is to be implemented. This may be an acute care, home health care, or long-term-care system. The core elements that help describe the organizational context include the prevailing culture of the system (e.g., patient centered); the nature of human relationships in the system including the leadership styles that are operational (e.g., team work; clear role delineation); and the organization's approach to routine monitoring of performance of systems and services within the organization (e.g., routine use of audit and feedback) (Kitson, Harvey, & McCormack, 1998).

Outcomes Effectiveness The ability of an intervention or care processes to produce (or fail to produce) desired outcomes (e.g., decreased pain intensity, decreased length of stay) in the typical practice environment with a variety of patients, many of whom have other factors that may affect the amount of benefit or outcome of the intervention (Brown, 2002). This often is used to denote the application of an intervention in the real world of practice. Evaluation of an EBP project is a type of outcome effectiveness. Evaluation of an EBP is important to determine (1) if the intervention can be used successfully in day-to-day practice and (2) if application of interventions in the real world of practice results in outcomes similar to those achieved in efficacy studies of the intervention.

Outcome Evaluation A quality improvement technique that monitors outcomes, usually of patients, to determine if the outcomes from application of the EBP are similar to those intended, such as a decrease in pain intensity scores. Staff and fiscal outcomes also might be used in outcomes evaluation.

Outreach/Academic Detailing Outreach and academic detailing are terms often used synonymously to convey the use of a trained individual who meets one-on-one with practitioners in their setting to provide information about the EBP. Information conveyed during outreach may include data on provider performance, information about the EBP, and consultation regarding specific issues in use of the EBP. Studies have demonstrated that outreach visits alone or used in combination with other translation interventions result in positive changes in practice behaviors of nurses and physicians (Titler, 2002).

Performance Gap Assessment Performance gap assessment is baseline evaluation of practice performance that informs members of an organization about a particular practice, and opportunities for improving performance related to a specific indicator (e.g., frequency of acute-pain assessment) or set of indicators (e.g., acute-pain management of hospitalized elders) (Oxman et al., 1995; Schoenbaum et al., 1995). This is a data-driven strategy/intervention used early in the implementation phase of translating evidence into practice to convey to individuals the congruency or incongruency between their current clinical practice and recommended practices from evidence-based guidelines, EBP reports, or systematic reviews.

Point Estimation A mean of a sample is only a guess of the true population mean. As such, it has a degree of error associated with using it, because we are only using a fraction of the elements of the population in deriving it. So if we were to calculate the mean of a sample and the answer was 35, we would say that our best guess of the population mean is 35, but realize that it probably is slightly higher or lower than 35. This guess is called a point estimation.

Process Evaluation Process evaluation is a quality improvement technique that monitors specific indicators directly related to the EBP. Monitoring nurses' use of a standard pain intensity scale for pain assessment is a type of process monitor to determine if nurses' processes of acute-pain management are aligned with the evidence on this topic. Process evaluation is usually undertaken to determine if the EBP is being used and implemented consistently by care providers.

Protocol "A detailed plan of scientific or medical experiment, treatment, or procedure" (*Merriam-Webster*, 1996, p. 939). A protocol may be even more specific than a guideline, as it is not only disease focused but can be tailored to a specific population and practice situation.

Randomized Controlled Clinical Trial A group of patients is randomized into an experimental group and a control group. These groups are followed up for the variables/outcomes of interest (NHS, 2001).

Reference or Gold Standard Diagnostic Test This is the most accurate diagnostic test possible for determining the presence of a disease or condition.

Relative Risk Ratio The relative risk ratio or index is just the opposite of the odds ratio. This index relates to the probability of risk (or lack of success) to that of success. Therefore, the ideal value of this index is less than 1. In other words, we want the probability of failure (the numerator) to be less than the probability of success (the denominator). Therefore, we want a very small fraction of less than 1.

Strength of Evidence This is an overall grade of the strength of evidence on a specific topic. Although various grading schemas are used, practice recommendations are usually graded using A, B, C, and so forth, with A being consistent findings from several randomized clinical trials and D or E grades used to convey conflicting research results, and/or use of expert opinion, case reports, or consensus (Agency for Healthcare Research and Quality [AHRQ], 2002).

Surrogate Diagnostic Tests Surrogate diagnostic tests are an alternative diagnostic test used because the reference standard test incurs an increased cost or risk to the patient, or is not available.

Sustainability Sustainability is the ability of an organization or individual to continue the use of EBP in routine clinical care following initial implementation.

Systematic Reviews Systematic reviews are a summary of past research on a topic of interest. The summary is arrived at through a rigorous scientific process similar to methods used in primary research. The scientific process used in systematic reviews includes: the review question(s), how studies will be located, the methods used for critical appraisal of the primary studies, criteria for inclusion and exclusion of studies, synthesis methods (e.g., meta-analysis, narrative summary across studies), and summary recommendations for practice and future research. The final product is a summary of the best available scientific evidence following application of the aforementioned process (AHRQ, 2002; Joanna Briggs Institute, 2000, 2001).

Translation Research Translation research is the scientific investigation of methods and variables that influence rate and extent of adoption of EBP by individuals and organizations to improve clinical and operational decision making in the delivery of health care services. This includes testing the effect of strategies and interventions for promoting the adoption of EBP, with the outcomes being the rate and extent of health care providers' use of these practices. (Titler & Everett, 2001).

REFERENCES

Agency for Healthcare Research and Quality. (2002). *Systems to rate the strength of scientific evidence. Summary*. Bethesda, MD: U.S. Department of Health and Human Services. Agency for Healthcare Research and Quality, Evidence Report/Technology Assessment Report Number 47, Publication No. 02-E015.

Brown, S. J. (2002). Focus on research methods. Nursing intervention studies: A descriptive analysis of issues important to clinicians. *Research in Nursing and Health, 25*, 317–327.

Davis, D. A., Thomson, M. A., Oxman, A. D., & Haynes, R. B. (1995). Changing physician performance: A systematic review of the effect of continuing medical education strategies. *Journal of the American Medical Association, 274*(9), 700–705.

Jamtvedt, G., Young, J. M., Kristoffersen, D. T., Thomson O'Brien, M. A., & Oxman, A. D. (2004). Audit and feedback: Effects on professional practice and health care outcomes (Cochrane Review). *Cochrane Library, Issue 1*, Chichester, UK: Wiley.

Joanna Briggs Institute. (2000). Appraising systematic review. *Changing Practice, 1*(1).

Joanna Briggs Institute. (2001). An introduction to systematic reviews. *Changing Practice, 2*(1).

Kitson, A., Harvey, G., & McCormack, B. (1998). Enabling the implementation of evidence based practice: A conceptual framework. *Quality in Health Care, 7*(3), 149–158.

Mateo, M. A., & Kirchhoff, K. T. (1999). *Conducting and using nursing research in the clinical setting* (2nd ed.). Philadelphia: Saunders.

Merriam-Webster's collegiate dictionary (10th ed.). (1996). Springfield, MA: Merriam-Webster.

Mount Sinai Hospital-University Health Network: Centre for Evidence-Based Medicine. (2001). Retrieved from http://www.library.utoronto.ca/medicine/ebm/glossary/NHS Research and Development: Centre for Evidence Based Medicine, 2001.

Oxman, A. D., Thomson, M. A., Davis, D. A., & Haynes, R. B. (1995). No magic bullets: A systematic review of 102 trials of interventions to improve professional practice. *Canadian Medical Association Journal, 153*, 1423–1431.

Sandelowski, M., Docherty, S., & Emden, C. (1997). Qualitative metasynthesis: Issues and techniques. *Research in Nursing and Health, 20*, 365–371.

Schoenbaum, S. C., Sundwall, D. N., Bergman, D., Buckle, J. M., Chernov, A., George, J. et al. (1995). *Using clinical practice guidelines to evaluate quality of care: Vol. 2. Methods*. Rockville, MD: U.S. Department of Health and Human Services, Public Health Service, Agency for Health Care Policy and Research.

Titler, M. G. (2002). Developing an EBP. In G. LoBiondo-Wood, & J. Haber (Eds.), *Nursing research* (5th ed.). St. Louis, MO: Mosby-Year Book.

Titler, M. G., & Everett, L. Q. (2001). Translating research into practice: Considerations for critical care investigators. *Critical Care Nursing Clinics of North America, 13*, 587–604.

Annotated Bibliography

Paule V. Joseph

Brown, C., Kim, S. C., Stichler, J., & Fields, W. (October, 2009). Predictors of knowledge, attitudes, use and future use of evidence-based practice among baccalaureate nursing students at two universities. *Nurse Education Today, 30,* 521–527.

A cross-sectional survey design was used to study a group of more than 400 students of baccalaureate programs from two different universities to identify predictors of knowledge, attitudes, and current and future use of EBP. The authors concluded that confidence in clinical decision making and preparedness for clinical practice can be predicted by knowledge and attitudes of students about the current and future use of EBP.

Butler, K. D. (2011). Nurse practitioners and evidence-based nursing practice. *Clinical Scholars Review, 4*(1), 53–57.

The author presents a study in which nurse practitioners' (NPs) beliefs and attitudes about evidence-based nursing practice (EBNP) and its implementation were assessed. Five research questions were developed to direct the study and an explanatory descriptive model to attain stated goals. The demographics of the participants were also assessed. The Evidence-Based Practice Beliefs and the Evidence-Based Practice Implementation Scale were used to collect data. The author concluded that NPs who worked in urban settings tended to use EBNP more than those who worked in rural or suburban areas. Although NPs had mainly positive beliefs and attitudes about EBNP, results indicated that NPs were inconsistent in the implementation of EBNP in the clinical setting.

Christie, J., Hamill, C., & Power, J. (2012, March). How can we maximize nursing students' learning about research evidence and utilization in undergraduate, preregistration programmes? A discussion paper. *Journal of Advanced Nursing*. Article first published online: 30 MAR 2012 DOI: 10.1111/j.1365-2648.2012.05994.x. pp. 1–13.

Christie, Hamill, and Powers discussed how to capitalize on nursing students' learning of research for use in practice. The authors highlight the importance of nursing research and its application as evidence-based nursing. They argue that understanding and engagement of nursing students in the research process is essential. By learning the research utilization process, nursing students learn how to value the importance and utility of nursing research. The authors conclude that in order to maximize students' learning of nursing research and its utilization, it must be embedded throughout the curriculum.

Cronje, R., & Moch, S. (2010). Part III. Reenvisioning undergraduate nursing students as opinion leaders to diffuse evidence-based practice in clinical settings. *Journal of Professional Nursing*. *26*, 23–28.

The authors looked at the application of Rogers's Theory of Innovation and Social Learning in promoting EBP for nursing students and practicing nurses. One of Rogers's hypotheses is that innovations are accomplished at the grassroots level. Including nursing students from early on in their academic career is contrary to the top-down approach that is used in many institutions to promote EBP. The author concluded that it is imperative for both nursing administrators and educators to empower students and nurses at the grassroots levels to promote practice change using an EBP approach.

Kenny, D., Richard, M., Ceniceros, X., & Blaize, K. (January– February, 2010). Collaborating across services to advance evidence-based nursing practice. *Journal of Nursing Research*, *59*(1S), S1–S21.

The project described in this article was part of the TriService Nursing Research Program (TSNRP) grant to develop an evidence-based program for injured soldiers. The Navy Medical Center and Army Medical Center served as primary sites for the project. Seminars were provided to active military nurses about developing and implementing EBP. The authors highlight some of the barriers and facilitators of this military-based project. Despite the challenges outlined by the authors, the EPB project was successful and attained the goal of creating three evidence-based guidelines.

Krainovich-Miller, B., Haber, J., Yost, J., & Jacobs, S. K. (April, 2009). Evidence-based practice challenge: Teaching critical appraisal of systematic reviews and clinical practice guidelines to graduate students. *Journal of Nursing Education*, *48*(4), 186–195.

The authors discuss the TREAD EBP model. TREAD is a tool for faculty to use in graduate courses. The model emphasizes the use of appraisal tools that facilitate rapid appraisal of systematic reviews. The article addresses challenges faced by nurse educators in modeling a new paradigm shift to graduate students. They concluded that the TREAD EBP model supports the importance of teaching using appraisal guidelines that are specific to this type of evidence.

Kruszewski, A., Brough, E., & Killeen, M. (June, 2009). Collaborative strategies for teaching evidence-based practice in accelerated second-degree programs. *Journal of Nursing Education, 48*(6), 340–342.

The authors addressed the challenges found in teaching accelerated second-degree students, especially in the short period of time in which their education is delivered. The article described the implementation of a curriculum redesign to meet those challenges. The program was shortened from a 19-month to 12-month format. In both the new and redesigned curricula, educators identified learning activities that enable students to participate in EBP, taking into consideration the diverse backgrounds of the specific populations. Collaborative teaching strategies were found to help students achieve EBP and translate it to practice.

McConnel, E., Lekan, D., Bunn, M., Egerton, E., Corazzini, K., Hendrix, C., & Bailey D. (2009) Teaching evidence-based nursing practice in geriatric care settings: The geriatric nursing innovations through education institute. *The Journal of Gerontological Nursing, 35*(4), 26–35.

The article highlights the gaps found in the educational preparation of nurses and the application of evidence-based care for older adults. The author explains the partnership created between the faculties at the Duke University School of Nursing and key stakeholders throughout North Carolina to develop an intensive continuing education (CE) series known as the Geriatric Nursing Innovations through Education (CNIE) Institute. The institute provides nurses with the most current scientific approaches to manage clinical syndromes experienced by the elderly population as well as the leadership skills needed to effectively care for residents with complex needs. The author acknowledges that outcomes at the individual patient level were not addressed; therefore, no data were gathered to support Improvement of patient outcomes. The authors concluded that the GNIE Institute represents a practical CE model for building RNs' capacity to implement evidence-based approaches in the care of the geriatric population.

McCurry, M., & Martins, D. (2010). Teaching undergraduate nursing research: A comparison of traditional and innovative approaches for success with millennial learners. *Journal of Nursing Education, 49*(5), 276–279.

The authors compare traditional methods and new approaches to teach undergraduate nursing research to the millennial nursing generation. The study was based on the needs of millennial learners or, "Y" generation, Echo Boomers, the Nintendo generation, or the digital generation (Raines,

2002). Previously investigated learning preferences of the millennial students were taken into consideration when revamping the syllabi for the research course. During the study, a Likert scale was used for students to identify the effectiveness of both the innovative assignments and traditional ones. The authors concluded that by combining new and traditional assignments millennial students were able to articulate the importance of evidence-based nursing practice. The authors defined traditional methods as using textbooks, didactic lectures with or without PowerPoint slides, and students' critique of published studies. On the other hand, the authors referred to innovative methods the inclusion of technology, in-class demonstration, and experiential project and team assignments.

Melnyk, B. M., Fineout-Overholt, E., Feinstein, N. F., Sadler, L., & Green-Hernandez, C. (January–February, 2008). Nurse Practitioner Educators' perceived knowledge, beliefs, and teaching strategies regarding evidence-based practice: Implications for accelerating the integration of evidence-based practice into graduate programs. *Journal of Professional Nursing, 24*(1), 7–13.

A descriptive survey was conducted with a sample of 79 nurse practitioner educators who were members of the Association of Faculties of Pediatric Nurse Practitioners (AFPNP) and the National Organization of Nurse Practitioners Faculties (NONPF). The survey used was guided by Prochaska and Velicer's Transtherotical Model of Organizational Change and Carver and Scheier's Control Theory. The authors also provided a list of books that faculty can use to both teach and learn EBP, and be part of national/international workshops that offer intensive training on how to implement and teach EBP. The authors concluded that the hypotheses tested were supported in that knowledge of EBP was correlated with EBP beliefs, comfort of educators teaching EBP, and whether their practices were evidence based. The authors also acknowledge the limitations of the study based on the survey response rate.

Moch, S., & Cronje, R. (January–February, 2010). Part II. Empowering grassroots evidence-based practice: A curricular model to foster undergraduate student-enabled practice change. *Journal of Professional Nursing, 26*, 14–22.

This article illustrates curriculum changes that have been successful in promoting EBP between nursing students and practicing nurses. The authors proposed an integrated curricular system called "Student-Enabled Practice Change Curricular Model." Within this curriculum, nursing students are leaders of new knowledge discussion groups that involve partnering with practicing nurses to gather evidence that informs their practice and facilitates learning EBP. The authors concluded that implementation of a new curriculum had a positive effect on both students and practicing nurses, fostering a greater understanding of EBP.

Moch, S., Cronje, R., & Branson, J. (2010). Part I. Undergraduate nursing evidence-based practice education: Envisioning the role of the students. *Journal of Professional Nursing, 26*, 5–13.

This review of literature focuses on the pedagogy used to teach EBP in undergraduate nursing schools. The authors focused on how both the role of the faculty and the students have been envisioned in promoting EBP in nursing. An extensive search was done in the Cumulative Index to Nursing and Allied Health Literature (CINAHL) database, and articles were chosen that met the inclusion criteria described by the authors. Nursing-related textbooks or books on EBP were also reviewed. The authors provide a table with a helpful and detailed review of both articles and books dedicated to EBP learning and teaching strategies. The authors suggest that there is evidence in the literature of a paradigm shift in which educators are foreseeing students not just as receivers of EBP education but also as active promoters of EBP in the clinical setting.

Stichler, J., Fields, W., Kim, S., & Brown, C. (2011). Faculty knowledge, attitudes, and perceived barriers to teaching evidence-based nursing. *Journal of Professional Nursing Practice, 27*, 92–100.

The author highlights faculty attitudes about EBP and strategies for teaching EBP. The study addressed three research questions: (1) What is the faculty's level of knowledge, attitudes, and practice of teaching EBP?; (2) What do faculty identify as barriers to teaching EBP?; and (3) What are the relationships among demographic characteristics, perceived barriers, and faculty's level of knowledge, attitudes, and practice of EBP? The study took place at public and private schools with baccalaureate and master's level programs. A group of 125 faculty participated in the study. The authors concluded that the study's findings helped to enhance the understanding of faculty knowledge, attitudes, and perceived barriers to teaching EBP.

Stiffler, D., & Cullen, D. (September–October, 2010). Evidence-based practice for nurse practitioner students: A competency-based teaching framework. *Journal of Professional Nursing, 26*(5), 272–277.

The authors explore EBP competencies for advanced practice nurses, especially NPs, utilizing a corresponding teaching framework. The authors identified three competencies for NPs: (1) understanding what EBP is and how to follow the EBP process; (2) synthesizing all evidence while integrating patient concerns, clinical experience, and judgment into clinical decisions; and (3) critically judging evidence appropriate to clinical management of patient conditions and issues. The authors explained how the implementation of the three identified competencies will provide NPs with the ability to inform their practice. The authors addressed the inconsistencies found on the NP certification exam, where students are tested on research utilization rather than EBP.

Whitmer, K., Auer, C., Beerman, L., & Weishaupt, L. (2011). Launching evidence-based nursing practice. *Journal for Nurses in Staff Development*, 27(2), E5–E7.

The article describes the effort of the administration in a university hospital to establish the Evidence-Based Practice Council (EBPC) to promote EBP within a shared governance model. The authors described the evolution of the model and the essential role of staff development. To get such a project off the ground, the chief nursing officer from the hospital partnered with the dean of the College of Nursing of Cincinnati University. The College of Nursing provided the institution with a nurse researcher who was also an associate member of the Institute of Nursing Research. This partnership allowed for the hospital to have direct access to the resources of the Institute. The EBPC was interdisciplinary council that included nurses, social workers, lactation consultants, and dieticians. The authors concluded that the incorporation of such a program in the institution provided nurses with the necessary tools to learn how to find the literature, evaluate their practice, and initiate change for best practice.

Zhang, Q., Zend, T., Chen, Y., & Li, X. (2011). Assisting undergraduate nursing students to learn evidence-based practice through self-directed learning and workshop strategies during clinical practicum. *Journal of Nursing Education Today*, 1–6.

The article describes a pilot study to provide undergraduate nursing students with the knowledge and skills to promote EBP during the clinical practicum. The purpose of the study was to assess the knowledge, attitudes, beliefs, and behaviors of undergraduate nursing students about EBP. The study included students from seven different universities in Hubei, China who had clinical assignments in the same teaching hospital. The interventions used were Self-Directed Learning (SDL) process of EBP and workshops for learning strategies to appraise the literature. The authors concluded that the integration of SDL and workshops during students' clinical assignments provided them with the necessary beginning skills in EBP and promoted better attitudes about EBP.

INDEX